Mental Disorders of the New Millennium

MENTAL DISORDERS OF THE NEW MILLENNIUM

Volume 1
Behavioral Issues

Edited by Thomas G. Plante

Praeger Perspectives

Abnormal Psychology

7/07

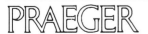

Westport, Connecticut
London

Library of Congress Cataloging-in-Publication Data

Mental disorders of the new millennium / edited by Thomas G. Plante.
      p. ; cm.—(Praeger perspectives. Abnormal psychology, ISSN 1554–2238)
  Includes bibliographical references and index.
  ISBN 0–275–98781–7 (set)—ISBN 0–275–98782–5 (v. 1)—
  ISBN 0–275–98783–3(v. 2)—ISBN 0–275–98784–1 (v. 3)   1. Psychiatry.
2. Mental illness. I. Plante, Thomas G. II. Series.
  [DNLM: 1. Mental Disorders. WM 140 M548326 2006]
  RC454.M462   2006
  616.89—dc22   2006015096

British Library Cataloguing in Publication Data is available.

Library of Congress Catalog Card Number: 2006015096
ISBN: 0–275–98781–7 (set)
      0–275–98782–5 (vol. 1)
      0–275–98783–3 (vol. 2)
      0–275–98784–1 (vol. 3)
ISSN: 1554–2238

First published in 2006

Praeger Publishers, 88 Post Road West, Westport, CT 06881
An imprint of Greenwood Publishing Group, Inc.
www.praeger.com

Printed in the United States of America

The paper used in this book complies with the
Permanent Paper Standard issued by the National
Information Standards Organization (Z39.48–1984).

10 9 8 7 6 5 4 3 2 1

Dedicated to my family matriarchs—
Marcia Plante, the late Anna McCormick, the late
Margaret Condon, and Marilyn Goldfarb—who have taught
me much about the human condition and who have well-
modeled compassion for others.

Contents

Preface

Tragically, the daily news is filled with stories about significant and remarkable problems in human behavior. Each morning we are greeted with news reports about murder, suicide, terrorist acts, drunken driving accidents, child molestation and abduction, drug abuse, gambling troubles, gang violence, various criminal behavior, and so forth. Other frequent stories reported in the press involve the betrayal of trust among highly respected and regarded members of society. These stories include the legal, sexual, financial, and general ethical lapses of politicians, leading sports celebrities, and movies stars. Some reports include the sexual abuse perpetrated on children and teens by school teachers, coaches, and members of the clergy. Other stories focus on the stress-related troubles soldiers experience following their duty in war. Still others focus on more and more reports of what appear to be mental problems such as autism, dementia, attention deficit disorders, panic, eating disorders, and depression, among both children and adults.

These troubles are reflected in recent cover stories in magazine news weeklies such as *Time*, *Newsweek*, and *US News and World Report*. Problems such as attention deficit hyperactivity disorder, autism, Alzheimer's disease, depression, panic disorder, murder-suicide, eating disorders, and child sexual abuse, among others, have been featured many times over as cover stories in these and other popular media outlets. The fact that these topics appear frequently on the covers of these news weeklies means they must impact significant numbers of people.

Perhaps just about everyone in the United States is affected by mental illness and abnormal behavior to some extent. Many people either suffer from one or more of the various mental disorders or live with those who do. It is likely that almost everyone in our contemporary society knows someone in his or her immediate family or circle of close friends and relatives who suffers from a significant abnormal behavior, psychiatric condition, or behavioral pattern that causes the person and his or her loved ones a great deal of stress.

Consider just a few of these statistics from our chapter contributors:

1. About 1 million people will die by suicide every year. The worldwide mortality rate of suicide is 16 per 100,000, or one suicide every 40 seconds. Fifty-five percent of suicides occur before age 44. Suicide is the third leading cause of death for both sexes.

2. About 1 million older Americans (1 in 35) is a victim of elder abuse each year, and between 3 and 5 percent of older adults over the age of 65 are or will be victims of abuse and/or neglect.

3. Epidemiological studies suggest the prevalence rate of child and adolescent depressive disorders ranges from 2 to 9 percent.

4. Over 18 million Americans suffer from some type of depression each year, and about 20 percent of the U.S. population will experience a significant depressive episode in their lifetime.

5. The number of probable adult pathological gamblers varies from just under 1 percent in the United Kingdom to between 1 and 2 percent in the United States and about 2.5 percent in Australia.

6. About 20 percent of all American women and 15 percent of all American men report being sexually abused by an adult while they were still a child.

7. About 4 percent of Catholic priests and 5 percent of school teachers have had a sexual encounter with a minor child in their care.

Clearly, mental illness and abnormal behavior touch the lives of just about all of us!

What's going on? How can it be that so many highly problematic psychiatric disorders, abnormal behaviors, and problems in living impact so many people? It wouldn't be an exaggeration to state that the vast troubles of the world stem from abnormal behavior. From ignoring global warming to terrorism, from murder to suicide, from divorce to gambling, from autism to dementia, it seems that abnormal behavior is at the root of so many challenges of our day.

Sadly, most of the books available in the field of abnormal psychology are not especially useful for the average educated lay reader. Much of the literature currently available tends to fall into two categories. The first includes academic books written by academics for an academic or scholarly audience. These books are often written in a very dry, jargon-filled, data-driven manner that is challenging for the general reader to get through. In fact, these books are often challenging for professionals in psychology and related fields to understand as well. The second category includes trade books that tend to be very simplistic and often tell the story of someone suffering from a particular problem. These books are often located in the self-help or inspirational section in a bookstore. Books of this type are written by those who experience the particular disorder, mental health professionals who treat the problem, or journalists who tell a remarkable story about a particular case that made news. Very few books are written for the educated lay reader that balance academic, scholarly, and clinical information with a readable, engaging, and user-friendly style.

The purpose of this series on mental disorders is to help bridge this gap between academic and self-help /inspirational books written on abnormal psychology topics that impact society—those topics that potential readers see on the covers of weekly news magazines or in daily newspapers. The series focuses on contemporary abnormal behavior topics and is compiled from contributions by experts for an educated lay audience. Leading experts who study, treat, evaluate, and reflect upon these troubles and issues have been asked to write chapters for you to help you better understand these contemporary problems. The chapters are based on the most up-to-date research and practice evidence and go well beyond the information provided in popular media outlets. Hopefully, you will find that the books are highly informative, contemporary, and readable.

If we better understand the factors that contribute to these contemporary abnormal behaviors and patterns, then perhaps we can find better ways to prevent some of these problems from emerging and better evaluate and treat those who suffer from these experiences. In an effort to create a better world for ourselves and our children we must do all that we can to prevent abnormal behavior and help those who are troubled by abnormal behavior in themselves, their loved ones, and their communities. In doing so, we will be better able to create an improved world.

Acknowledgments

Many people other than the author or editor assist in the completion of a book project. Some contribute in a direct way while others help in a more supportive manner. I would like to acknowledge the assistance of the people who worked to make this book idea a reality and who have helped me in both direct and indirect ways.

First and foremost, I would like to thank the contributors to this volume. Leading experts who represent the very best that the professional community has to offer graciously agreed to contribute quality chapters to this book project. Second, I would like to thank my associate editors, Drs. DeLeon, Kaslow, and Plante, for agreeing to serve as associate editors for this book and all the books in the abnormal psychology book series. Third, it is important to recognize the wonderful people at Greenwood who published this book. Most especially, many thanks go to Debbie Carvalko, our editor at Greenwood. Fourth, I would like to thank Santa Clara University, which has supported me and allowed me many opportunities to pursue my scholarly academic activities and interests.

Fifth, I would like to acknowledge the anonymous persons who are referred to in this book, who have allowed their life experiences and traumas to become instruments of learning for others. Sixth, I would like to thank my family patriarchs (Bernard Plante, the late Henry McCormick, and Eli Goldfarb) and matriarchs (Marcia Plante, the late Anna McCormick, the late Margaret Condon, and Marilyn Goldfarb) and my sisters (Mary Beauchemin and Leeann Sperduti), all of whom have taught me much about the human condition. Finally, I would like to thank my wife, Lori, and son, Zachary, for their love and support while I worked on yet another compelling book project.

Chapter 1

The Psychopathy of Everyday Life

Martin Kantor

Who is the psychopath in your life?

Is it the motorist who is an aggressive, narcissistic, remorseless, selfish individual without kindness, empathy, altruism, or regret? The driver who honks remorselessly, bends a fender then leaves the scene, and grabs a parking space right out from under you? Is it the motorist who blames you for her mistakes? Can't we relate to the story of the individual who describes being stopped at a red light when he was hit from behind by a driver? Instead of apologizing, the driver emerged from her car and severely chastised this individual for impeding the flow of traffic. "It's my fault" and "I am truly sorry" were no more in her vocabulary than they were in the vocabulary of the lawyer who absconded with his client's escrow money or the CEO who bankrupted his company so that he could gratify his personal, very expensive, appetites.

Is it the dentist who for fame, money, and power evolved crazy theories with more gusto and greater ease than sensible ones, and who even came to believe in his theories himself? This man was able to build a busy practice and was more than able to pay the mortgage on his beach house by revising old fillings made of mercury, claiming that they caused blood poisoning that showed up in the form of Chronic Fatigue Syndrome. When the regulatory agencies caught up with him, and when his patients read the adverse publicity about the questionable scientific basis of mercury filling poisoning, he lost most of his practice. So he had to find another way to make money. He then started recommending that all his patients undergo what he called preventive dentistry, which involved grinding down a whole tooth instead of simply filling a cavity, giving as his reason, "That way, the tooth will never become decayed again." His motivation was not to preserve teeth. His motivation was to enhance his bottom line.

Is it your psychiatrist? When in residency a particular psychiatrist often made up cases for presentation at a conference. Afterwards he got through the licensing exam by paying for the answers available on the underground. When in private practice, he allowed himself to be bought with cheap gifts and free lunches by those attempting to convince him to prescribe certain medications and not others. Also, he would only prescribe a medication made by a drug company in which he had a financial stake. He worked on a panel deciding which drugs were safe without recusing himself, as he should have, on the grounds that he received money from the drug companies that made the drugs he was recommending. When referring his patients out he would send them not to the best person available but to his golfing buddies. While he himself refrained, he turned a blind eye when his colleagues had sex with their patients, in private agreeing with them that that was sometimes justified as a form of therapy. At times he would sleep during the session and report his revealing dreams back to the patient claiming that that was a form of therapy. One of his specialties was treating anxiety, but really what he was doing was pushing drugs, for he would write literally hundreds of prescriptions for benzodiazepines without first taking a complete medical history or doing the requisite mental and physical examinations. Many times he cheated the insurance company by lying about the amount of time he spent with a patient. He also practiced alternative forms of medicine where he inappropriately prescribed nutritional supplements alone for ailments that required conservative medical treatment then deified his essentially trivial interventions as powerful curatives, and to ice the cake, lobbied politically to have his treatment approach formally recognized and legitimized so that the insurance companies would pay for it.

Is it your spouse? A consumer registered his car to a phony out-of-town address in a state with lower car insurance, tapped into the cable line to get free cable, and when the cable company gave him premium channels without charging him for them never mentioned it so that he could continue to get the service without having to pay the bill. He would often buy things, use them, and then when he no longer needed them return them to the store. For example, once when he was boarding his brother's dog, he bought a cage from a pet store, used it for the few days that the dog was with him, and then brought it back. When he bought electronic equipment and dropped it he would return it to the store claiming that it was defective, and he often brought back plants he had himself killed saying that they simply had died because they were defective. When a store had a big sale he would buy several items then resell them on eBay. When a policeman caught him speeding, making an illegal turn, or using a cell phone when driving, he would falsely claim an emergency that required his immediate presence. Joining the paying crowd at intermission he would sneak into a show or concert for the second act. In bookstores he would peel back the shrink wrap from books so that he could read them without buying them, and he would borrow CDs from the library then make copies of them and sell them to his friends. He would send letters without stamps, using as the return address the address of the recipient, hoping that the letter would arrive at its proper place as "returned." He would regularly drop his personal garbage in a public bin, use the supermarket as a smorgasbord—eating his way through the olive bar, underreport his income on his tax forms, purchase stolen goods after buying into the excuse that they fell from the back of the truck, and sneak into the gym—after telling the person at the front desk that he was just there to meet someone at the cafeteria he would go into the bathroom, remove his outer clothes revealing his gym clothes underneath, then unabashedly proceed to the work floor. He would alter a medical insurance form after his doctor filled it out so that he could increase the benefits due him, substitute stickers on super-market items so that an item would check out for less, and on more than one occasion, he deprived a real estate agent of an earned commission by teaming up with the buyer to purchase the property behind the agent's back.

Or is it you? A psychopathic consumer gave the lie to the maxim that the customer is always right. For he lied, cheated, and stole from the merchants he dealt with, which he did for any number of financial and personal reasons. He not only wanted to pay as little as possible for desirable merchandise, he also liked the fun and excitement of putting something over on the establishment. He borrowed many a book from the library then "forgot" to give it back. When leaving a hotel he would regularly steal the towels, and when leaving a restaurant he would frequently try to nab any souvenir dishes he could lay his hands on. He would often say he had a dinner or hotel reservation he hadn't actually made, hoping to get the restaurant or hotel to correct an error they didn't make by offering him space he didn't reserve. He always corrected waiters or waitresses when they overcharged him on a check, but he never corrected them when they made a mistake in his favor. When he thought he could get away with it he would eat dinner at a restaurant then complain about the food or service (the old-time comedian's "Waiter there's a fly in my soup") to get comped, to leave a lesser tip, or both. He frequently sent out letters of complaint about a product in order to get the company to apologetically send him free coupons good for purchasing more of the same. When applying for a job he regularly omitted negative information about his past work history, and on credit applications he would significantly inflate his income. In other circumstances he would under-report his income, as he once did in order to gain admission to a middle-income housing project. Eventually he put all his assets into a corporate name so that he would be eligible for benefits available to those with a low income, and once he even tried to apply for Supplemental Security Income benefits on the grounds that he was completely impoverished.

Most of us will recognize friends, family, acquaintances and strangers we read about in the daily news in these composite examples. Yet the extant scientific literature on psychopathy hardly mentions such individuals at all. When it comes to psychopathy, the available literature reveals only a few of its faces. It tends to focus exclusively on seriously ill, truly evil people like John Wayne Gacy, David Berkowitz, and Saddam Hussein, but it neglects the lawyer for whom winning a case is more important than discovering the truth; the ad writer who uses fragments of information to put a good face on a bad product; the doctor who, because he owns stock in the company that produces the drug, touts a costly medication over one that is less expensive but equally effective; the politician who sells out for a mess of concrete in the form of the new driveway for her house, installed in exchange for voting for the contractor's new construction project before the planning board; and the CEO of a major corporation who decides not to insure his employees, knowing that the taxpayers will have to pick up the bill for their medical care, so why spend the extra dollars?

These are the individuals I call "the psychopaths of everyday life." Though their problems are both widespread and devastating in their effects, to date they belong to a poorly understood group whose emotional difficulties are barely recognized, hardly fathomed, and rarely treated. To the best of my knowledge, with the exception of Martha Stout's recent book *The Sociopath Next Door*,[1] written more for the layperson than for the therapist, these individuals have been almost entirely neglected by the scientific establishment. When they are mentioned at all, they are referred to in passing, whereupon the focus predictably shifts rapidly to seriously disturbed psychopaths, and especially to those seriously disturbed psychopathic individuals that form that subgroup of patients we diagnose as having an antisocial personality disorder.

To understand and treat the psychopaths of everyday life we first must distinguish them from the severe psychopaths, from whom they differ significantly in style, causation, incidence, and effect. *Descriptively*, while mild psychopathy closely resembles a personality disorder, severe psychopathy more closely resembles a psychosis. *Dynamically*, mild psychopaths are less aggressive and more guilt-ridden than their more severe counterparts. *Therapeutically*, mild psychopathy has both a much more benign course and a better prognosis than psychopathy that is severe. Also, unlike the more severe forms of psychopathy, which are often treatment resistant, mild psychopaths can, with the right approach, often be helped significantly through psychotherapy.

Not all observers believe that such an entity as mild psychopathy even exists. For example, Hans Toch says that being a mild psychopath is like being a little bit pregnant (p. 144).[2] Along similar lines, Henry Pinsker (personal communication,

2004) suggests that the term psychopath has become too broad and dilute to the point that it has lost its specificity, having been applied to anyone who is an opportunist or a criminal.

Other observers do recognize mild, partial psychopathy. The blurb in the back of Donald W. Black's book *Bad Boys, Bad Men* includes under the rubric of psychopathy "black sheep ... con men, or misfits [who] shirk everyday responsibilities, abuse drugs and alcohol ... and lash out at family members," and in the book itself Black speaks of "successful bad boys." As Black says, "Antisocials are not just muggers, rapists, and violent assailants. They sometimes are embezzlers, tax evaders, fraudulent business men, corrupt stock brokers, and conniving attorneys ... who habitually commit white-collar crimes" (p. 152).[3] Robert D. Hare calls mild psychopaths "white-collar psychopaths" and says of them, "These individuals are every bit as egocentric, callous, and manipulative as the average criminal psychopath; however, their intelligence, family background, social skills, and circumstances permit them to construct a façade of normalcy and to get what they want with relative impunity" (p. 102).[4] Although the psychopaths described in Hervey Cleckley's *Mask of Sanity* are almost all severely ill, on occasion, without much focus or elaboration, Cleckley discusses mild psychopaths who "are able to make some sort of adjustment in life" (p. 211).[5]

I believe that the mild psychopaths like the ones about which these observers speak are still psychopaths, and they are more numerous and in some ways even more dangerous to society than severe psychopaths. For by lying, cheating, and swindling on a massive scale their mayhem deprives many victims of a great deal. While it is true that these individuals are rarely violent to persons, they can do a great deal of violence to the dignity, identity, and bank accounts of many people. They rarely take lives, but they do often ruin them.

I continue my discussion of the *psychopathy* of everyday life with a general discussion of the *psychopathology* of everyday life.

THE PSYCHOPATHOLOGY OF EVERYDAY LIFE

By the term "psychopathology of everyday life" I mean thought and behavior centered somewhere near the middle of a continuum where "normal" is on the left of the mean and pathological is on the right. However, especially when it comes to personality disorder, it is often difficult to answer the question "What is normal and what is pathological?" The *DSM–IV* (The American Psychiatric Association's *Diagnostic and Statistical Manual*) notes that "Personality Disorders represent maladaptive variants of personality traits that merge imperceptibly into normality and into one another" (p. 633)[6] and John M. Oldham and Lois B. Morris note that personality disorders are "exaggerations of ... personality styles that are present to varying degrees

within every individual. It is the *quantity* of each personality style along a continuum, not its quality, that tends to spell problems in life" (p. 21).[7] When it
comes to psychopathy, I believe that "normal" opportunistic individuals who
place personal gain in importance above truth or the collective good, consider
winning the only thing worthwhile, and twist logic into obtaining personal
advantage by so skillfully selecting and misrepresenting facts that even they
themselves come to believe in the truth of their distortions are on the left of
the continuum, where on the right are those "pathological" individuals we formally identify as full psychopaths based on their having crossed the border
into the realm of serious lying, cheating, and criminality completely unfettered by anxiety and totally unbounded by conscience.

In differentiating abnormal from normal we have to leave room for personality
differences. All of us are not alike, so behavior such as introversion, or even
deviousness, is more pathological for some than it is for others. It is also
important to distinguish abnormal behavior from behavior that looks abnormal but is normal, because under the circumstances it is both predictable
and universal—for example, on vacation or at a special time of the year for
which we have coined such terms as "spring fever," "midsummer madness," and
"winter doldrums," suggesting that cultural allowances are made for intermittent, for example, seasonal, deviation from year-round norms. Specific
external (situational) circumstances also can make a substantial difference.
For example, if you are an accountant, a checking ritual makes sense in your
job (i.e., is reactive to or part of the job). If you are an FBI agent, a formal,
unbending, controlling, ungiving personality with paranoid features can represent
not a style of illness but an appropriate or even   creative manifestation of
health. Additionally, defining social deviance is always difficult because variations exist from society to society. For example, what would be abnormal in
a collectivistic society might in an individualistic society pass for perfectly
acceptable behavior.

Determining motive helps us distinguish between abnormal and normal. For
example, it helps us distinguish between the serious psychopath—the bad bank
robber who intends to be an enemy of the state—and the nonpsychopath—the
latter-day good Robin Hood who by stealing from the rich and giving to the poor
intends to be a friend of the people.

Differentiating adaptive from maladaptive personality traits also helps us
distinguish abnormal from normal. Personality *traits* are the building blocks
of both (normal) personality *style* and (pathological) personality *disorder*.
Personality traits can be compared in subject matter and style to proverbs and
other related sayings, such as maxims, and we can think of them as a lifetime
overvaluation and realization of a proverb or maxim that takes the form of

an overvalued idea that grabs hold and guides thought and behavior. Because personality traits are like proverbs and maxims, proverbs and maxims can serve as headlines to the story of one's personality traits, and ultimately of one's personality type or style. As such, these apt, pithy headlines, summaries of the core attitude of an individual, are a good indication of the individual's personality style. Thus the individual who lives by the formulations "Cleanliness is next to godliness" and "Never postpone to tomorrow what you can do today" tends to be an overly scrupulous but still normal obsessional type. "We have nothing to fear but fear itself" describes the propensity for denial found in those with a hypomanic bent. The maxims "There's no business like show business," "A sucker is born every minute," and "Caveat emptor" are the rallying cries of the individual with a psychopathic personality style.

The personality traits of the normal individual are more adaptive than the personality traits of the individual who is abnormal. An example of an adaptive personality trait might be ambitiousness, and an example of a maladaptive personality trait might be self-destructiveness. Depending on context and content, the same trait can be either adaptive or maladaptive. The personality trait of *adaptive* evasiveness is illustrated by the behavior of the familiar political figure with a psychopathic bent who evaded one question by answering another. When asked, "When is this war we are in going to be over?" he answered, "We have to persevere and pursue the enemy for as long as it takes to win." This individual ducked by answering not the question he was asked but instead a somewhat related question: "Should we give up now or persevere and fight to the end?" In contrast, the personality trait of *maladaptive* evasiveness is illustrated by the behavior of the individual at the center of a widely publicized case who was punished not for her initial misdeeds but for lying about them to the government.

Statistically speaking, few individuals look markedly abnormal. The vast majority of the *abnormal* individuals that we run across in our daily lives are suffering from mild psychopathology, making them *seminormal*. In the case of psychopaths, seminormal or mild psychopaths have to be differentiated on the one hand from normal individuals who are merely somewhat morally challenged and on the other hand from individuals suffering from severe psychopathy who have a diagnosable antisocial personality disorder.

Theodore Millon gives the name "nonantisocial aggressive personality" to a category of individuals who fit the description of seminormal psychopathic individuals (p. 181).[8] Hare, as previously noted, refers to mild psychopaths as "white-collar psychopaths" and speaks of "subcriminal psychopaths" and "successful psychopaths."[4] Robert I. Simon calls mild psychopaths "passive psychopaths," whom he goes on to describe as "individuals who] tend to be parasitic and exploitative of others [unlike the] aggressive psychopaths [who] commit major crimes" (p. 27).[9] Stout speaks of the sociopaths next door.[1] I call these individuals variously mild or partial psychopaths or the psychopaths of everyday life.

Seminormal individuals are rarely salt of the earth people, and their personality traits are mostly negative and maladaptive. This rule, however, has exceptions, notably the fact that being excessively clean occurs perhaps as often as being excessively dirty.

In seminormal individuals the past and present manifestations of the disorder, while still overt, are moderately attenuated. For example, speaking of the past manifestations of psychopathy, the *DSM–IV* suggests that as adolescents adult psychopaths routinely present with signs and symptoms of a conduct disorder.[6] But while seminormal psychopaths may have been dishonest adolescent girls and boys who lied, cheated, and stole, they were probably not recklessly impulsive truants who ran away from home, serious brats who regularly acted in an intimidating aggressive manner, devilish fire setters, or sadists who seriously hurt and maimed animals. If they were arrested it was more for misdemeanors than for felonies, and if they were punished it was not by being jailed but by being fined.

As for now in the 21st century, as adults seminormal individuals may have almost as many difficulties as those people we officially recognize as disordered. Negative thoughts and behaviors such as selfishness prevail over positive ones such as caution, honesty, and altruism. These individuals do make waves, ruffle feathers, and call significant attention to themselves. However, their difficulties, for one reason or another, are undeveloped or otherwise held in abeyance. For example, seminormal psychopathic individuals retain some capacity to feel love, and even pity. These emotions can kick in at the last minute to slow the process down and keep it from taking over completely, as these individuals feel sorry for those they are about to hurt, and in response, they go a bit easy on them. Seminormal psychopaths also retain a modicum of guilt. For example, they might apologize to those they wronged, even though the apologies have no practical effect on their subsequent behavior. Furthermore, their deviant behavior is not persistent and repetitive. One episode might subside long before another appears. One year a seminormal psychopath cheats on his final exam. Later in life he cheats at cards, still later on his taxes, and later still on his wife, so that the individual traits even when serious in and of themselves do not completely deform, distort, and usurp the entire personality by becoming a regular and predictable behavioral feature.

Seminormal individuals also display pathological traits selectively, in some areas but not in others, with the result that their disorder is not characterized by a full expression. Consequently, their problems, only showing in certain facets of their thoughts and behaviors, are limited to certain arenas and involve only one or two parameters of functionality. For example, one seminormal psychopath stole from work in order to better provide for his wife and children at home, making him an embezzler who was also, however, a loving husband and father.

Seminormal individuals manage to turn a maladaptive trait such as cheating into an adaptive trait such as getting ahead regardless of the cost. Indeed, when it comes to seminormal psychopathy, being successful may be as much the rule as the exception. Successful seminormal psychopathic individuals still function effectively and creatively within the mainstream, but they do so in a clearly psychopathic mode.

Seminormal individuals also have a disorder that is reactive, that is, it is a more or less transient response to external, often traumatic, life events. Included here are those seminormal psychopaths who steal not for fun and excitement or because they are so insatiable that they want it all even though they already have enough but because they have little to eat. In cases like this the psychopathic symptoms can be transient and are likely to improve with an improvement in circumstances.

Finally, seminormal individuals retain a measure of control over themselves to the extent that they can keep their worst aspects from emerging and taking over their personality completely and destructively. For example, a seminormal psychopath's professed goal was to be more like a saprophyte than like a parasite. To this end he used people for his nefarious ends but deliberately steered clear of harming them seriously. He would cheat on his expense account at work and embezzle from his company, but though he could have embezzled his company dry, he stopped short of that. In his interpersonal relationships he was narcissistic and lacked empathy, but he would never destroy relationships completely. Instead he would deliberately set out to maintain them, although he did that only for purposes of manipulating them.

My discussion next turns from "What is normal, and what is seminormal?" to "What is psychopathy?" (Psychopathic Personality Disorder), whether mild, moderate, or severe.

PSYCHOPATHY

One can define psychopathy according to its generally accepted core dynamics: antisocial behavior in the presence of a relative or absolute absence of anxiety and guilt and an inability to experience remorse; an incapacity for feeling empathy and an inability to be altruistic; and an absence of clear and understandable human motivation.

Alternatively, one can, as does the *DSM–IV*,[6] define psychopathy behaviorally, more in terms of social deviance than in terms of core personality difficulties. Behavioral constructs emphasize maladaptive behaviors such as unpredictability, impulsivity, irresponsibility, ruthlessness, and criminality. The major advantage of defining psychopathy behaviorally rather than dynamically is that interrater reliability is greater, for it is easier to agree about what constitutes criminality than it is to agree about what constitutes lack of empathy. However, there are several disadvantages to using strictly behavioral criteria. They tend not to go to the heart of the matter, they tempt the making of value judgments, and they are highly dependent on social standards that vary both from society to society and within one society, leaving us without a fixed platform in space from which to measure deviation: bad from good, acceptable from unacceptable, social from antisocial. Who is the psychopath? The individual who sneaks across the border through the dessert to get into the United States, the posse patrolling the borders and mercilessly hunting down the trespassers, or the person who puts water out so that the "illegal immigrants" don't die of thirst in the hot sun? Who is the psychopath? The gang member in a crime-ridden neighborhood or the person who refuses to go along and join the gang? Technically speaking, as bizarre as it sounds, in Nazi Germany the SS guards would not, according to strictly social definitions, be the psychopaths. The psychopaths would be the people who, in defiance of regime policy, failing to conform to social norms, tried to save the Jews. For most teenagers, and in the teenage societies that they, and some of their adult compatriots, form, being countercultural is not a problem but a goal. The *DSM–IV* criterion "disregard for and violation of the rights of others"[6] is especially awkward because to a great extent rights are culturally dependent. In a totalitarian, collectivistic society, it is not antisocial but prosocial to deprive others of the right to speak freely, and those who insist on demanding their rights in such a place are the ones most likely to wind up branded as psychopathic enemies of the state. The Boston Tea Party would in some circles today be considered to have epitomized antiauthoritarian acting out, and it is ironic that according to legend the repressive dictator Joseph Stalin considered the modernistic composer Dimitri Shostakovich to be the one who was the psychopath!

Another disadvantage of using behavioral criteria to define psychopathy is that actual psychopathic behavior is often hidden. After all, these are individuals who are famously untruthful. They also know how to manipulate mental health professionals, and the entire system, to create the impression that they behave well, or that, if they behave negatively, that their bad behavior is justified by circumstances.

Perhaps the most serious problem associated with defining psychopathy behaviorally is that behavioral definitions by nature tend to emphasize the negative over the positive features of a disorder, for example, psychopathic criminality over psychopathic cleverness. But the socially valued behavior of the doctor who speaks euphemistically (that is, who lies) in order to put a good face on a bad prognosis is in a way just as psychopathic as the behavior of the quack healer who uses sophistic skills to sell the public an entirely worthless nostrum. It would appear that emotionally disordered behavior has its beneficial side and that not all aspects of a personality disorder, or even the personality disorder itself, are self-destructive and maladaptive. Therefore, the concept of positive psychopathy does not actually challenge our basic concept of what constitutes a personality disorder.

It is not surprising then that many people who are considered successful in business are actually suffering from what can be termed a "temporally effective" psychopathy—one in which well-defined sadistic and amoral elements are efficiently controlled because out of control they could compromise everything that has been gained. When psychopathy takes this form, not of negative actions but of positive interpersonal, social, and creative display, it begins to look more like a virtue than a vice. Indeed, psychopathy is so often able to be harnessed for the appropriate service of self in a socially useful activity that many of us wish we were more psychopathic than we already are. Conversely, we all sometimes need to think and act a bit like a psychopath, for not being a little psychopathic can constitute an impediment that makes it harder for us to protect our well-being and to get ahead in the world. Not being able to tell a white lie to spare others' feelings or to save our own skins when we are cornered can, after all, be detrimental to our ability to function—personally, socially, professionally, and politically. It is not surprising then that many of us, secretly identifying with psychopaths, admire and want to become like them. At least in our dreams we find ourselves enjoying being hardhearted. Now, as we see it, with fewer scruples holding us back we could reach the highest pinnacles of achievement. Now, as we see it, we could achieve more by functioning in a less than guilty fashion, unconcerned about our wrongdoing, able to victimize others with little or no regrets—for now we are thoroughly rid of our inhibiting scruples and completely unfettered by our retrospective regrets.

Examples of positive psychopathy in our society include the pleasant, harmless, acceptable, and even fun psychopathy of Fritz Kreisler, the violinist and composer who wrote music in the olden style and then, rather than attributing it to his own hand, said he had found it; and that of the composer Charles Ives, who, otherwise not obviously psychopathic, may have backdated his compositions to make them seem more avant-garde. Less acceptable but still within the realm of what is generally tolerated is the psychopathy of the realtor who becomes rich and successful by selectively underplaying the flaws of subpar properties in order to inflate their prices. For example, in calculating the amount of rent a small apartment complex brings in, this realtor simply "forgot" to say that one of the tenants was a nun who paid considerably less than market-value rent, had a lifetime lease, and had no plans to leave. Many successful salesmen can point to their psychopathy as the real reason for their success. This was the case for a patient of mine, a life insurance salesman, someone who had previously signed himself into a mental hospital just to beat a drug rap. During treatment with me he tried to take out a life insurance policy on my life to protect his investment in his therapy in case I died or was killed—a clever, though self-serving, and, for me at least, potentially dangerous, idea, but one that illustrates the close relationship that often exists between narcissism, psychopathy, and creativity.

After discussing psychopathy in this general way I focus my discussion on mild psychopathy—the psychopathy of everyday life.

THE PSYCHOPATHY OF EVERYDAY LIFE

Mild psychopaths, the psychopaths of everyday life, appear to the casual observer to be upright, honest citizens whose reputation is "merely" marred by a touch of dishonesty. They can be differentiated from patients suffering from severe psychopathy, particularly Antisocial Personality Disorder, as follows:

> Patients with an antisocial personality disorder resemble hardened criminals. Their crimes often involve directly aggressive acts to individuals and go beyond mayhem to murder.

In contrast, mild psychopaths are more like ordinary schemers and conners. Their crimes tend to fall into the gray area of criminality, such as the crimes of opportunity of ad writers who speak part truths that effectively mask whole falsehoods, emphasizing the positive and eliminating the negative to sell a nearly worthless product—quite possibly still stealing more overall from an unsuspecting and gullible public than all the armed robbers of this world collectively take from banks or than crooked CEOs steal from large companies.

> Patients with an antisocial personality disorder are commonly found in jail or in forensic psychiatry units.

In contrast, mild psychopaths are often found in the courts. If they go to jail it is often because they miscalculated or experienced a run of very bad luck.

> Patients with an antisocial personality disorder mostly lack discernible anxiety, are short on empathy, and are incapable of feeling guilt or remorse, either now or after the fact. When convicted of a crime they do not show guilt or remorse because they so lack the ability to know what guilt and remorse feel like that they cannot even fake it.

In contrast, mild psychopaths often become somewhat anxious, are capable of feeling some guilt and remorse, and retain some ability to empathize. In court mild psychopaths have enough residual empathy and ability to feel guilt and remorse to allow them to figure out how to apologize to the people they hurt—although they usually do so less because they really mean it and more because they want a shorter sentence.

Patients with an antisocial personality disorder tend to be extremely impulsive individuals.

In contrast, mild psychopaths are often quietly and resolutely calculating and retain the desire and the ability to plan ahead.

Patients with an antisocial personality disorder completely lack loyalty.

In contrast, mild psychopaths often retain a sense of loyalty to select groups— the familiar "honor among thieves."

Patients with an antisocial personality disorder tend to be completely oblivious to feedback, without audience sensitivity or much if any concern about the effects of their actions on others—all part of their tendency to show poor conditionability.

In contrast, one can often approach, get through to, and influence mild psychopaths, at least to an extent. While they could care more, it's not entirely true that they couldn't care less.

Patients with an antisocial personality disorder hurt people for the sheer fun of it.

In contrast, mild psychopaths often hurt people as much for profit as for fun. They are more opportunistic than sadistic. They may enjoy making their victims writhe but they also enjoy making themselves rich. (An important caveat, as the DSM–IV notes, is that "Antisocial Personality Disorder must be distinguished from criminal behavior undertaken for gain that is not accompanied by the personality features characteristic of this disorder."[6] Thus while a psychopath would by definition be an opportunistic crook, an opportunistic crook would not necessarily by definition be a psychopath.)

Patients with an antisocial personality disorder usually show little or no improvement as they get older.

In contrast, mild psychopaths may, and often do, grow up and out of their psychopathy. They frequently have an epiphany later in life where they suddenly and often unexplainably begin to feel guilt and remorse for their past actions to the point that they actually achieve a measure of reform. This rule also has its exceptions, for mild psychopaths can stay the same or get worse. For example, the "mere" antics of Truman Capote's youth seem to have hardened into a serious mistreatment of his best friends, whom he badly hurt by criticizing and exposing them—virtually, it would appear, for a combination of professional and personal gain, and perhaps also to have some great immoral fun at their expense.

> Patients with an antisocial personality disorder produce mainly negative responses in us. We invariably dislike, refuse to tolerate, and are afraid of the serious psychopath.

In contrast, we (too often) tolerate, embrace, and even love the mild psychopath, taking him or her into our hearts and homes—one reason why we call these individuals "confidence men" and view them not as subhuman but as superior life-forms.

> Patients with an antisocial personality disorder often live as outsiders in society.

In contrast, mild psychopaths are often "insiders," in many senses of the term, including its use in the phrase "insider trading." Instead of removing themselves from people and society, mild psychopaths keep close relationships going with others, mainly, however, so that they can manipulate them for their own ends. We might say that while patients with antisocial personality disorder, as well as all serious psychopaths, remind us of (dangerous) outlaws, mild psychopaths remind us of (troublesome) in-laws. That is, they are less like hard-core criminals and more like those difficult people we all know who live among us spitting on the floor, throwing apple cores out of the windows of moving cars, blasting their horns at drivers who don't get moving when the light changes, turning up their personal stereos on public conveyances, yelling into their cell phones—calculatedly oblivious to the discomfort of others around them, or putting their dogs to sleep because they bark too much. In a typical difficult behavior of a mild psychopath, a man breaks into a line of people waiting to check their coats. When his wife reminds him, "There is a line," he retorts, totally oblivious to her concerns or the feelings of the others he has cut off, "I know. I'm on it."

> When patients with an antisocial personality disorder are caught and exposed, they make things worse for themselves by becoming angry, vindictive, and reflexively even more confrontational.

In contrast, mild psychopaths seem to know how to avoid being chastised and punished and know just what to do to get out of a difficult spot. When caught in the act they tend to become reflexively more ingratiating.

Mild psychopaths are not, however, entirely benign. Behaviors characteristic of the antisocial such as selling drugs to children or joining murderous gangs are not entirely unknown in the mild psychopath, and some mild psychopaths even wind up being admitted to mental hospitals. While mild psychopaths are rarely extremely violent or maim or kill with knives and guns, they can, and often do, murder people, although they usually do so indirectly. For example, in a not atypical scenario they might skim money off a project and put up a building that ultimately collapses, injuring or killing its occupants.

Mild psychopaths can also be inhumane in the extreme. As con artists and confidence men, they can fool, and even destroy the lives of, millions. In the ranks of the widely destructive we find the ad writer who fleeced hoards by touting the superiority of one aspirin over another based on an elusive purity or another value falsely claimed to be exclusive, doing so in terms carefully calculated not to break the law; the ad writer who got the poor to spend more than they could afford by convincing them to overspend during a discount sale, persuading them that they would save more if they spent more; and the ad writer who compromised many people's eyesight by promoting a cure for nearsightedness based on the following flawed hypothesis presented as scientific truth: glasses never cured anyone's eyesight; since the myopia of people who wear glasses invariably gets worse, it follows that glasses cause myopia, so throw away your glasses and, for a price, I will show you how you can see perfectly well without them. Belonging here too are the actions of the politicians who ultimately harm us all by destroying perfectly good opposition candidates with attack ads that make victims not only of their opponents but also of the truth; reporters and book reviewers who destroy reputations by omitting facts that might save or enhance them; realtors who steal other realtors' exclusive listings then offer customers cut-rate commissions to make the switch to them; crooked telemarketers who sell worthless products; Internet phishers who empty bank accounts and steal identities; shady corporate CEOs who fake balance sheets to artificially enhance the value of their stock; office workers who regularly call in sick when they are well, rationalizing their behavior as taking a mental health day, or who cheat on their time cards by leaving early then getting someone else to stamp the cards for them, or who steal large amounts of office supplies then resell them on eBay; and used-car salesmen who turn the odometer back or sell cars that have been in a wreck or flood without even mentioning their background.

In conclusion, however unfortunate, a certain amount of psychopathic opportunism, greed, distortion of reality, bullying, and cheating must be taken for granted in the world. Even the most "normal" individuals among us are mildly psychopathic. This is because to some extent we all use psychopathic methods to cope, achieve, and succeed. All of us have the potential to be aggressive when that suits us, and all of us have a lax enough conscience structure to make us selectively morally reprehensible—selfish, unloving, and unempathetic, guilt free and at will, when that suits our purposes. All of us can be unreliable when we see an opportunity to feed ourselves a little pleasure or ill-gotten gain. All of us can be much too willing to compromise our ideals, for, as they say, "Every person has his price." However, while when the lure and prospect of instant gratification looms we can all become evasive, tricky, and dishonest, some of us, the normal individuals and milder psychopaths among us, recognize and control our potential for deviltry better than others. Either a compulsive morality kicks in to set limits on how evil we permit ourselves to be or our better judgment kicks in and we watch what we do simply because we are afraid of getting caught.

THERAPY OF THE MILD PSYCHOPATH

Individual Therapy

Most clinicians view psychopathy as an untreatable disorder that responds neither to traditional therapeutic methods nor to untraditional treatment approaches. For example, Cleckley states that "I do not have any dogmatic advice as to a final or even a satisfactory way of successfully rehabilitating psychopaths,"[5] and Hare says that "with few exceptions, the traditional forms of psychotherapy . . . have proved ineffective in the treatment of psychopathy. Nor have the biological therapies, including . . . the use of various drugs, fared much better."[4] Hare even suggests that treatment can sometimes actually make these individuals worse.

In a dissenting view, Otto F. Kernberg outlines a psychoanalytically oriented method he believes to be effective for treating psychopaths.[10] Black suggests a specific method that focuses not on "why behaviors developed" but on "how they can be eliminated" and recommends cognitive therapy that focuses on exposing and challenging cognitive distortions such as my "desires are adequate grounds for [my] actions" (p. 152).[3]

I believe that while severe psychopathy can be at best very difficult to treat with any form of therapy, mild psychopathy is treatable using traditional individual approaches, so long as these are specifically adapted for dealing with the special problems these patients present.

That does not mean that even the mildest of psychopaths are easy to treat. Even mild psychopaths tend to be uninsightful individuals who deny their illness. What awareness they have of the nature, depth, and extent of their disorder tends to be dim at best. So they might say, "I am not sick" or "If I am sick it's because of what the world did to me." Many also have an aggressive side to them that puts some therapists off, as well as a narcissistic character structure that leads them to believe that they do not have to change because they are just fine the way they are. Many hesitate to do the hard work that effective therapy entails, and few willingly relinquish the pleasures, rewards, and excitement of acting out, such as the fun they get from defeating authority as they sadistically watch their do-gooder therapists squirm and fail in their crusades to help them become more socialized.

However, the outlook improves somewhat when:

1. Unsuccessful by chance or self-destructive by design, they find themselves in trouble with society or the law and have to attend and show progress in therapy.
2. They retain a modicum of guilt and self-loathing.
3. They are lonely because material gain has come at the expense of the loss of friends and family—those fleeced and those critical of the individual's antisocial behavior.
4. They have finally become aware of the inefficiency involved in attempting to get something for nothing.
5. They have finally become aware of how they have failed to meet their potential and now want to go from being social misfit to pillar of society.
6. They have been coping psychopathically with a series of unfavorable circumstances that are now behind them.

In my opinion, these individuals can benefit the most from an *eclectic* form of treatment that emphasizes both early and here-and-now issues and employs a combination of psychodynamic, cognitive-behavioral, and interpersonal approaches—simultaneously resolving unconscious conflicts; recognizing and correcting cognitive distortions; correcting behavior by both positive and negative enforcement, that is, with both encouragement and admonition; and working through interpersonal difficulties. Some therapists have noted that mild psychopaths get better on their own upon becoming depressed, which they may do after getting into trouble with other people in their lives or with the law. These therapists have therefore set out to convert psychopathy into depression and to then use the depression as an impetus for change and a focus of treatment. One therapist successfully induced depression in a psychopathic patient by treating him nonaffirmatively. She undermined the patient's narcissistic defenses by asking him such confrontational questions as "Who do you think you are that you are entitled to get something for nothing?" or an even harsher "What makes you feel that you are really a special somebody, not a big nobody?"

Other therapists, disagreeing, prefer to use a more supportive approach. Their goal is to build a positive, long-term, therapeutic relationship that will at a minimum tide these individuals over the rough spots in their lives. These therapists may be satisfied to just keep the patient alive and out of trouble while waiting for the disorder to remit spontaneously. Such therapists affirm the patient. They view him or her not as bad but as troubled, and instead of responding to the inevitable flare-ups and relapses with negative behavioral correctives such as "You'll be discharged from (i.e., thrown out of) therapy if you continue this way," they focus on offering the patient positive feedback and special incentives and rewards for doing well, such as a day pass from the hospital to go shopping as a reward for sticking with and doing well in occupational therapy.

An important caveat is that therapists who respond to the usual psychopathic cons and manipulations by becoming morally judgmental and punitive are not likely to help their patients. More likely they are going to make them worse.

Milieu Therapy

Briget Dolan, while holding out little hope for individual therapy, feels more sanguine about group and milieu therapy taking place in a democratic therapeutic community without a hierarchical structure.[11] This community emphasizes group therapy, and most of the discipline is taken over by a governing body made up of patients, of course always under staff supervision.

Family Therapy

Working with the family is an integral part of treating psychopathic patients. The therapist can double-check the patient's history and monitor the patient's progress with a view to making certain that he or she isn't continuing to behave badly and then covering up. The therapist can also help the family recognize, learn about, and accept the diagnosis of psychopathy. Most families can use useful therapeutic advice on how to deal with and cope with the psychopath, in particular on how the family members can protect themselves from the psychopath's abusive verbal, emotional, physical, and financial assaults. The therapist can also help the family plan for a situation that doesn't improve. For example, the therapist might advise the family that it can be a bad idea to leave a psychopathic child an inheritance outright and that a much better idea is to provide him or her with an annuity.

Black, emphasizing the importance of helping those "who [every day] live with ASP . . . in someone they love," stresses the importance of having the family "take . . . a stand against antisocial behavior" (p. 152).[3] Families of adolescent children with a conduct disorder often need to be helped to strike a healthy balance between being too permissive and being too punitive with the child. Overly permissive parents need to strongly and unambivalently set limits that discourage their children from acting out antisocially. They should avoid treating their children like infant kings and queens to the point that they bring their children up believing that their parents, and the world, owe them everything. As examples, parents should discourage their children from faking being sick in order to stay out of school, forbid their children to associate with bad companions, and make certain that their children are not hiding drugs or bomb-making equipment in their rooms. They should avoid reflexively rescuing their children each time they get into trouble and instead allow them early on to get a taste of the negative consequences of their antisocial actions so that they do not grow up believing that they can get away with just about anything.

However, parents should not go to the opposite extreme and deprive their children unduly. Parents who do that can turn their children into adults chiefly or only concerned with making up for previous lacks by any means whatsoever. I have seen cases where children became rebellious as their way to cope with excessively controlling, punitive parents. Such children first parentalized society then behaved antisocially to get back at their parents—by keying cars, destroying their neighbor's lawn ornaments, egging their neighbor's houses, defacing property with graffiti, or driving through gay neighborhoods shouting anti-gay epithets out of car windows.

This said, I do not fully buy into Black's suggestion that a central therapeutic task is to help families "recognize that it's not your fault" (p. 152)[3] if a loved one is psychopathic. I strongly believe that parents, other family, and friends can and frequently do enable psychopathy, which they often do as a way of solving their own problems or as an indirect way of getting exactly what they long for. Some parents have done their enabling by encouraging the child to act out for them either subtly or openly. In the realm of subtle encouragement, one mother did this by wishing for a bouquet of flowers within earshot of the child each time the family passed a neighbor's garden. In the realm of overt encouragement, a mother took her child out of school in order to begin home schooling. Her real motive was not to provide the child with a better education but to avoid having her unruly child properly disciplined by the authorities. I have had more than a few cases of enabling spouses, such as a spouse who is a crook at heart enjoys and profits from having a thief in the family.

Enabling families need to start setting firm rules and enforcing them strictly. They need to stop rewarding psychopathic behavior and to instead start responding in a therapeutic way by setting limits on those family members who lie, cheat, steal, and otherwise behave psychopathically. In particular they need to stop undermining the therapist in order to defeat therapy. A therapist was doing well with a psychopath patient—until the patient's parents saw the therapist with his lover at the opera and informed the patient that the therapist was most likely gay. They did this deliberately to disrupt therapy so that the patient could resume his pathological ways, ways that served his parents' dynamic needs and practical purposes.

SOCIAL REMEDIES

Those who propose social remedies for psychopathy fall into two camps: those who blame an increasingly liberal society for the present-day rise in the incidence and severity of psychopathy, and those who suggest that the real problem lies with the ultraconservative point of view, because that predictably leads to the reactive rebelliousness and defiance characteristic of the psychopathic way of life.

Benjamin B. Wolman, a psychologist whose view of the causes of and cures for psychopathy reveals a conservative bent, suggests that psychopathy is caused at least in part by a permissive society. He specifically blames a "flimsy, inconsistent, overpermissive, and procrastinating judicial system" for creating "a social climate conducive to sociopathic, antisocial acts." Focusing on the problem of unlimited freedom, he insists, "Democracy does not mean unlimited freedom to organize self-righteous sociopathic gangs." He then suggests (in text he underlines for emphasis), that "democracy means the same freedom for all, [not as the] dictators and terrorists practice all freedom for some" (p. 158).[12]

H. J. Eysenck concludes that psychopathy is the product of faulty conscience development and that "conscience . . . is a conditioned response," suggesting that treatment that does not focus on conditioning is likely to be ineffective, so that "traditional psychodynamic and non-directive client-centered therapies are to be avoided within general samples of offenders." Eysenck also suggests getting serious about punishing crime. As he notes, while "caution should be given on the occasion of the first offense . . . serious punishment should follow the next offense" and should consist of "the restricted use . . . of prison [as] rehabilitation" (p. 46).[13]

Society needs to stop enabling psychopathy. The attitudes of our individualistic (as opposed to collectivistic) society are to an extent mirrored in the psychopath's concern for his or her own rights over the rights of others and of society as a whole. In our society we as individuals not only tolerate but also encourage individual psychopathy, and we do so for a number of reasons. One is our generally overly permissive attitude that unconsciously stays our hand when it comes to stopping others' psychopathic behavior, so that we find ourselves coming up with one reason after another to figuratively, and sometimes even literally, let psychopaths get away with murder. Another is our tendency to ourselves be frustrated psychopaths who want to act psychopathically but due to laudable self-restraint can do little more than provoke others to act out for us. Also, not surprisingly, those of us who secretly want to behave psychopathically ourselves hesitate to condemn psychopathic behavior in others. To illustrate, writing about street vendors selling fakes, Tracie Rozhon and Rachel Thorner, two *New York Times* reporters, asked someone buying from the vendors if they are concerned about legal consequences of their behavior.[14] The revealing and all-too-typical dismissive response was: "'Whatever . . . I'm not the one who is going to get into trouble'" (p. C5).[14] Finally, too many of us have a competitive sadistic streak that prompts us to indulge our appetite for Schadenfreude, so that we stand by and watch with glee as psychopaths bring our rivals down and get sinful pleasure from being able to say to ourselves, "I am smart, not like those dummies."

However, there are flaws in the hypothesis that overpermissiveness is the root of all psychopathy. For one thing, the possibility exists that the punitive behavior of one breeds the sneaky, aggressive, rebellious, retaliative behavior of the other. Many of my patients became and remained psychopaths in part in order to get revenge on an establishment they felt had, and indeed sometimes actually had, wronged them. Certainly, sending adolescents to reform school for psychopathic criminality can backfire when, instead of reforming, the individual learns even more psychopathic ropes.

Another flaw in Eysenck's theory is one Eysenck himself suggested. Since these individuals show poor conditionability, they won't learn from any kind of experience, good or bad, which means they will learn little or nothing from being condemned, controlled, and punished. As one patient said about himself, "I am like a dog that pulls right through its choke collar to be able to continue as before, testing limits even though I know how unpleasant or dangerous the consequences of my actions are likely to be."

What can we all do? As therapists and related professionals we can take pains to avoid self-serving actions that set a bad example, such as giving corrupt testimony in court, cheating on Medicare, or touting idiosyncratic therapy based on ill-considered theories that cross over into the realm of quackery.

As laypeople, all of us can help our children, parents, neighbors, and coworkers, superiors and underlings on the job, become healthy, balanced people. We can set a good example for all concerned by being neither excessively punitive nor excessively overpermissive. We can become more empathic and altruistic as well as more generally affirming, the latter by seeing and acknowledging the other person's point of view, understanding his or her motivation, even or especially when his or her actions are not to our liking, and treating others not as objects to be pushed around and toyed with like chess pieces but as intelligent, sentient individuals with human desires and needs, to be understood, respected, loved, and, whenever reasonable and possible, gratified.

All concerned, whenever possible, can and should use personal and professional influence and political clout to inject rationality and fairness into a world where presently passion replaces perspective and dishonesty triumphs over accountability. For example, we should all speak out against social hypocrisy. In particular we should all work toward a society that does not send mixed messages that are the product of, and in turn create, a severe crisis of morality. Those of us in authority must avoid on the one hand saying, "Do as I say" and on the other hand saying, "Do as you wish." It strikes me as maladaptive and counterproductive that we now condemn drunk driving and yet build bars on the highway, and on the one hand condemn computer hacking and on the other hand fail to pursue and punish hackers, or, pursuing and finding them, first let them off easy then reward them with a job working for us as consultants, side by side as allies in the fight against computer crime. To me it is just common sense that our society, which today condemns spyware for clogging computers and stealing personal information and tomorrow catches but fails to punish those who write the programs, needs to do one of two things, and to do neither of them halfway. It needs to either change its attitudes and ways, or it needs to just accept the fact that sooner or later psychopaths, both mild and severe, will be in the majority, and that psychopathy will come to constitute not an emotional disorder that needs to be vanquished but a standard of normalcy that needs to be accepted, and even respected. If we are not careful, I predict that we will find ourselves in the position of being unable to answer with certainty Dr. Raeleen Mautner's (personal communication, 2005) perceptive and troubling question: "Is psychopathy abnormal, or is it normal to be a psychopath?"

REFERENCES

1. Stout, M. (2005). *The sociopath next door*. New York: Broadway Books.
2. Toch, H. (1998). Psychopathy or antisocial personality in forensic settings. In T. Millon, E. Simonsen, M. Birket-Smith, & R. D. Davis (Eds.), *Psychopathy* (pp. 144–158). New York: Guilford Press.
3. Black, D. W. (1999). *Bad boys, bad men*. New York: Oxford University Press.
4. Hare, R. D. (1999). *Without conscience*. New York: Guilford Press.
5. Cleckley, H. (1955). *The mask of sanity*. St. Louis, MO: C. V. Mosby.
6. American Psychiatric Association. (1994). *Diagnostic and statistical manual of mental disorders*, (4th ed.). Washington, DC: Author.
7. Oldham, J.M., & Morris, L. B. (1995). *The new personality self-portrait*. New York: Bantam Books.
8. Millon, T. (1981). *Disorders of personality: DSM–III, Axis III*. New York: John Wiley and Sons.
9. Simon, R. I. (1996). *Bad men do what good men dream*. Washington, DC: American Psychiatric Press.
10. Kernberg, O. F. (1998). The psychotherapeutic management of psychopathic, narcissistic, and paranoid transferences. In T. Millon, E. Simonsen, M. Birket-Smith, & R. D. Davis (Eds.), *Psychopathy* (pp. 372–392). New York: Guilford Press.

11. Dolan, B. (1998). Therapeutic community treatment for severe personality disorders. In T. Millon, E. Simonsen, M. Birket-Smith, & R. D. Davis (Eds.), *Psychopathy* (pp. 407–430). New York: Guilford Press.
12. Wolman, B. B. (1999). *Antisocial behavior.* Amherst, NY: Prometheus Books.
13. Eysenck, H. J. (1998). Personality and crime. In T. Millon, E. Simonsen, M. Birket-Smith, & R. D. Davis (Eds.), *Psychopathy* (pp. 40–49). New York: Guilford Press.
14. Rozhon, T., & Thorner, R. (2005, 26 May). They sell no fake before its time. *New York Times,* pp. C1, C5.

Chapter 2

Narcissism: Greek Tragedy, Psychological Syndrome, Cultural Norm

Jerrold Lee Shapiro and Susan Bernadett-Shapiro

Most people know the story of the youth Narcissus, who became so enamored with his own image in a reflecting pond that he ultimately eschewed all romantic relationships with others, pined away, and died. Lesser known is the precursor to that final episode: Narcissus's fear of finding an imperfection and his cruelty to maidens. The nymph Echo was one who felt his disdain. She became enamored with young Narcissus, "a youth, whose beauty surpassed all others,"[1] but when she agreed to meet with him, his rejection was most cruel. When she endeavored to "throw her arms around his neck, he started back, exclaiming, 'Hands off! I would rather die than you should have me!'"[2] Echo slunk away to live in the wilderness, suffering in grief until she died. As legend has it, only her voice remained, even to this day, to reply to anyone who calls over canyons to her. Narcissus's cruelty to Echo was hardly unique. When he shunned another maiden, she prayed to an avenging goddess that he should suffer the same fate of rejection as she. Her prayers were answered. One day, Narcissus, tired and thirsty, knelt down to drink from a fountain and glistening pool. Seeing his own image reflected in the water, he believed it was a beautiful water spirit. In that moment, he fell in love with his own image. Of course his attempts to kiss and embrace the beloved object were unsuccessful. Each time he tried to feel it,

> it fled at the touch, but returned again after a moment and renewed the fascina-
> tion. He could not tear himself away; he lost all thought of food or rest, while
> he hovered over the brink of the fountain gazing upon his own image. He talked

with the supposed spirit: "Why, beautiful being, do you shun me? Surely my face is not one to repel you. The nymphs love me, and you yourself look not indifferent upon me. When I stretch forth my arms you do the same; and you smile upon me and answer my beckonings with the like."[3]

As he pined away, his tears fell into the water and disturbed the image. As he saw it depart, he exclaimed, "Stay, I entreat you! Let me at least gaze upon you, if I may not touch you."[4]

Thus exist two major components of a modern day affliction: (1) obsessive self-involvement, including fear of defects and feelings of grandiosity and entitlement and (2) a lack of empathy (leading to cruelty) toward others.

The term narcissism describes both a psychiatric relational disorder and perhaps an evolving cultural norm.

As early as the turn of the 20th century, Theodore B. Veblen warned of "conspicuous consumption"—the elevation of form over substance.[5] In 1979, Christopher Lasch depicted a serious decline of social justice and a corresponding increase in competitive individualism.[6] Historians such as Richard L. Rapson have also noted the evolving imbalance between collectivism and individualism in American culture.[7] As rampant individualism becomes dominant in a culture, image takes on a higher priority than internal substance and narcissism becomes normative. Several questions emerge from these observations.

- Where are the boundaries between creative self-involvement and pathological relating?
- Is narcissism becoming the norm in modern-day America?
- Is narcissism a cultural phenomenon or a psychiatric syndrome?

To answer these questions, we explore both the psychological disorder and the cultural enhancement of narcissistic behavior.

A WORKING UNDERSTANDING OF NARCISSISM

It is important to recognize the common misconception that narcissists are in love with themselves. Just as for the Narcissus of myth, the narcissist is not in love with himself.[8] *He is in love with his reflection.* This is an important difference and is an essential piece in understanding the narcissistic syndrome. Rather than being in love with himself, he often fears at a deeper level that he is quite unlikable. Because his yardstick for lovability is observed perfection, he lives in how others see him. He lacks an objective or realistic measure. Instead, he becomes lost in whether, and how much, his reflection (also known as his "public self" or "persona") is appreciated. In short, the narcissist doesn't know or strive to know who he truly is. He is obsessed with his appearance.

This is the essential flaw. Because he loves only image or reflection, the narcissist must constantly strive to project an idealized image of himself. He becomes obsessed with perfecting the facade. In doing so, he may well deplete his energy, making him emotionally vulnerable. So depleted by putting all this energy into his appearance, he is often deeply hurt by others who either criticize or ignore his highly crafted image.

To the narcissist, love is indistinguishable from admiration, fear, or even awe. When he feels feared or "respected" by others, he believes that he is loved. Sadly, because the image is what draws the respect, he must constantly live up to this projection. In this way, he becomes progressively divorced from his inner self and married to the illusion. Any "true self" that he may have becomes solely a slave to the image.

Is a True Narcissist "Selfish"?

Because his image is paramount, it is easy to consider him selfish and egotistical. Yet there is an inherent conflict in that supposition. The narcissist is driven to please others, if, for no other reason, to be seen as a truly wonderful person. In this way, paradoxically, he becomes unattuned to his personal needs, aside from his need for admiration. Instead of putting himself first, he ends up putting last his true self, which becomes increasingly submerged. Meanwhile, his craving for the love and admiration of others forces him to serve only his childlike illusions of omnipotence and omniscience. Thus, because his very existence is ruled by how others respond to his image, his personal needs for growth, self-development, and intimacy are submerged or lost.

With so much of his energy focused on image enhancement, he has little left to give to others, which, combined with his inability to love flawed human beings, ultimately dooms him to a life of emotional loneliness. Although he is lonely, he presents the aura of a fierce individualist, zealously protecting his turf from others' dependency. This perfectionistic illusion of emotional independence is a "defensive" stance, which allows emotional nourishment for neither self nor others.

Entitlement: The Appearance of Extreme Selfishness

The combination of an illusion of caring and an illusion of extreme selfishness comes from a unique aspect of this personality: the belief in entitlement. If the image is so positive, surely he deserves to be treated better than normal people. As we will see later in this chapter, when the narcissist is treated as if he were an equal to others, he takes that as a betrayal, often feels cheated, or feels as if he is the object of discrimination. As an entitled person, he believes that he should get more than a fair share, and his anger at such a slight can be quite formidable.

Having a superior (entitled) air is tied closely to a sense of grandiosity. Of course, some narcissists are quite dynamic, extraverted, and successful. Yet it is quite rare that their actual level of success matches their inflated self-image.

Thus, the paradox. He believes he should have special status, based on the quality of his image, but at another level, the substance of his true self goes unnoticed.

Because he lives primarily through a projected idealized self-image, the narcissist must constantly receive praise from others. This is the "evidence" of his superiority, and in the need for ever-increasing praise, he often exploits others as little more than instruments for personal gratification. Because of the belief that he is not accountable to mere average people, he will easily justify the consequences his behavior has on others' lives.

It is important to note that he is not unaware of the impact on others. He doesn't care, because he doesn't value nonfunctional, caring relationships with others. His experience and understanding of relationships is limited to one-way or mutual adoration, which enhances his perceived standing in a group. This quality is often perceived as a lack of empathy: a telling symptom of narcissism.

The Perils of Narcissism

Any personality that is so dependent on reflected glory is constantly vulnerable. A simple negative perception or minor criticism can be grounds for devastating threat. When Robert, an engineer at a software company, received his annual evaluation from his boss, it contained all "1's" and a single "2." Robert could not accept or tolerate the second highest category for one item, without risking a complete crumbling of his perfectionistic facade. A classic narcissist, he considered the objectively reasonable evaluation as an attack, which he believed had to be met with a show of great force to "right this terrible wrong." Robert's boss and coworkers were quite surprised by his extraordinary reaction.

Narcissists like Robert have a dichotomous experience of the world. Because there is no possibility of accepting a less than perfect evaluation, his psyche cannot allow for any shades of gray. In this way, the narcissist lives his life on the emotional edge. The narcissist is responding to extreme danger—emotional life threats—and his reactions seem extraordinary to others who fail to see the threat. One cannot have even a minor disagreement without tapping into his "fight or flight" response.

This level of reactivity leads to an almost paranoid quality in the way the narcissist relates to others. He must constantly question their motives and look for criticism or disapproval. His extreme responses to minor or even absent slights often come across as bullying and blaming.

He cannot accept blame personally. It would constitute an injury to his image. Once wounded, the narcissist will accept no apologies, unless they are accompanied with humiliation, full acceptance of all responsibility by the other person, and extraordinary recompense. Forgiveness is not part of the narcissistic life. Often relationships are permanently broken over a perceived slight.

Narcissistic wounds can particularly be delivered by others who have previously held high status (for their successes, position, or what they can offer). Once hurt by an individual who he had initially idealized, the narcissist's fury has barely any bounds. His devaluation of the person is often quite public and destructive. Falling from the narcissist's grace renders a person "unsupportive" and useless in providing resources. Because such a fall presents a glimpse of a frightening picture of the narcissist's personal vulnerability, it is greeted by him with abhorrence, denigration, and rage.

Because the flip from idealizing to denigrating is so dichotomous and because it takes so much to fill up the narcissistic need, long-term relationships are likely to fail, and new people need always to be brought in continuously to pick up the slack.

NARCISSISM AS A CLINICAL SYNDROME

It is not always easy to distinguish between narcissistic character traits, cultural-centric narcissism, and narcissistic personality disorder. Only the last is a clinical syndrome. Narcissistic Personality Disorder is defined in the *DSM–IV* (*Diagnostic and Statistical Manual* published by the American Psychiatric Association). The syndrome is diagnosed on Axis II and represents one of the disorders of personality. Primarily, these diagnoses are descriptive of relational rather than thought, mood, or anxiety disorders. Generally, they are considered to be based on developmental deficits in relationship development.

As can be seen in Table 2.1, the narcissist is characterized as a selfish, uncaring, ruthless, and exploitive person. This is in quite sharp contrast to his internal experience, which is more one of anxiety, a deep lack of confidence, and often dissatisfaction. In short, the internal and external experiences of a narcissist are quite discrepant. Feelings of superiority and entitlement are matched unconsciously by insecurity and the need to constantly prove himself. His successful demeanor is often a single step away from instability. Propriety and the need for acceptance can give way to tantrums and bullying. How could he get this way? What could produce a Narcissistic Personality Disorder?

Table 2.1
***DSM–IV* Diagnostic Criteria for Narcissistic Personality Disorder**

According to the DSM–IV, Narcissistic Personality Disorder is characterized
as follows:

A pervasive pattern of grandiosity (in fantasy or behavior), need for admiration, and lack of
empathy, beginning by early adulthood and present in a variety of contexts, as indicated by
five (or more) of the following:

1. has a grandiose sense of self-importance (e.g., exaggerates achievements and talents,
   expects to be recognized as superior without commensurate achievements)
2. is preoccupied with fantasies of unlimited success, power, brilliance, beauty, or ideal
   love
3. believes that he or she is "special" and unique and can only be understood by, or
   should associate with, other special or high-status people (or institutions)
4. requires excessive admiration
5. has a sense of entitlement, i.e., unreasonable expectations of especially favorable
   treatment or automatic compliance with his or her expectations
6. is interpersonally exploitative, i.e., takes advantage of others to achieve his or her
   own ends
7. lacks empathy: is unwilling to recognize or identify with the feelings and needs of
   others
8. is often envious of others or believes that others are envious of him or her
9. shows arrogant, haughty behaviors or attitudes

Source: American Psychiatric Association, Desk Reference to the Diagnostic Criteria from *DSM–IV*
(Washington, DC: American Psychiatric Association, 1994), 282.

THE ETIOLOGY OF NARCISSISM

It is important to note that all theorists who address this syndrome agree
that narcissism is a healthy and appropriate stage of childhood development.
Sigmund Freud originally viewed it as the normal developmental stage between
the autoeroticism of the infant and capacity for the developing child to love
others.[9]

Heinz Kohut's theory of the self perhaps best illuminates both normal and
clinical narcissism.[10] *The self,* defined as the "center of the of the individual's
psychological universe,"[11] forms through relationships with primary caregivers. The child's sense of self evolves as a result of the interaction between
the child's innate potentials and the empathic responses of adult caregivers.
To develop effectively, a child's budding self has two distinct needs: mirroring
and availability of an ideal adult image with whom the child can identify and
internalize.

Mirroring. When a caregiver attends to a child, listens to him, reflects his accomplishments, extols his positive qualities, and generally spends quality time with

the child, it is referred to as *mirroring*. It involves noticing the small things a child does well, such as smiling, walking, coming when called, or treating a pet kindly. When this happens, the child feels appreciated and experiences himself as a valued person who can then begin to appreciate himself.

Another aspect of mirroring involves the child reflecting his mistakes in a manner that promotes healthy self-knowledge and self-esteem. For parents, this means acknowledging the error without disparaging the person. Such non-traumatic failures foster development of the child's self. He grows emotionally as he internalizes these parental functions, and he successfully meets new challenges through reliance on his budding internal self (ego structure). Once this base is in place, the self grows further in the absence of direct parental responses, when the challenge is within the child's developing capacity.

In healthy development, the child's normal initial sense of grandiosity ("when I cry, milk is produced") is gradually modified and transformed into energy, ambition, and self-esteem.

Furthermore, as the child experiences the parents as reliable empathic figures, he is able to internalize a reliable ideal self with which to guide behavior and empathize with others.

> **Internalization.** In addition to the parental reflection of the child's appropriate grandiose-exhibitionistic self, there is an equivalent need for the parents to be mature persons for the child to emulate. As the parents exhibit ethical behavior, justice, and compassion, the child begins to find and develop those qualities in his self. In short, the caregivers provide an ideal adult image with whom the child can identify and subsequently internalize as his own idealized self.

Narcissistic Disorders

Narcissistic disorders are believed to arise when there is a consistent failure of either of these parental characteristics that normally promote psychological growth.

Thus they can arise when the child does not receive appropriate mirroring during early childhood. When the child experiences repeated failure to applaud and admire his emerging accomplishments, his grandiose self goes underground and becomes unavailable for continued development and modification. The child experiences a split in which his grandiosity remains unintegrated into his personality. This produces a paradoxical combination of bravado and low self-esteem. The mirror hungry child is compelled to attract the attention of others to bolster his low self-esteem, often through a spiraling series of empty accomplishments.[12]

Similarly, the child who lacks a parent who can provide a proper ideal image for identification will engage on a search to find such an idealized "other" with whom he may identify for the purpose of building internal psychic structure, specifically the ideal self. This seeking can take the form of joining pro-social groups or joining gangs and cults. In a milder form it can be the naive trust in powerful charismatic leaders and the need for our celebrities and politicians to be perceived as royalty.

Narcissistic pathology results from the repeated empathic failure of the caregivers. Usually, these failures are the result of the parents' own pathology and inadequately developed self. Such parents may be preoccupied with their own needs for grandiosity and may even expect that the child would provide the parents with satisfactory mirroring. These parents may also need the child to be ideal as a way of fulfilling their own needs for ego strength. In this way, the children are seen as mere extensions of their parent's selves rather than as separate beings with their own needs.

Many authors have argued that the extreme neglect that comes from a failure of mirroring and ideal parent internalization could constitute a form of emotional abuse: a precondition for most personality disorders. It seems clear that the dehumanization that results from sexual, physical, or psychological abuse represents extreme forms of repeated empathic failure.

A child who is frustrated and/or abused learns quickly that the only "object" he can trust, the only one who is reliably available, and the one person he can love without risk of abandonment is himself.

Once a child eschews the untrustworthy others, his development of a model/ideal self is severely limited. Instead, he adopts the more primitive grandiosity and begins to feel omnipotent and omniscient. Unchecked by reality, he believes himself superior, worthy of adoration, and entitled to special treatment as an adult. The relational traits of a mature person, such as empathy, compassion, working hard toward a goal, fair comparisons with others' skills and boundaries, and especially the ability to postpone gratification are simply not learned. Often he feels as if he has a birthright and is preordained to be part of the ruling class.

Of course, faced with the vagaries of the real world, this feeling and presentation is quite vulnerable. Indeed, his emotional susceptibility to criticism is brittle. Having failed to develop a realistic self from interactions with caregivers and later, other adult figures, he is "struck to the core" with even slight disagreement. This is so because at a deep level, he fears that he has been exposed as a phony. All narcissists are besieged by unconscious feelings of inadequacy and low self-worth (fluctuating with exaggerated, yet fragile, overvaluation of self-worth) that result directly from the (often unconscious) fears of another emotional abandonment. In short, having suffered from repeated empathic failure by his caregivers, he replicates this lack of empathy to others as an adult.

Craig is a good example of this phenomenon. At 38, he had a long history of relationships with women but no long-term commitments. His primary means of interaction involved looking for praise for his myriad successes as a real estate salesman and a consistent debasing of his current lady friend. He would frequently treat his partner, Denise, as stupid and beneath him. On his 37th birthday, he criticized the special meal she cooked for him, the wine she chose, her manner of dress, her weight, the way she talked to his friends that she invited, and finally, aspects of her love making. Months later, after several repetitions of humiliation, she left him. He reacted with fury at being rejected and was deeply hurt. Emotionally, he experienced a replication of his childhood trauma, when his mother left him with his stepfather and did not return for over a year. His fury was magnified a year later when he heard that Denise had married another man, Carl. On the surface he saw her new husband, who was far less successful financially than he, as unworthy of a woman who had been with him at one time. He could not comprehend that Carl offered Denise empathy and compassion—something he could not.

Craig's failing with Denise did not lead him to self-reflection or a revised sense about how to treat others, especially significant others. Indeed, his theories of what occurred were primarily confirmations of his initial conclusion that she was inferior to him. Of course, his pain about this loss lingered for years, doubtlessly compounded by several subsequent similar experiences.

The disorder from which he suffered was developmental and historical. To repair it in the present, he would have to experience a relationship in which he received the mirroring he missed as a child. He would need an emotionally corrective relationship to supersede the failure of the original parental one. Craig was fortunate. He was able, over time, to develop such a relationship with a therapist, and by the time he was in his mid forties, he was able to transform the mirroring and internalization of that relationship into a more complete sense of himself and subsequently a successful relationship with a woman, to whom he is now married

What constitutes good enough parenting to avoid the development of a narcissistic personality disorder? Parents need to be mature enough to focus on their children's needs for appropriate limits. They need to be present and engaged with enough integrity to be experienced as an ideal other. Parents cannot be perfect. In fact, being, or striving to be, perfect could hinder their children's development. Parents who demonstrate through words and deeds that they are worthy of respect and esteem will provide a "good enough" figure for identification.

WHY DO WE SEE AN INCREASE IN NARCISSISTIC PATHOLOGY?

Parents who lack an empathic capacity or consistency have been with us for a very long time. Yet it seems that narcissistic personality disorders are increasing in the modern world. There are many potential reasons, both psychological/familial and sociocultural:

1. We may see an increase in narcissistic personalities due to *advances in assessment and diagnosis.* We may better understand the normal development of the psyche and the specific failures in the normal developmental processes that can result in the manifestation of clinical narcissism.

2. Our *culture and family structure have also evolved* in directions that might result in a greater incidence of empathic failure in child rearing and consequent narcissistic pathology. The diminution of physical proximity to extended family and close-knit communities can result in added pressure on parents and children to negotiate interactions without traditional supports. This, combined with busy or absent parents, may contribute to a lack of appropriate mirroring and available adult figures for idealization and identification.

3. *Divorce and other trauma* may expose children to an early rupture in their need to idealize parents. Exposure to breech of commitment, betrayal, infidelity, parental abuse of drugs and alcohol, and parental decompensation during a divorce can be traumatic for the child's budding self-development and identification with parents. Divorce ushers in an abrupt loss in idealization that disrupts the children's trust, both in their parents and in their selves. It can inhibit or reverse a more gradual awareness of parents' imperfections, during which the child can retain his own idealized self and idealized other even as these are modified appropriately over time into "good enough" self and other. Whatever the traumatic event, it is the comfort and caring that the parent provides during the event that is important. A divorce handled well can be less traumatic than simply parents' busy schedules, where the parents miss the empathic connection, understanding and attunement necessary for the child's developing psyche. Repeated empathic failure, not imperfection, is the problem.

4. *Fear* may be another factor that contributes to parental empathic failure. We have more fear these days about preparing our children for the future. We know they will compete in a global society for limited resources. We have increased fears for their safety as we are exposed to media coverage

of every disaster imaginable. Because of these fears, parents may be more demanding of their children academically, expect more independence at an earlier age, and yet try to shelter them from perceived dangers. In this regard, they may miss their child's developmental needs in favor of their own needs for him to do well in life and be prepared for what appears to be an increasingly uncertain future. We may miss our children's need for listening, understanding, and empathic responding in our own hurry to get things done and provide a better life for them.

Narcissism is a normal stage in child development and does not entirely vanish in adulthood. In a healthy individual, infantile narcissism is gradually transformed to energy, ambition, self-care, self-growth, and the extension of self to family and community. Pathological narcissism is the result of repeated empathic failure during childhood and the lack of adult figures for idealization, identification, and internalization. Specific factors contributing to empathic failure may include the isolation of the nuclear family, single-parent families, lack of social supports such as high quality affordable child care, preschools, and elementary schools, and cultural values such as individualism and materialism.

THE CULTURE OF NARCISSISM

Consider the characteristics of the narcissist. He exudes a sense of belief in his own specialness and associates primarily with others of special or high status. He requires a certain level of admiration. He is comfortable with interpersonal exploitation, discarding former supporters and spouses as they ascend or maintain status. He is envious of those above him in wealth, public recognition, or influence and expects and suspects that others envy his fame.

Such qualities are common to many of the notable successes in American culture. Our stars and modern heroes are remarkable for their larger-than-life images and public presentations. Can we not view many of our sports heroes, movie stars, supermodels, and titans of industry as grandiose, arrogant, and in consistent need of unlimited admiration?

Cultural Royalty

The expectation of special treatment for stars is quite strong. In 2005, film superstar Tom Cruise, on a promotional tour to promote both his new film and his new engagement, expressed outrage that interviewers did not accept *unquestioningly* his views on Scientology. The question is not about Mr. Cruise's craft, nor his box office appeal. It is about the hubris of expecting that his skill as an actor will make him a valid religious spokesman.

Professional athletes, the gladiators of our times, are paid and encouraged to be uniquely narcissistic. Football star Terrell Owens has insisted for the second time in two years that his legal contract be revised upward. Last year, he refused to report to one team to which he was traded, forcing a more favorable trade. In Mr. Owens's mind, he is larger than his team, larger than his sport. Mr. Owens is not alone.

When future hall of fame baseball pitcher Pedro Martinez left the Boston Red Sox for the New York Mets, his stated reason for making the move was "respect." To him and his stardom, the Red Sox were willing to reward him insufficiently for the level of his personal image.

Professional basketball player Latrell Sprewell, who unfortunately is best known for choking his former coach in a practice, expressed his deep hurt and sense of being "disrespected" (a key term for narcissistic injury) when he was offered *only* $14 million in his most recent annual contract. When the media jumped on his "arrogance," he reportedly replied, with supreme self-justification, that he had a family to feed.

He Who Dies with the Most Toys Wins

Of course, Mr. Sprewell's salary is minimal compared to compensation for CEOs in some large corporations. Their remarkable salaries compared to those of their workers can only be explained by greed or narcissism.

According to *Forbes* magazine's (2004) annual review of top packages for CEOs, Terry S. Semel of Yahoo! "earned" $230.6 million; Barry Diller of IAC/InterActiveCorp, $156.2 million; and William W. McGuire of UnitedHealth Group, $124.8 million.[13] Mr. McGuire's success was generated in large part by reducing health benefits to subscribers and compensation to health care providers.

Other notables include Oracle's Larry Ellison and his three-quarters of a *billion* dollars in 2001; Apple's Steve Jobs's nearly $400 million in 2000; Michael Eisner's roughly $1 billion since becoming CEO of Disney; and former Tyco CEO Dennis Kozlowski's $100-million-a-year pay package. Apparently Mr. Kozlowski deemed this compensation insufficient. When he was indicted for stealing $600 million in company funds and for evading sales taxes, he resigned with generous severance. Of course, the gold standard of severance/retirement packages went to former GE CEO, Jack Welch. As came to light in his highly public divorce, he received, in addition to a substantive pension, lifetime tickets to New York's Yankee Stadium and Boston's Fenway Park, a Manhattan penthouse, a plane at his disposal, a chauffer and cars, and numerous other perks.

It could be greed alone that allows these individuals to take compensation that goes so far beyond "feeding their family," but from a psychological perspective, it is something else as well. Such remuneration enhances the comparative image of the recipients. If they compete successfully with others, they somehow do not have to reflect on an inner sense of insecurity and fears of rejection. Of course, a couple of million dollars annually can purchase any number of sycophants in an entourage.

What is particularly interesting from a cultural standpoint is that the media and many in the culture see these salaries and egos as admirable, or at least justifiable. What else can explain that the oft-expressed belief that a CEO is *worth* the $100 million annual compensation packages. According to Harvard professor Rakesh Khurana, MBA students believe these salaries justifiable, doubtlessly in the hope that they too will catch lightning in a bottle.[14]

Success is not the criterion for such reward. Rather, it is the appearance. Indeed, failure is often rewarded with personal retirement packages that could clothe and feed all the residents of some nations. Two grand examples of the significance of form over substance appeared in a mid-July 2005 *Wall Street Journal* article.

On July 14, the *Journal* reported on the 25-year sentence for former WorldCom CEO Bernard Ebbers for his role in the $11 billion fraud during the late 1990s.[15] Mr. Ebbers was charged with ordering employees of the company to "hit the numbers"; to falsely report earnings to meet Wall Street analysts' expectations. On July 15, the paper had a feature article on image consultants, in which was stated, "In a world where people are finding no end to the pressure to be stylish, the booming market for upscale personal services has spawned a new even more rarified creature: the self described lifestyle designer."[16] Such lifestyle experts are dedicated to the image—often quite at odds with the person. In psychological terms, they are focused on the public rather than the real self.

CULTURAL NARCISSISM AND THE MEDIA

There is always a heavily debated question of the extent to which the media reflects a culture and the extent to which it creates one. As is the case with most long-standing heated debates, there is truth to both positions. In the case of narcissism as a cultural phenomenon, the media clearly plays a significant role.

One example of the media expectations of a cultural royalty that stands above all the rules was a recent incident in Paris. Oprah Winfrey, one of the most famous and successful women and one of the most recognizable person-alities in the world, was denied entrance to Hermes, a luxury-goods store in Paris, when she arrived just after closing. Miss Winfrey reportedly expressed disappointment, because there were still shoppers visible within. For the media, however, it went far beyond disappointment; it was an international incident. News coverage around the world speculated on the possibility of racism and ubiquitously pondered why a store would not reopen its doors for such a notable. The sense of the stories was clear: someone of Oprah's fame and fortune *should not* have to follow rules and *should* always receive special treatment.

Perhaps popular cultural values are espoused and manipulated by their prime purveyor, U.S. network television. Many of the most popular programs are of the reality genre. These are almost always characterized by contests in which there is one supreme winner and many losers. *The Apprentice* is but one example in which the key words are uttered by Donald Trump: "You're fired," he roars from his special boardroom as another contestant is confronted with the fact that he or she can no longer play in "The Donald's" field. Mr. Trump's image is exemplary of the culture of narcissism: he refers to himself in the third person as "The Donald" and is primarily well known as the developer whose name must appear on each edifice and on his array of highly publicized marriages, divorces, and prenuptial agreements. He is the sole purveyor of winning and losing.

Similarly, the show *Survivor* involve less popular individuals being "voted off the island"—a term for banishment—in primitive cultures, the worst of all rejections. *American Idol* is a talent show, similar to the old Ted Mack's *Original Amateur Hour*, but with a mean-spirited quirk. Poor performers (or those who show insufficient amounts of skin) are not just losers or runners-up. They are ridiculed by the host.

Whether the narcissism inherent in popular culture is potentially harmful or just distasteful is still in question. When narcissism enters the political realm, the harm is evident.

The Form of Politics

Cultural narcissism has reached well beyond staged reality programs. It has reached into the political realm as well. "Will it play in Peoria?" the mantra of the Nixon administration, has held sway long after Mr. Nixon was forced to leave office for substantive sins. The phrase was an index of how well a particular political maneuver appeared rather than whether it actually reflected deeper truth. Our politicians are "packaged" by Madison Avenue for television and radio sound bites and targeted to specific audiences with the same slick style that is used to sell soft drinks, beer, soap, deodorants, cars, or, increasingly, prescription medications. Teams of speechwriters, clothes designers, and image consultants present an illusion of the person that may or may not truly represent the candidate or office holder. Using charged language, image makers may even alter the nature of issues. Thus, in dealing with the most divisive issue of legalized abortion, what one political faction calls "right to choose," their opponents refer to as "right to life."

The current George W. Bush administration is especially adept at such image control. When he ran for president, his history with substance abuse was somehow declared "not for consideration." His desired reduction of the tax on large estates was refashioned as a "death tax," to garner support from millions who would never benefit personally from such a tax break. Indeed, the money ultimately will come out of their pockets and benefits.

At their extreme, the image makers have been able to create labels for their desired programs that are diametrically opposite their actual impact. A social program such as the No Child Left Behind Act, promoted to enhance education, is, upon closer scrutiny, a reduction in some teaching budgets. The Clean Water Act has provisions that allow for continuing pollution of our water sources. Indeed, we invaded Iraq to protect America from "Weapons of Mass Destruction" that indeed never existed. This seems like a painful déjà vu to President Lyndon Johnson's use of the Gulf of Tonkin incident in 1965. In that case, a purported attack on U.S. vessels was deliberately misconstrued yet served as the reason for increased U.S. military involvement in Vietnam. Just like the Bush administration's misrepresentations in Iraq and remarkable leeway given by Congress, Congress also gave Mr. Johnson unprecedented power in Vietnam. Johnson was authorized to "take all necessary measures to repel armed attack against the forces of the United States and to prevent further aggression."[17]

How is all this related to narcissism? How has our culture gone from a substantive to an image orientation, the way that Narcissus lost sight of anything but his reflection? The answers are both sociocultural and psychological.

ENTITLEMENT OR ENTROPY?

It has been noted by many social commentators that over the past century in the Western world there has been a drift toward disintegration of human relationships and institutions. The individual is honored above the group. Despite much greater access to information, there appears to be a concurrent deterioration in quality parenting and child rearing within our society.

Much of this shift dates to the beginning of the Industrial Revolution. Men were forced from their small family farms and businesses to work in larger centers for increasingly larger corporations. Communities became less efficient in supporting their members. Rather than an equity-based, caring, compassionate ethic that fosters emotional development, we find increasing competitiveness. The "me" generation of the 1970s was never supplanted by the anticipated "we" years. Even the current revival of religious and political interest in the country appears less ecumenical and more segmented, primitive, exclusionary, and fundamental in nature. A mode of business increasingly present since the late 1970s is defined by "eat what you kill" or "I got mine, you get your own!"

When a culture begins to value greed and form over substance, historians are drawn to the insights of Edward Gibbon in his 18th-century classic *The Decline and Fall of the Roman Empire*.[18] A narcissistically oriented culture is vulnerable. It takes but a single misstep to bring it crashing down. When we look behind the curtain at the great Wizard of Oz, we see an old man with smoke and mirrors, trying to protect his image rather than his constituents or his self.

Many observers believe that Western culture is heading into this special form of oblivion. One characteristic of decline that parallels Gibbon's perception is described by Aaron Stern as a strident demand for increasing rewards and a concomitant "unwillingness to accept responsibility for government, family and other social institutions."[19]

In 1899, Thorsten Veblen commented on the loss of social connection in his *Theory of the Leisure Class*.[20] In this influential tract, he postulated that "conspicuous consumption" served only form. It benefited neither society nor the individuals who experienced it. It was simply a new competition, in which the greatest show of economic largesse was the victor. It was show, not substance.

Christopher Lasch describes the alarming growth of ego in our culture, contrasting that growth with the necessary loss of ego inherent in true maturating.[21] He attributes this in part to the corruption of the American Protestant ethic. The Horatio Alger self-made man was in Lasch's terms the "archetypical embodiment of the American dream, [who] owed his advancement to habits of industry, sobriety, moderation, self-discipline, and avoidance of debt." Focused on delay of gratification for greater goals in the future, he made investments in business, family, and community that could grow slowly over time. His gratification came from his good works. For Sigmund Freud, *Arbeit* (work) was a cornerstone of personal human growth.[22] For Lasch, "the self-made man took pride in his judgment of character and probity; today . . . practices the classic arts of seduction, with the same indifference to moral niceties, hoping to win your heart, while picking your pocket."[23]

Goodbye, Horatio Alger. Hello, P.T. Barnum!

Since the turn of the 20th century, social commentators have been decrying a definition of success based on salesmanship and personal magnetism rather than good works. This notion expanded in the 1940s and 1950s with Dale Carnegie's *How to Win Friends and Influence People*[24] and the popularity of radio preacher Norman Vincent Peale.[25] The appearance of success began to supplant hard work as the source of social acclaim.

Today, we are inundated with social imperatives to "dress for success" and to "look your best." Periodicals are filled with suggestions for better living by hiding physical faults. One has only to view the first 50 pages of a women's magazine such as *Seventeen* (which is read primarily by 13-year-olds) or *Cosmopolitan* to discover that a woman's hair, lips, weight, odor, teeth color, bust line, complexion, and so forth, are all defective but correctable with some over-the-counter product. Surely, happiness will follow.

On TV this is carried further to the extreme with "makeovers" or "extreme makeovers" or even "ambush makeovers." These shows take in the "ugly duckling" and transform (typically) her into a beautiful swan in appearance. As part of these image transformations, we have seen a frightening increase in plastic surgery in an industry that has shifted its focus from disfigurement to seemingly commonplace "beauty adjustments." Elective procedures were up 44 percent in the year 2004 alone.[26]

Of course, the underlying assumption is most narcissistic. It is not about the person per se; it is about how she appears to others. What about a person's psychological or spiritual makeover? That is not for the media. That is not about narcissism, because that involves self-reflection and admission that a person wishes to change to be a better person.[27]

Lasch continues,

> In a society in which the dream of success has been drained of any meaning beyond itself, men have nothing against which to measure their achievements except the achievements of others. Self-approval depends on public recognition and acclaim, and the quality of this approval has undergone important changes in its own right. The good opinion of friends and neighbors, which formerly informed a man that he had lived a useful life, rested on appreciation of his accomplishments. Today men ... wish to be not so much esteemed as admired.... They want to be envied rather than respected. Pride and acquisitiveness, the sins of an ascendant capitalism, have given way to vanity.[28]

In a narcissistic world, there is great vulnerability. Fame is a fleeting phenomenon like the daily news. Today's heroes are tomorrow's answers to a trivia question. When our fame, or notoriety, is so dependant on glamour and publicity, the individual's self-esteem is at the mercy of fads and vagaries of public opinion. Lasch concludes, "When policy making, the search for power, and the pursuit of wealth have no other objects than to excite admiration or envy, men lose the sense of objectivity, always precarious under the best of circumstances. Impressions overshadow achievements."[29]

Being a celebrity has become an end unto itself. In the 1950s and 1960s, Zsa Zsa Gabor was a seemingly ubiquitous celebrity for the accomplishment of nothing more than being a celebrity. Similarly, relatively meaningless acts such as Janet Jackson's exposed breast at the 2004 Super Bowl halftime show or the action of a streaker at any sports event create media feeding frenzy. As Daniel Boorstin opined in 1972, "People talk constantly, not of things themselves, but of their images."[30] These he refers to as "pseudo events," or, nonevents and images that receive a lot of attention.

For the narcissist, or indeed for the narcissistic culture, there are only two categories: (1) the rich, great, important, and famous and (2) the hoi polloi, or masses. Otto Kernberg, a prolific authority on narcissism, notes that the narcissistic individual is so fearful of belonging to the mediocre that he worships heroes and yet viciously turns against them when they dissapoint.[31]

One example of this duality can be found in the profoundly disturbed individuals who murder for fame's sake. Thus the assassin attaches himself to his victim with a deadly intimacy. Thus it was for John Hinckley, who shot President Reagan in a belief that this would impress Jodie Foster, an actress he admired after watching her role in the film *Taxi Driver*. Curiously, Mark David Chapman, who shot John Lennon a year earlier in 1980, also mentioned Ms. Foster as the object of his fantasies.

For Christopher Lasch, these individuals go far beyond egoism. Indeed, for them, the self loses its boundaries and merges with its surroundings. This is the embodiment of pathological narcissism.

COLLECTIVISM AND INDIVIDUALISM

The cult of personality or charisma, as many have described such phenomena, is quite a dramatic shift from the "organization man" so eloquently described by William Whyte in 1956.[32] Modern successful executives are a far cry from Whyte's self-sacrificing "company man." Corporate advancement today is accomplished through the ability to use others, to change companies regularly for incremental advancements up the corporate ladder, and, more than anything, by convincing others that you are a winner. For Kernberg, such persons are forever searching for external omnipotence from which they can finally derive strength.[33] Historian Richard Rapson attributes many of these changes to broader cultural patterns.[34] He describes a major revolution in Western culture from collectivism to extreme individualism over the past three centuries.

The American Founding Fathers made a strong point that each individual had a natural right to the *pursuit* of happiness: a great change from the class-bound European models of the day. For narcissists, this is interpreted as an individual *entitlement* to happiness and a scramble for wealth and notoriety, with an attendant lack of empathy for others.

Not all Western countries follow the American extreme. Many European countries honor individualism but pay greater attention to social rights. Typically, this means that they tax themselves at twice the U.S. rate to support social programs. Asian cultures typically are far more collectivistic. Individual needs are subordinated to the needs of family, village, or other identification group. These cultures emphasize conformity, harmonious interdependence, and attending to and fitting in with others.

Hazel Markus and Shinobu Kitayama argue that in most Western independent cultures, there is a belief in the inherent separateness of people.[35] These cultures value individuality, uniqueness, and independence. Most non-Western interdependent cultures, on the other hand, insist on the fundamental connectedness of human beings. The self is defined in relation to ancestors, family, friends, and workmates. In the West, there is a greater focus on independence than interdependence.

Harry Triandis and his colleagues note that individualists are good at meeting strangers, forming new groups, and getting along with a wide range of people.[36] They are less good at managing long-term relationships. Collectivists, on the other hand, make a sharp distinction between in-group and out-group members. With family and friends, they are warm and cooperative. With out-group members, they are formal and non-cooperative.

Although cultural patterns provide generic stereotypes, most people in developed cultures are almost always faced with a balancing act between the needs of the one and the needs of the many. The narcissist cannot balance these needs, because in part, he is unaware of them. Thus he is plagued with both demands—Western needs to look superior and Eastern focus on others' impressions. For Rapson, American individualism has edged into selfish narcissism; he believes that, for all of us, a balance with the collective concerns would make life infinitely richer.

CAN NARCISSISM BE ACQUIRED?

The question remains as to whether narcissism can be culturally conveyed or whether it is inevitably the result of what Heinz Kohut called "repeated empathic failure" or an emotional developmental disability. Psychiatrist Robert B. Millman defined the concept of *acquired situational narcissism*, a temporary psychological dysfunction that often accompanies fame. Dr. Millman believes that his celebrity patients may act awful because of the situations in which they find themselves. He argues that they acquire their narcissism by being fed their image by the entourage and media around them. In an interview with *New York Times* reporter Stephen Sherrill, Millman notes, "They're not normal. And why would they feel normal when every person in the world who deals with them treats them as if they're not? We're all complicit in acquired situational narcissism. . . . We've created it. They're just responding to us."[37] Millman also notes, as for all narcissists, "Their marriages fall apart, they make lousy parents, they take copious quantities of drugs, they get into trouble with the law. Because they truly don't believe the world is real, they begin to think they're invulnerable. Some even risk their lives, since the world can't hurt them if it's not real."[38]

Sam Vaknin, a prolific writer on this subject, disagrees. He argues that because every human being—regardless of the nature of his society and culture—develops healthy narcissism early in life, it becomes pathological only by abuse. For Vaknin, acquired situational narcissism is merely an amplification of earlier narcissistic conduct, traits, style, and tendencies.[39] Not only are narcissists drawn to celebrity, but once powerful, rich, or famous, they gain immunity from social sanctions for expressing the underlying disorder.

Whether or not cultures can create narcissism is an interesting question. What is not in doubt is how cultures support narcissism.

THE DOWNSIDE

In many ways, narcissism is sexy. Flash is appealing. The very possibility that anyone may become a star and receive the spotlight treatment is enticing. Being noticed for looking good and gaining high praise seems to many the antidote to their childhood rejections and painful social exile during junior high school years. Asked about their dreams, many Americans will answer "fame and fortune," in that order. So what's wrong with this picture?

1. It is only a picture; a Dorian Gray kind of reality.
2. The cultural toll is quite heavy. In a world with few big winners, the many losers have to support the excesses of these larger-than-life characters. Not only are there clear distinctions between the haves and have-nots, the enticing illusion for all those at the bottom is to somehow rise to this elite class. Of course, this pressure encourages those in the winner's circle to continually resist others from joining their ranks. In short, a narcissistic culture is rife with class warfare. Indeed, a Gallup Poll taken right after the now-famous tax cuts of the first George W. Bush administration showed wide support for the cuts in estate taxes by people unlikely to ever benefit from such reductions. The poll results were stark: over 20 percent of the voters believed that they were in the top 1 percentile in income; another 20 percent believed that they would be in the top 1 percent. That, more than anything, represents a narcissistic illusion.
3. Those who are so focused on preserving their image have little left with which to do the work of the society that they presumably are leading.

4. Individualism carried to the extreme produces losers rather than winners. The U.S. men's and women's teams at the 2004 Olympic Games are exemplary of narcissism's downside. Although the players on the men's basketball team were individually the most talented on a man-by-man basis, they lacked the teamwork necessary to win more than a bronze medal. By contrast, the women's soccer, basketball, and softball Olympic teams were paragons of teamwork and collective work. They all decisively won gold medals. Similarly, the Los Angeles Lakers professional basketball team featured four future Hall of Fame players on their roster. Yet they lost decisively in the NBA Finals to the Detroit Pistons, a team with no star power but much team play.

Bill Bellichek's New England Patriots startled the football world by winning three Super Bowls in four years. They so eschewed individual notoriety that they insisted on being introduced not as starters or stars but as a whole team. Red Auerbach, one of the most successful basketball coaches in NBA history, was fond of observing that regardless of each person's shooting ability, there is only one ball. His success was predicated on individuals playing roles and subverting their egos for the good of the team.

An interesting picture of individualism running amok is portrayed by James Poniewozik.[40] He describes a ride in the family car (SUV) in which each member of the family is plugged into different entertainment during the drive. With the freedom afforded by TiVo, we have ceased to experience cultural events simultaneously. No longer is a phenomenon like the TV miniseries *Roots* able to catch the hearts and minds of the populace as a whole and provide so much to share. Instead, now we each watch a program at our own private time. Just as for the SUV ride, family and community take a back seat to the media input. As Poniewozik states, "Through niche media, niche foods and niche hobbies, we fashion niche lives. We are the America of the iPod ads—stark, black silhouettes tethered by our brilliant white earbuds, rocking out passionately and alone. You make your choices, and I make mine. Yours, of course, are wrong. But what do I care?"[41]

It's not surprising that we would apply the same principle to politics. Do I tune into a "red" or "blue" state perspective on TV or the Internet? We no longer get The News; we choose the news and the slant we desire. There is a great danger here. Narcissism in politics leads to major failures. To maintain its image of righteousness, a narcissistically based political administration has to block dissenting views, require fierce loyalty, prefer propaganda to objectivity, and sell the notion of their religious or moral superiority.

False representation is no problem for narcissists. It is the image speaking. For example, the totalitarian regimes of USSR politics, ushered in by Joseph Stalin, were reported by a large propaganda machine, always represented by the

Soviet controlled newspaper *Pravda* (which is the Russian word for "truth"). Thus it is that programs such as No Child Left Behind, supposedly geared to better educational opportunities, expend funding on testing rather than on educating, or that "saving the rainforest" means burning it down.

The world is getting better and worse for narcissists. Rampant individualism comes with increasing independence and freedom. The commensurate decline in social civility and institutions is beneficial to the image side of the narcissist, who can be less deterred by social bonds. Yet even as his fame increases and the star image is enhanced, there is an increase in isolation and attendant opportunity for abandonment and rejection. Without the more collective social props, no clear reparative social fabric, and more likely replications of early losses, there is simply less chance to correct the rejections of the past.

IS THERE A CURE FOR NARCISSISM?

Although theorists differ on the approaches to treating narcissism, there are several points in common. Almost all therapists who treat individuals diagnosed with personality disorders (Axis II in the *DSM–IV*) agree that the relational deficits have some genesis in childhood. Most, like Kohut, believe that narcissism, in particular, is caused by repeated empathic failure and a splitting off of a "false self" from the real self.[42]

Thus, treatment for narcissists involves the rediscovery and support of the real self. This is no easy task. When his softer, more vulnerable self (versus his image) is exposed, the narcissist is likely to flee from therapy, often with great derision for the therapist. The therapist must first find a way of creating a supportive environment in therapy, within which the narcissist can feel safe enough to explore slowly his vulnerable sides.

Complicated Therapy

A number of factors make treatment of narcissists quite difficult.

- Treatment is necessarily long-term (over a year).
- Treatment entails an open-ended verbal contract that the therapist will be available for the duration of treatment. This consistent availability helps relax somewhat the narcissist's fears of abandonment if they feel vulnerable.
- Narcissism is a disorder of personality. Unlike many behavioral or anxiety disorders, it is always present.
- Many characteristics that make relationships most difficult (lack of empathy, grandiosity, entitlement, and extreme vulnerability to slight with resultant rage) also inhibit the therapeutic relationship.

+ Narcissism is also commonly compounded with allied disorders, such as paranoia, obsessive-compulsive disorder, and impulsivity.

The Style of Treatment

Most therapists who directly treat personality disorders are psychodynamic in orientation. Essentially, the goal is to create an opportunity for the true self to resume the growth that was inhibited in childhood. The therapist tries to do this by offering a holding environment: fertile ground rich in safety, predictability, justice, nurturance, and re-parenting, such as mirroring and an ideal self with which to identify. In this emotionally corrective environment, the narcissist may learn that his past experiences with rejection are not immutable; that some relationships may in fact be nurturing and supportive.

Therapy typically begins with listening and accurate empathy. It is normal during the early sessions for the therapist's comments to be ignored or noted only as supportive. Gradually, the therapy proceeds with a combination of eliciting the narcissistic (false self) defenses and then supporting them to help the narcissist use the strength of his psyche to attend to the weaknesses. Thus the therapist will not challenge directly the omnipotence. Conversely, she will appeal to that very grandiosity to work assiduously on ridding the narcissist of self-defeating and counterproductive thoughts and behaviors. In short, this may reinforce the narcissist's feeling of power while underscoring the need for change.

It's a tenuous balance. Any challenge to a narcissist may be perceived as wounding and may result in an extraordinarily angry response. Direct confrontations could lead to a power struggle with no possible victor. If the narcissist wins, he devalues the therapist; if he loses, he feels humiliated, persecuted, and exposed—these situations do not create a ripe environment for effective therapy.

Consider this report from a narcissistic patient who was in the process of switching "to a competent therapist." The following phone conversation was precipitated when the therapist announced that she would be taking a three-week vacation a month hence.

I mean, who the hell does she think she is? What kind of professional credentials does she have . . . Ph.D. from the University of Kansas? Kansas, for Christ's sake . . . and that office, could it have been furnished worse? It was beyond even those guys from "Queer Eye"! Plus, you can't imagine the shoes she wore with that dress. How in hell could she help me? I am a success; not someone hidden away in a small office, with no support staff. I should ask for my money back for all those wasted sessions, maybe I should sue her for malpractice, just for the waste of my valuable time.

To the client, the therapist's vacation plans underscored that he was not the only important person in that relationship. This realization served to reactivate the pains of abandonment he suffered as a child; hence the childlike level of rage at this wound. The upcoming separation was simply too much like a deep personal rejection. In a shockingly swift turnaround, the therapist went from a position of overvaluation (my therapist, who is, by definition, the best) to devaluation (another inferior mortal, who, of course, let me down).

A great deal of the therapy involves uncovering the past—especially painful childhood memories. The patient gets to relive psychologically the slights, conflicts, and trauma in an environment of acceptance. It is assumed that in order to survive the failure of the original caregivers to mirror and provide a model for identification, the child represses his needs and develops this protective grandiose image or false self rather than his true self. Once the unconscious (repressed) issues begin to emerge in a safe environment, the therapist interprets them gently for the client. Through the lengthy process of uncovering, support, and interpretation, the client begins to gradually learn to live more in his real self and drops the accoutrements of the "image."

The relationship with the therapist (often referred to as the transference relationship) then becomes the testing ground for the client's healthier and more real future relationships.

Although other forms of therapy have been used in treatment, the brief outline above coordinates most closely to psychodynamically oriented therapies, the source of the bulk of the work over the years.

Hard Therapy

Some question whether Narcissistic Personality Disorder is curable at all. Most authors caution that, at best, it is very difficult. Sam Vaknin comments on the importance of early detection and treatment.[43] Most psychiatric textbooks warn therapists to be modest in their expectations and alert to potential harm to their own mental health.

Focusing on these difficulties for therapists, Howard Goldman warns that people with personality disorders "cause resentment and possibly even alienation and burnout in the healthcare professionals who treat them."[44]

There are also some indications in the literature that a therapist is sometime fooled into believing that his or her narcissistic patients are cured. Narcissists are consummate actors who can in role deceive both therapists and themselves. In addition, because these patients are often so difficult as clients and sometimes abusive to therapists, there is a definite impulse for therapists to overestimate the therapeutic gains.

A particular challenge for therapists is the undeniable fact that a narcissist's life in the fast lane is more exciting than a "normal" life. As one patient observed, "For me, getting better is like being neutered." Such individuals usually do not seek therapy for anything less than a major life crisis.

The Other Side of the Coin

Narcissism is among the mental disorders that sometimes moderate with age. Occasionally, around the midlife years, the antisocial aspects of the disorder seem to spontaneously improve.

Therapists who believe in Acquired Situational Narcissism or cultural narcissism naturally see positive results with major shifts in the environment. Thus, Jennifer, a woman known even among her most competitive colleagues as a "heartless litigator and shameless self-promoter," found herself in a crisis when a disaster threatened the lives of her parents and siblings. Although it was with great regret and some anger, she "temporarily" returned to the small town in British Columbia to which they had relocated, to "see to their affairs and *protect my inheritance*." Out of the San Francisco legal environs, she experienced a "new world" in which she didn't have to prove herself at all. In the course of her six-month stay, and the deaths of both parents, she found, for the first time, an ease with herself and a relationship with a man who "should have been beneath me." She decided to remain in British Columbia, transition to a far less aggressive career, and was reportedly happy for the first time in her 45 years. Ironically, that spring, her name appeared on a magazine touting the toughest ten lawyers in California. For the first time in her life, the accolade was unimportant.

CONCLUSION

Narcissism is both a set of character traits and a personality disorder. It is characterized by an intense focus on form over substance. Whether it appears in its grandiose, entitled form or as a constant fear that the true needy self within will be discovered, it can be devastating to an individual, to those around him, and indeed to a whole culture.

We need to work to prevent the lack of empathy within our families and institutions. The remedies include education, social safety nets, universal health care, including mental health care, and social support through our churches, schools, corporations, and government. The quality of parenting that our children receive as well as the institutions and environments in which they live have a profound impact on the psychological health of these future adults—our future culture and world community. A better balance between individualism and collectivism is essential, as is a focus on more substance. As any novice engineering student can describe, *form follows function*, not the reverse.

NOTES

1. Thomas Bullfinch, *Bullfinch's Mythology* (New York: Avenal, 1978), 101.
2. Ibid., 102.
3. Ibid., 103.
4. Ibid., 104.
5. Theodore B. Veblen, *The Theory of the Leisure Class* (1899; repr., New York: Modern Library, 1934).
6. Christopher Lasch, *The Culture of Narcissism: American Life in an Age of Diminishing Expectations* (New York: Norton, 1979).
7. Richard L. Rapson, *American Yearnings: Love, Money and Endless Possibility* (Lanham, MD: University Press of America, 1988).
8. For purposes of clarity only, in this chapter, narcissists are referred to by male pronouns. Therapists are presented as female. In reality, there seems to be a slightly greater number of male narcissists and an equal number of therapists of each sex who treat them.
9. Sigmund Freud, *Totem and Taboo*, standard ed., vol. 13 (1913; repr., London: Hogarth Press, 1955).
10. Heinz Kohut, *How Does Analysis Cure?* (Chicago: University of Chicago Press, 1984).
11. Heinz Kohut, *The Restoration of the Self* (New York: International Universities Press, 1977), 17.
12. Michael St. Clair, *Object Relations and Self Psychology: An Introduction* (Belmont, CA: Brooks/Cole Publishing Co., 1986).
13. S. De Carlo, "CEO Compensation," *Forbes*, April 21, 2005, http://www.forbes.com/2005/04/20/05ceoland.html.
14. Rakesh Khurana, interview by Paul Solman, *Newshour with Jim Lehrer*, July 5, 2004, http://www.pbs.org/newshour/bb/business/july-dec02/ceo 3_12–04.html.
15. Dionne Searcey, Shawn Young, and Kara Scannell, "Ebbers is Sentenced to 25 years for $11 Billion WorldCom Fraud," *Wall Street Journal*, July 14, 2005, A1.
16. Robert J. Hughes, "Who Did Her Personality?" *Wall Street Journal*, July 15, 2005, W1.
17. Thomas G. Paterson and Dennis Merrill, eds.., *Major Problems in American Foreign Relations*, vol. 2, *Since 1914: Documents and Essays* (Lexington, MA: D.C. Heath and Company, 1995), 539.
18. Edward Gibbon, *The Decline and Fall of the Roman Empire* (London: Wordsworth, 1776–78).
19. Aaron Stern, *Me: The Narcissistic American* (New York: Ballantine, 1979), 1.
20. Veblen, *The Theory of the Leisure Class.*
21. Lasch, *The Culture of Narcissism.*
22. Sigmund Freud, *Group Psychology and the Analysis of the Ego*, standard ed., vol. 18 (London: Hogarth Press, 1921).

23. Lasch, *Culture of Narcissism*, 53–54.

24. Dale Carnegie, How to Win Friends and Influence People, reissue ed. (1937; repr., New York: Pocket Books, 1990).

25. Norman Vincent Peale, 1898–1993, was on the radio for over 50 years preaching a message of positive thinking. Growing up with strong inferiority feelings he developed and refined the message that anyone could overcome such a childhood with faith and positivity.

26. American Society for Aesthetic Plastic Surgery, "11.9 Million Cosmetic Procedures In 2004," American Society for Aesthetic Plastic Surgery, February 17, 2005, http://surgery .org/press/news-release.php?iid = 395.

27. There are media doctors with credentials that are somewhat related to counseling (Ruth, Laura, Phil), but they also focus on observable rather than inner shifts.

28. Lasch, *Culture of Narcissism*, 59.

29. Ibid., 60.

30. Daniel Boorstin, *The Image: A Guide to Pseudo Events* (New York: Atheneum, 1972), 204.

31. Otto F. Kernberg, *Borderline Condition and Pathological Narcissism* (New York: Jason Aronson, 1975), 234.

32. William H. Whyte, *The Organization Man* (New York: Simon and Schuster, 1956).

33. Kernberg, *Borderline Condition and Pathological Narcissism*, 234–36.

34. Rapson, *American Yearnings: Love, Money and Endless Possibility*.

35. Hazel R. Markus and Shinobu Kitayama, "Culture and Self: Implications for Cognition, Emotion and Motivation," *Psychological Review* 98 (1991): 224–53.

36. Harry C. Triandis, Christopher McCusker, and C. Harry Hui, "Multimethod Probes of Individualism and Collectivism," *Journal of Personality and Social Psychology* 59 (1990): 1007.

37. Stephen Sherrill, "Acquired Situational Narcissism." interview with Robert B. Millman, *New York Times*, December 9, 2001.

38. Ibid.

39. Sam Vaknin, Malignant Self Love: Narcissism Revisited, 2005, http://samvak.tripod .com/cv.html. Also available in hardcover, Lidija Rangelovska, ed. (Skopje, Macedonia: Narcissus Publications, 2005).

40. James Poniewozik, "The Age of Ipod Politics," *Time*, September 27, 2004, 84.

41. Ibid.

42. Heinz Kohut, *How Does Analysis Cure?*

43. Vaknin, *Malignant Self Love: Narcissism Revisited*.

44. Howard H. Goldman, *Review of General Psychiatry* (East Norwalk, CT: Appleton and Lange, 1995), 318.

Chapter 3

Anger Disorders: Diagnosing an Unrecognized Mood Disorder

Heather C. Lench

Every day we are presented with bad news—men beating their wives, spouses killing each other, teenagers with guns at school, a father who shoots his son's coach for kicking the son off a high school football team. Media, video games, television, and parenting are all blamed for these tragic events. But these situations share another common factor. The perpetrators of violence were probably all angry for some reason. Some of these people may have suffered from a mental disorder characterized by chronic or intense anger. Although societal factors and parenting no doubt affect whether a person will become violent, anger disorders are treatable, and such treatment may reduce rates of violence.

Identifying who has an anger disorder is complex and difficult for the average person and for trained clinicians alike. Above are extreme examples, but what about instances from everyday life? A normally calm woman becomes an angry whirlwind behind the wheel of her car—a driver who pulls in front of her is likely to be cursed, given obscene hand signals, and honked at repeatedly while she drives a foot from the bumper. A man regularly becomes angry with his closest friend and punishes the friend by refusing to talk to him or to show up for their carpool in the morning. A woman is frustrated that a coworker may get promoted before her and begins to spread nasty rumors about the coworker. Which, if any, of these people has an anger disorder? Who would benefit from treatment for anger?

Unfortunately, relatively little is known about anger disorders or their treatment. There is evidence that a significant portion of the population may suffer from anger disorders and that people with anger disorders are more likely to be violent. In the past decade, there has been a surge in the number of people referred for anger management treatment by the legal system and various programs. People are frequently mandated to attend treatment after committing domestic violence or child abuse offenses or after causing significant disturbance at work. Yet clinicians do not have guidelines to treat these individuals, and there is no official set of diagnoses for anger disorders.[1] The lack of a diagnosis for people suffering from anger disorders translates into fewer studies on the disorders and their treatment. It also means that researchers and clinicians cannot compare notes on what qualifies as an anger disorder. Often it is not clear if people in anger management treatment actually have an anger disorder that would benefit from treatment. This chapter will review existing and proposed anger diagnoses, issues related to diagnosis, and treatment strategies.

WHAT IS ANGER?

Multiple dimensions are used to describe how people experience anger. Anger is accompanied by physical reactions. These include changes in arousal, increased muscle tension, and changes in hormone and neurotransmitter functioning. These physiological reactions lead to the "pumped up" or "flushed" feeling people often have when angry. The heart beats faster, adrenaline releases, and the body prepares for action.[2] Anger is also related to changes in cognition. Essentially, anger leads people to attend to, process, and remember information related to their anger. A husband and wife arguing about finances are likely to notice new clothes on the other person, think about their spouse's spending habits, and remember past occasions when their spouse failed to be frugal. These cognitions often lead to even more anger, potentially creating an escalating cycle. Anger includes a phenomenological component as well, which is the subjective awareness and labeling of angry feelings. Physiological, cognitive, and phenomenological components of anger are internal—the person experiencing anger is aware of them, but an outsider would not be. The final component often described in definitions of anger is behavioral. Behavioral expressions of anger include facial changes, verbalizations, and behaviors. An observer often determines if someone is angry using these behavioral cues.

EXISTING ANGER DISORDERS

Anger is a part of several existing psychiatric disorders defined in the *Diagnostic and Statistical Manual of Mental Disorders (DSM–IV–TR)*.[3] This is the official manual used for the diagnosis of mental disorders by every clinician who diagnoses or treats clients. Intermittent explosive disorder most resembles an anger disorder, but it is focused on behavior, not emotion. It is defined as an impulse control disorder not classified elsewhere in the manual, and its defining feature is aggression out of proportion to the situation. Essentially, it is characterized by discrete episodes where the person "fails to resist aggressive impulses and this failure of control results in assaults or property destruction" (p. 663). The diagnosis cannot be given if the person also demonstrates depression or anxiety. Irritability and rage are explicitly mentioned as possible affective symptoms, but they are not required for diagnosis. The manual suggests that these outbursts of anger and aggression are the result of an underlying personality disorder.

Anger is explicitly mentioned in several personality disorders listed in the *DSM–IV–TR*. This is potentially problematic for people with anger disorders because treatment for personality disorders is not usually covered under insurance plans. Personality disorders are considered difficult to treat, often requiring years of therapy and resulting in little or no change. There is no evidence that problems with anger necessarily result from personality disorders, and, as will be discussed shortly, anger can be effectively treated. Three personality disorders include anger or anger-related cognitions. Paranoid personality disorder is described as "a pattern of pervasive distrust and suspiciousness of others such that their motives are interpreted as malevolent" (p. 690). In other words, paranoid personality disorder is associated with an exaggerated tendency to read threats into situations, a tendency that is also associated with anger. Antisocial personality disorder is associated with disregard for and violation of the rights of others. The *DSM–IV–TR* lists "irritability and aggressiveness, as indicated by repeated physical fights or assaults" (p. 706) as one of the primary symptoms. One of the primary symptoms of borderline personality disorder is unstable mood and mood reactivity, including intense periods of sadness, anger, or anxiety. Anger is also listed separately as a symptom when it is inappropriate and intense or the person has difficulty controlling the anger, as evidenced by frequent anger episodes, constant anger, or recurrent physical fights.

In practice, problematic anger is conceptualized as a subtype of existing mood disorder diagnoses. For example, a person who meets criteria for a depressive disorder and is also suffering from frequent anger and aggression would be diagnosed as having a depressive disorder not otherwise specified. This practice creates a barrier to the proper treatment of people suffering from anger disorders. If anger is considered a minor part of other presumably more pressing symptoms, clinicians may not address issues related to anger, and these problems may go untreated or cause attempts at therapy to fail. When angry people decide (or are forced) to attend therapy, they either are not diagnosed or are given a diagnosis that does not capture the emotional quality of their disorder—insurance will not pay for treatment of a disorder that does not exist. This misdiagnosis can lead to increased feelings of being misunderstood and not connected to the therapist and may lead to the wrong treatments. Imagine a man who is primarily angry all the time and seeks therapy. The therapist tells him he is depressed with irritable mood, but the man does not feel depressed—just angry. Is he likely to be invested in treatment? Is he likely to feel that he is being treated correctly, and will he have faith that he can improve if the therapist does not even seem to understand his issues? The problem of diagnosis is compounded by the fact that depression, anxiety, and anger frequently present together in the same patient as comorbid disorders.[4] There is pharmacological and psychological evidence, however, that dysfunctional anger exists in people who do not have symptoms of anxiety or depression.

PROPOSED ANGER DISORDERS

Eckhardt and Deffenbacher have proposed several anger diagnoses and criteria.[2] Generally, they propose diagnoses for anger disorders that include angry affect, physiological responses, cognitive indices of anger, and verbal or physical aggression. Adjustment disorder with angry mood is characterized by an angry mood in response to a specific stressor that occurs within three to six months after the stressor. Situational adjustment without aggression is characterized by an intense reaction to a specific event that lasts longer than six months and is accompanied by physiological arousal and minimal aggression. Eckhardt and Deffenbacher also propose a situational adjustment with aggression, which is similar to the previous diagnosis with the addition of persistent aggression. General anger disorder without aggression is characterized by chronic and pervasive anger that occurs more days than not for at least one year, and the person is not without anger for more than one month. A similar category is proposed for general anger disorder with aggression. In sum, the proposed anger disorders include acute reactions, intense reactions out of proportion to the situation, and chronic anger.

Several additional factors may need to be included in anger diagnoses. For instance, people may experience intense anger in response to specific stimuli.[5] Just as someone with a specific phobia may experience intense anxiety in the presence of spiders, people may experience intense anger in the presence of certain cues. The cues that cause anger episodes may be consistent enough to be generalized into broad categories, as is the case with phobias, or they may be specific to each person. More research is needed, but one can imagine categories of situations that might elicit inappropriate anger responses—perhaps including jealousy, driving, or competition.

Multiple anger diagnoses have been proposed, but there is currently little evidence for or against these diagnostic categories. They are based on the factors associated with anger and the framework for diagnosing the other mood disorders of anxiety and depression. Researchers are currently developing evidence for the diagnostic categories, but it will be a long and difficult process unless public interest turns to understanding anger disorders. Work in this area may also be slowed by fears that diagnosing anger as a mental disorder could make people feel less responsible for controlling their anger and could be used in court to reduce legal culpability. The latter fear is related to a phenomenon already present in the legal system. "Crimes of passion," which are for the most part episodes of intense anger, are already a mitigating factor in the legal system. For instance, a man who kills his wife and her lover in a fit of rage upon discovering them in bed is held less responsible than a man who killed his wife in order to receive a large insurance check.

WHY DO PEOPLE BECOME ANGRY?

Part of the reason that there is disagreement about whether anger disorders should be a diagnoses is ongoing debate about what causes anger. Some researchers describe general determinants of anger. For example, Berkowitz argues that the presence of aversive conditions increases the likelihood of anger.[6] Other approaches attempt to identify the circumstances that cause anger and the results of anger in those circumstances. Appraisal theories of emotion consider anger to occur when several circumstances are met in the environment, although there is disagreement about the exact nature of these circumstances. The most inclusive explanation is that anger results when a goal is blocked but still attainable with additional effort.[7] For example, children judged that a boy with an injured leg would feel angry if he had to rest until it was better and would feel sad if he would never be able to use the leg again, irrespective of whether the leg injury was intentionally caused or not.

When people appraise that a goal is blocked, resulting anger motivates additional effort to attain the goal. This additional effort can increase the likelihood that the goal will be attained. This explanation of anger can explain why people often feel angry at other people.[2] If someone is intentionally blocking a goal, the goal can still be reached with additional effort if the person is removed. For example, if you are late for work and the person in front of you is driving at 25 miles per hour, it is likely that feeling angry and speeding around him or her will get you to work faster. Anger serves a similar motivating function even if there is no one to blame. If your computer crashes, feeling angry can motivate you to quickly take your computer to be fixed and perhaps invest in recovering the lost hard drive material. Viewing angry people as striving for blocked goals has not yet influenced research on anger disorders, but it is possible that anger disorders are caused by tendencies to see goals as obstructed or to see failed goals as attainable. Angry people may have impossible standards for other people, and, when they cannot reach these standards, those with an anger disorder may believe others are responsible.

IS ANGER ALWAYS BAD?

Anger has a bad reputation—it has a long history of being blamed for many of the ailments of society and incidents of tragic violence. Anger is often equated with the loss of control and reversion to animal instincts.[8] Ancient Roman writers described it as a madness that impaired rationality and civility. The Stoics, known for their military dominance, regarded anger as a useless emotion, even in war or competition. Although anger often precipitates violence and aggression, people are often angry without being aggressive and people are often aggressive without being angry. People can be aggressive when they want to pressure someone to do their wishes, even if they are not angry.

In fact, aggression follows very few anger episodes. Averill asked a large number of people to describe anger in their own lives.[9] They reported that physically aggressive behaviors followed only about 10 percent of angry episodes, and nearly one-third of these were incidents of spanking a child to correct behavior. There was a relatively higher rate of verbal aggression in nearly half of all the reported angry episodes. However, both types of aggression were reported less often following anger than talking things over and doing something calming. Aggression may be an attempt to deal with blocked goals when other attempts to resolve the problem have failed, and it is only one of the possible behaviors that follow anger.

Anything more than mild irritation is sometimes described as inappropriate and a result of irrational thinking. However, the evidence does not seem to support this view.[10] Aristotle regarded anger as a useful emotion, if properly controlled, because it prevents injustice.[8] Anger motivates change, which is sometimes needed. People who described angry incidents reported that anger often led to positive outcomes. Both the angry person and people who were targets of anger reported positive consequences, including resolution of problems and social sharing.[9] People often feel empowered, in control, and potent when they are angry, which can lead people to resolve problems when needed.[11] People who do not become angry, even when it is appropriate, are in many cultures regarded as pushovers inviting more punishment.

HOW DO YOU TELL IF ANGER IS DYSFUNCTIONAL?

One way to identify dysfunctional anger is to look at how well it serves the needs of the person.[12] If anger leads to discussing a problem and reaching a positive conclusion, then it is functional. If anger leads to attacking someone and facing legal or social consequences, then it is not functional. An example of the same situation that results in functional and dysfunctional anger may help make this point clear. Fred and Roger both take a date that they really want to impress to a local restaurant. Both men encounter an acquaintance that proceeds to tell embarrassing jokes about their personal hygiene. Both are having their goal of making a good impression on the date threatened by this intrusion, and, as a consequence of this blocked goal, both become angry. Fred proceeds to make an intelligent quip about the other man and asks the man to excuse them, after which he and his date laugh about the intrusion. Roger becomes red in the face, rudely insults the man, and violently pushes the man away from his date, after which his date is embarrassed and frightened and Roger is asked to leave the restaurant for causing a disturbance. People with dysfunctional anger may not be able to deal effectively with stress and may become frustrated, which can lead to increased anger.[12,13] In the example, Roger did not cope effectively and created an even more stressful situation—not only has he failed to impress his date but he has been publicly embarrassed and frightened his date. Roger becomes frustrated at his terrible failure and experiences even more anger the next time he is embarrassed.

Another sign that anger is not serving the needs of the person is if it has health consequences. Anger can be expressed outward toward others or inward toward the self. It was once believed that expressing anger could be cathartic and reduce internal suffering, but the evidence does not support this suggestion. Directing anger inward or outward is associated with serious health issues. People who frequently express their anger suffer from higher rates of mental and physical ailments than people who express anger less often.[14] This relationship might be due to the fact that frequent anger expression can cause conflict within social circles, leading to prolonged stress for the individual.

Although anger is experienced from early infancy, the overt expression of anger is very controlled compared to other emotions.[15] There are ways of expressing anger that are more likely to be labeled inappropriate in different cultures.[16] If others deem the way someone expresses anger to be inappropriate, anger is likely to result in more conflict and is unlikely to resolve the situation effectively. For example, Briggs visited an Inuit group that disapproved of the overt expression of anger—they believed anger was potentially destructive and dangerous in their environment, which required cooperation.[17] When

Briggs expressed anger toward outsiders on behalf of the group, she was ostra-
cized and viewed as dangerous. Her anger, though justified, did not have a positive effect because she expressed it inappropriately in the cultural context, and
therefore it was dysfunctional.

Men and women experience and express anger at similar rates, but what is
considered to be appropriate anger expression also varies by gender.[9] Some ways
of expressing anger may be viewed as inappropriate for women but appropriate
for men, and vice versa. Women are more likely than men to suppress anger or
express it through physical symptoms.[18] Men report more aggression.[19] These
gender differences in anger expression may be driven by what is socially appropriate, and violations may lead to negative outcomes. There is some evidence
that this is the case. Suppressing anger led to quicker recovery for women, but
in men suppression was associated with increased blood pressure and slower
recovery from anger.[20] Thus the same anger expression may be dysfunctional
depending on whether it fits with standards based on culture and gender.

While defining dysfunctional anger by actions and outcomes can be useful,
it does not offer a comprehensive definition that can be used to identify anger
disorders. Anger problems and anger expression problems often coincide, but
they are not equivalent.[2] If more attention were given to anger diagnosis, other
markers of anger could be identified and treated *before* someone is violent or
develops a serious illness. The most obvious sign of depression is suicide, but in
recent decades a clear set of markers has been developed to identify depression
before that point. Having negative effects is definitely part of any diagnosis of
mental illness, but it is not the primary component of most diagnoses—it is
necessary but not sufficient. Most likely, anger can be dysfunctional and have
the potential for negative effects if it is experienced too intensely in relation to
the situation, too frequently, or at a constantly elevated level. Anger may also be
dysfunctional if the person copes with and expresses anger poorly and thus is
slow to recover from an episode or damages social relationships.

WHAT MIGHT CAUSE AN ANGER DISORDER?

The causes of anger disorders are currently unknown because they are not
recognized as official diagnoses and therefore are not studied as such. There is,
however, evidence about what relates to dysfunctional anger. People who develop
an anger disorder may lack the coping or anger expression styles necessary to effectively deal with anger. Those who have effective coping skills can resolve a situation
that evokes anger in a positive and productive way. Without effective coping, people may experience an increase in anger as their attempts to resolve the situation
repeatedly fail. In addition, their maladaptive attempts at coping may cause social

conflicts as others are affected by their attempts. Over time, ineffective coping can strain the individual and increase conflict. The angry person is likely to experience more frequent and intense anger. Someone who is not coping effectively is likely to continue to feel frustrated by those situations. His or her family and friends are likely to be upset from prior incidents of anger, leading to a more stressful environment. Coping and anger expression likely determine whether people develop anger disorders.

Coping is an attempt to either alter the environment to make it less stressful or to increase personal resources to deal with the stressor.[21] Good coping skills are defined by their effects—those that create positive emotions by changing the situation or changing how one perceives the situation are considered healthy and effective. Coping strategies that are likely to resolve many situations effectively include problem solving, framing the situation into opportunity for positive outcomes, and giving positive meaning to events.[22] Ineffective coping fails to make people feel better and may actually increase negative emotions because the situation is not resolved. For example, Susan becomes angry with a coworker for failing to complete his work, which then falls on her shoulders. If Susan copes by focusing on the opportunity to learn from the task and to impress the boss, it is effective coping. If Susan gets in a screaming argument with the coworker and they are sent to resolve their problem with the boss, it is not effective coping and can prolong the stress of the original event.

Angry people report potentially problematic coping styles. They tend to focus on solving the problem less and use more aggressive and antisocial actions.[23,24] In other words, angry people are more likely to focus on retaliation and less likely to focus on developing ways to solve the problem. People referred for anger management treatment also report that they typically did not seek social support to help them cope.[23,24] People perceive friends and family as less supportive and less available when they are angry, and thus people with an anger disorder may be less likely to seek out people for support.[25]

Angry people also express their anger differently. Expressing emotion in ways that are not socially acceptable is likely to lead to social conflict and be dysfunctional. For example, in many societies physical violence and verbal abuse are considered dysfunctional, and in many countries there are laws prohibiting abuse. If the cultural rules indicated that anger should result in physical violence toward spouses, then it would not cause social conflict and would not be dysfunctional. Those with anger disorders are likely to express anger in ways that violate the cultural systems for expressing emotion. People high in trait anger reported that they express anger in a number of potentially problematic ways. These include directing anger toward themselves, physical assault on people, physical assault on objects, noisy arguing, verbal assault, and nonverbal negative action such as glaring or giving the finger.[23]

Angry people report fewer positive ways of expressing anger, including less reciprocal communication and fewer time-outs to calm down. They also maintain using fewer strategies to control their anger expression. As anyone who has ever been in a heated argument knows, it takes more control to understand the other person's views than to scream that they are wrong. The fact that angry people are less likely to control how they express their anger may underlie many of their expression problems. An intervention targeted at increasing control might also decrease negative expression and increase positive expression.

WHY IS DYSFUNCTIONAL ANGER BAD?

Anger disorders, like other mood disorders that significantly impair functioning, can be devastating for individuals, family, and friends. Although the exact prevalence of anger disorders is unknown and cannot be estimated without an official diagnosis, it is likely that a large portion of the population is affected by anger problems. In a recent survey, 25 percent of college students and 31 percent of people referred for court-mandated anger management treatment met criteria for chronic anger.[23] Anger in these surveys was related to reported problems with friendships, work, and romantic relationships. Therefore, it is likely that anger in this sample was dysfunctional.

Dysfunctional anger has negative effects on health. Anger has consistently been linked to hypertension and coronary problems, both when it is expressed toward others and the self.[2,14] People high in hostility have larger increases in blood pressure following an anger induction in the laboratory and are slower to recover from blood pressure increases.[26] This increased reactivity and slow recovery from anger may stress the physiological system. Anger is associated with increased blood pressure and adrenaline as well as release of other neurotransmitters and hormones. People who do not recover quickly from such episodes can experience damage to their organs and blood vessels. In addition to direct effects of anger on health, anger may change health habits. For example, people are more likely to smoke when angry or if they have an aggressive disposition.[27]

Probably the most devastating effects of anger disorders are on relationships. People with anger disorders are likely to feel alone, misunderstood, and disrespected by those closest to them. Anger, especially if it is out of proportion to what is justified, is likely to cause an angry reaction in others. This may cause conflicts, and potentially the person with a disorder will feel misunderstood and attacked as a result of the conflicts.[25] If angry persons feel that their anger is justified, they may think that others simply do not care enough to correct their wrongs. If they are aware that their anger is not justified, they may feel out of control and frightened of who they might hurt next time they become angry.

People who were chronically angry or in anger management treatment were less likely to be involved in a romantic relationship and reported fewer friends than people without chronic anger.[23] They experienced the relationships that they did have as poor in quality and conflictual, reporting that their relationships were filled with verbal and physical conflict. Angry people reported more friendships that ended due to conflict and more conflict in their current relationships. Anger also appeared to affect work—angry people reported changing jobs frequently, conflict at work, and less satisfaction with their current job. Angry people likely experience the most conflict in the relationships in which they spend most of their time—angry college students reported more work and school conflicts whereas the older anger management sample reported more conflict in their romantic relationships. This may in part be due to the fact that, over time, angry people strain their social networks, losing friendships and work relationships due to conflict.

People do not usually become angry at strangers—they more often direct their anger toward those they know and love.[9] Within relationships, anger appears to be scripted and well rehearsed.[15] If this script involves violence, it is likely to be repeated every time anger is experienced. Anger has been linked to homicide and domestic violence, as those who become violent are more likely to be high on measures of anger.[2,28] There is also evidence that anger can lead to excessive blaming within relationships. When married people become angry they tend to believe their spouse is intentionally causing the negative events.[15] Dysfunctional anger can lead to a cycle wherein the spouse is perpetually blamed for incidental negative situations. For example, a man who does not receive a promotion at work may blame his spouse because she was not friendly enough at a company lunch.

The prevalence of anger disorders and the effects of these disorders have implications for society as a whole. As mentioned, it is likely that a sizable portion of the population has an anger disorder. Anger is a risk factor for cardiovascular disease and illness. Anger is also associated with negative health behavior such as smoking, which has multiple negative health consequences. Thus, anger disorders are costing society financially for the treatment of those who become ill. In addition, society is affected financially and morally by the violence that can result from dysfunctional anger.

DOES ANGER CAUSE VIOLENCE?

The relationship between anger and violence is complex.[28] In a review of studies that examined the relationship between anger and intimate partner violence, there was evidence that anger was a factor in violence for men. Men who had become violent toward their spouse reported more anger and hostility than men who were not violent, even when their relationships were equally distressed, potentially indicating the presence of an anger disorder. The authors of this study conclude that men with a history of violence are angrier than men who had not become violent. However, they note that it is not clear whether anger precipitated violence in any particular conflict. In other words, the question of whether men felt angry at their partner before becoming violent remains unanswered. There is good reason that this question has not yet been addressed—it is difficult and unethical to follow potentially violent people and examine what happens when they beat their spouse. There is some evidence that men who become violent may have trouble labeling emotions, and so they experience *less* subjective anger than men who do not become violent.

Anderson and Bushman have proposed several ways that anger can influence violence.[29] First, anger may reduce normal restraints on violence by making aggressive responses feel justified to the person. Anger is intuitively compelling and difficult to ignore. For example, a woman who becomes angry at her child for drawing on the walls may feel that smacking the child is justified by the situation. She might say to herself, consciously or unconsciously, "If it weren't a serious situation, why would I be so upset?" Second, anger can also disrupt the ability to control cognitions and behavior, leading to more impulsive aggression. Anger and controlling its expression require cognitive resources. When resources are strained by anger there are fewer available to control behavior. A man who becomes angry at his wife, for example, is cognitively distracted by anger and is less likely to suppress his urge to hit her. Third, anger is an informational cue and can perpetuate people's focus on the anger-evoking situation, cause them to remember things that made them angry in the past, and prime them to act aggressively. The mother in the example above would be more likely to remember all the past instances when her child misbehaved. Fourth, anger can also influence aggression because it causes physiological arousal—it is much easier to become aggressive with adrenaline flowing, muscles tensed, and increased blood flow than without. The extent to which each of these pathways predicts whether a person with an anger disorder becomes violent is currently not known, but each of these pathways could lead to violence.

Although violence prevention is a top priority for many governmental agencies, there is a general reluctance to acknowledge anger as a potential risk factor for violence. This reluctance may stem in part from the fact that little is known about anger, how to measure it, or when it becomes dysfunctional.[28] In many states, anger management is prohibited as a treatment for domestic violence, partially because of fears that such treatments may not hold perpetrators responsible for their actions and may overlook other potential causes of violence, such as a need for control and societal tolerance for violence.[28] This is a legitimate concern but should not exclude the possibility that anger management could help at least some perpetrators. Not all men and women who become violent have an anger disorder, but treatment would be helpful for those who do. Dysfunctional anger makes others angry, which may lead them to want to punish violent perpetrators and ignore suggestions that anger treatment may be effective in reducing violence. Anger cannot be an excuse for committing a criminal act or hurting others, but there may be treatments that can effectively reduce violence by addressing anger as a treatable disorder.

CURRENT TREATMENTS FOR DYSFUNCTIONAL ANGER

What is anger management therapy? It's a popular phrase, but what does it mean? For a mental disorder, there is frequently abundant research on what works and does not work with which clients. Additionally, to administer therapy requires a professional license verifying appropriate training in relevant techniques and issues. Because anger is not currently recognized as a mental disorder, there are no guidelines for which therapy to give or who should give it. Anger management groups are conducted by clinicians, nurses, arbiters, and people with no professional licensing requirements. Treatment is often given in groups, and the number of sessions is often determined by courts or insurance. It frequently includes a variety of techniques that seem like they would work or have proven useful with other mental disorders, especially anxiety and depression. The focus is frequently on teaching the person to control his or her anger through various means, including counting to 10 before acting and thinking about the consequences of anger.

There is evidence about what works to treat dysfunctional anger, but it is limited. The research is often confusing and unclear, which may lead clinicians to reject reviewing the literature for guidelines.[30] Several specific problems make the research difficult to interpret. One discrepancy between research and practice is that most research uses volunteer populations, frequently college students, whereas most angry clients are forced to attend therapy. Another discrepancy is in the resources available for therapy. As a result, most therapy is conducted in a group format, despite evidence that individual therapy is more effective at reducing anger and promoting long-term behavior changes.

Despite the lack of clarity in the research, there is evidence that therapy improves the functioning of clients with anger problems. Anger management treatment lowers blood pressure rates.[31] There is also specific evidence about which therapies work from meta-analyses. A meta-analysis reviews all available studies on a topic, in this case the effects of treatment on anger, and analyzes all of the results collectively. Thus, it is a powerful technique to examine what works and what does not work. Several such reviews have been conducted and have generally found that multiple types of therapy have moderate to large effects in treating angry clients and were beneficial.[32,13]

Therapies that target multiple components of anger may be especially effective. As mentioned, anger is related to physiological responses, cognitions, subjective awareness of anger, and behavior. One multicomponent treatment is stress inoculation therapy. This therapy is one of the most frequently used to treat anger and appears to have a moderate treatment effect.[1] Clients with anger problems treated with this type of therapy are on average better off than 76 percent of clients not treated with the therapy. Novaco, the developer of stress inoculation therapy, views anger as a response to specific situations due to cognitive, emotional, and behavioral variables within the person.[33] For example, imagine a man who is overlooked for a promotion at work and has a dysfunctionally angry response. This response is determined by his thoughts (he's never treated fairly and it's probably the fault of that guy who always kisses up to the boss), his emotions (he's generally in a bad mood anyway and this is really the last straw—he can barely breathe he's so mad!), and behavioral repertoire (well, yelling at his boss is all he can think to do).

Stress inoculation therapy focuses on addressing these dimensions through cognitive preparation, skill acquisition and rehearsal, and application of learned skills during mildly stressful imagined or role-played situations. In therapy, the man above would learn to identify situations that typically make him dysfunctionally angry and address the cognitions that lead to an inappropriate response. To learn control over his angry behaviors, he would learn relaxation techniques and then use those techniques during increasingly stressful situations, either role-played with the therapist or imagined.

There is additional evidence of some strategies that may be useful during treatment, although they have not been systematically investigated. One such strategy is derived from dialectic behavior therapy, a technique developed for treating suicidal clients.[34] This strategy places specific emphasis on teaching clients to tolerate physical and emotional distress and targeting specific areas for change while accepting the person as a whole. These techniques may be particularly useful for people with anger disorders, who have difficulty tolerating distress and may feel more understood if attention were placed on changing specific behaviors instead of the whole self.

Another strategy that may be useful is to involve family and friends in the treatment process. People referred to anger management treatment reported seeking social support during stress less often than others.[23] Involving spouses, family, and friends in the treatment program may help to create a nurturing environment that could assist in reducing angry outbursts. Feindler has developed a treatment strategy for adolescents that includes family involvement.[35] A similar approach for adults may be useful. Physical exercise may also be a useful strategy because it may help alleviate the coronary heart risks associated with high anger as well as normalize physiological reactions during stress.

Another strategy that may be effective in treating anger is to tailor the treatment to the problem. In their review of treatments for anger, Del Vecchio and O'Leary found indications that the type of anger treatment that is most effective depends on the type of anger problem being treated such as road rage while driving.[36] While this makes intuitive sense, it is impossible to determine which therapies are effective for various problems without there being commonly recognized anger disorders. The type of treatment that is effective may depend on a variety of factors that have yet to be explored. For example, therapy with people who tend to blame others may require a different approach than with people who blame themselves. Likewise, people who physically assault others may require a different approach than people who use passive-aggressive strategies to retaliate against people.

ANGER PROBLEMS AND THE BRAIN: ARE THERE OTHER OPTIONS?

During the medieval ages, philosophers believed that people with angry temperaments had an excess of yellow bile.[8] Although this is no longer a plausible medical explanation, the exact physiological causes of anger are unclear. There are decades of evidence that dysfunctional anger can be caused by damage to the brain.[37] A case example of this influence is shown in Phinneus Gage. In the 1800s, he worked with the railroad laying track. He was regarded by coworkers as a gentle and good-humored man. During his work, a tamping iron was accidentally blown through his head. He recovered from the physical injury fairly well, but his personality underwent a drastic change. He became irritable and angry, often verbally assaulting others.[38] As with other emotions, anger is related to brain functioning, and serious organic injury can lead to dysfunction.

There is also evidence that dysfunctional anger may be related to specific neural dysfunction within the brain. Fava and his colleagues describe multiple case histories of people suffering from what they call "anger attacks."[39,40] These are brief episodes of anger out of proportion to the situation and accompanied by physiological symptoms. Anger attacks are similar to panic attacks, but people experience themselves as angry, not anxious. They treated clients who presented with these attacks with medication and saw significant improvements. The patients generally had no anger attacks after treatment but began having anger attacks within a few days if they stopped medication. Patients improved when treated with antidepressant drugs at lower doses than would normally be required to treat depression. Their findings and subsequent research indicate that anger attacks are likely caused by serotonin deficiencies. Serotonin is a neurotransmitter that is also implicated in depression.

It is unknown whether a similar treatment would be helpful for people with other anger disorders, but the findings thus far justify further investigation. Typically, people with anger disorders are taught to control their cognitions and behaviors during therapy. This therapeutic process could be facilitated by the use of medication to treat some of the potential neurological causes of anger problems. This step would require that anger disorders be recognized as treatable mental health disorders worthy of attention. If the use of medication could reduce violence and health consequences, it is likely worth further research into anger disorders and their potential treatments.

THERAPY RECOMMENDATIONS

Treating angry clients is difficult. Generally, clinicians attempt to build a therapeutic alliance, to ally themselves with the client so they are both working on the same issues. Angry clients are especially likely to be forced into therapy against their will and therefore may not recognize their anger as a problem and may be unwilling to address it. They may see their problem as caused by others, and they may seek the therapists' help to convince the others that they are wrong.[41] Nearly all recommended treatment packages for dysfunctional anger begin with developing a therapeutic alliance and identifying the client's specific motives for changing his or her anger.[30] To assist a client in becoming aware of and willing to change dysfunctional anger, Deffenbacher recommends several techniques.[42] Increasing awareness of the consequences of anger and identifying suppressed anger may help clients become cognizant that anger is central to their difficulties. Focusing on anger as a problem can be reinforced by reframing anger as contrary to clients' self-identity and reducing the tendency to blame others. Strategies that focus on external cues, such as behavioral therapy, may be more effective in the beginning stages of therapy. Such strategies fit with the clients' mind-set of blaming others or situations for their difficulties, and clients may be more willing to participate in a therapy with this focus.

Therapists are also at a disadvantage when dealing with angry clients because they are not trained to handle clients who become angry at them. Professional therapists report that clients often become angry in session, and they perceive anger directed toward them as a highly stressful experience, almost as stressful as suicidal statements.[43] Most clinicians report emotional reactions to a client who is verbally abusive in therapy.[44] Therapists are only human, and they are likely to become angry or afraid when someone is aggressive toward them. A therapist has to learn to manage his or her own emotional reactions in order to be effective working with angry clients.

CONCLUSION

Despite growing concern with societal violence and high rates of homicide and abuse, there is insufficient research on anger or how to treat it. It is likely that anger disorders are highly prevalent in our society, and the effects of these disorders are often devastating for the individual, the family, and society as a whole. There is no diagnosis for anger disorders, which hinders research on the disorders and treatments. The lack of diagnosis also makes it difficult for people with anger disorders to get therapy. They may be misdiagnosed and treated for the wrong disorder, or their insurance may refuse to pay for treatment. In order to establish a diagnosis, it is critical that the research community explore criteria for mood disorders in the *DSM–IV–TR* and whether anger disorders can be distinguished diagnostically from other mood disorders such as depression and anxiety.

After reading the descriptions in this chapter, can you identify whether the people at the beginning of the chapter have an anger disorder? What types of treatments do you think might be effective for each of these people? More than likely, it is still difficult to easily identify who has an anger disorder and how to treat them. Perhaps the 21st century will see the recognition of anger disorders and the development of appropriate treatments for them.

REFERENCES

1. Beck, R., & Fernandez, E. (1998). Cognitive-behavioral therapy in the treatment of anger: A meta-analysis. *Cognitive Therapy and Research, 22*, 63–74.
2. Eckhardt, C.I., & Deffenbacher, J.L. (1995). Diagnosis of anger disorders. In H. Kassinove (Ed.), *Anger disorders: Definition, diagnosis, and treatment. Series in clinical and community psychology* (pp. 27–47). Philadelphia: Taylor & Francis.
3. American Psychiatric Association (2000). *Diagnostic and statistical manual of mental disorders* (4th ed., text rev.). Washington, DC: Author.
4. Endler, N.S., & Parker, J.D. (1990). Stress and anxiety: Conceptual and assessment issues. *Stress Medicine, 6*, 243–248.

5. Eckhardt, C., Norlander, B., & Deffenbacher, J. (2004). The assessment of anger and hostility: A critical review. *Aggression and Violent Behavior, 9*, 17–43.
6. Berkowitz, L. (1989). Frustration-aggression hypothesis: Examination and reformulation. *Psychological Bulletin, 106*, 59–73.
7. Levine, L.J. (1995). Young children's understanding of the causes of anger and sadness. *Child Development, 66*, 697–709.
8. Kemp, S., & Strongman, K. T. (1995). Anger theory and management: A historical analysis. *American Journal of Psychology, 108*, 397–417.
9. Averill, J.R. (1983). Studies on anger and aggression: Implications for theories of emotion. *American Psychologist, 38*, 1145–1160.
10. Ellis, A. (1977). Rational-emotive therapy: Research data that supports the clinical and personality hypotheses of RET and other modes of cognitive-behavior therapy. *Counseling Psychologist, 7*, 2–42.
11. Scherer, K.R., & Wallbott, H.G. (1994). Evidence for universality and cultural variation of differential emotion response patterning. *Journal of Personality and Social Psychology, 66*, 310–328.
12. Grieger, R.M. (1986). Anger problems. In A. Ellis & R.M. Grieger (Eds.), *Handbook of rational-emotive therapy* (Vol. 2, pp. 121–140). New York: Springer.
13. Edmondson, C.B., & Conger, J.C. (1996). A review of treatment efficacy for individuals with anger problems: Conceptual, assessment, and methodological issues. *Clinical Psychology Review, 16*, 251–275.
14. Keinan, G., Ben-Zur, H., Zilka, M., & Carel, R.S. (1992). Anger in and out, which is healthier? An attempt to reconcile inconsistent findings. *Psychology and Health, 7*, 83–98.
15. Fitness, J., & Fletcher, G.J.O. (1993). Love, hate, anger, and jealousy in close relationships: A prototype and cognitive appraisal analysis. *Journal of Personality and Social Psychology, 65*, 942–958.
16. Tanaka-Matusumi, J. (1995). Cross-cultural perspectives on anger. In H. Kassinove (Ed.), *Anger disorders: Definition, diagnosis, and treatment. Series in clinical and community psychology* (pp. 81–90). Philadelphia: Taylor & Francis.
17. Briggs, J.L. (1998). Never in anger: Portrait of an Eskimo family. In J.M. Jenkins & K. Oatley (Eds.), *Human emotions: A reader* (pp. 45–54). Malden, MA: Blackwell.
18. Haynes, S.G., Feinleib, M., & Kannel, W.B. (1980). The relationship of psychosocial factors to coronary heart disease in the Framingham study: III. Eight year incidence of coronary heart disease. *American Journal of Epidemiology, 111*, 37–58.
19. Harris, M.B. (1993). How provoking: What makes men and women angry? *Aggressive Behavior, 19*, 199–211.
20. Lai, J.Y., & Linden, W. (1992). Gender, anger expression style, and opportunity for anger release determine cardiovascular reaction to and recovery from anger provocation. *Psychosomatic Medicine, 54*, 297–310.
21. Lazarus, R.S., & Folkman, S. (1984). *Stress, appraisal, and coping.* New York: Springer.
22. Folkman, S., & Moskowitz, J.T. (2000). Positive affect and the other side of coping. *American Psychologist, 55*, 647–654.

23. Lench, H.C. (2004). Anger management: Diagnostic differences and treatment implications. *Journal of Social and Clinical Psychology, 23,* 512–531.
24. Whatley, S.L., Foreman, A.C., & Richards, S. (1998). The relationship of coping style to dysphoria, anxiety, and anger. *Psychological Reports, 83,* 783–791.
25. Palfai, T.P., & Hart, K.E. (1997). Anger coping styles and perceived social support. *The Journal of Social Psychology, 137,* 405–411.
26. Fredrickson, B.L., Maynard, K.E., Helms, M.J., Haney, T.L., Siegler, I.C., & Barefoot, J.C. (2000). Hostility predicts magnitude and duration of blood pressure response to anger. *Journal of Behavioral Medicine, 23,* 229–243.
27. Whalen, C.K., Jamner, L.D., Henker, B., & Delfino, R.J. (2001). Smoking and moods in adolescents with depressive and aggressive dispositions: Evidence from surveys and electronic diaries. *Health Psychology, 20,* 99–111.
28. Norlander, B., & Eckhardt, C. (2005). Anger, hostility, and male perpetrators of intimate partner violence: A meta-analytic review. *Clinical Psychology Review, 25,* 119–152.
29. Anderson, C.A., & Bushman, B.J. (2002). Human aggression. *Annual Review of Psychology, 53,* 27–51.
30. Digiuseppe, R., & Tafrate, R.C. (2001). A comprehensive treatment model fornger disorders. *Psychotherapy, 38,* 262–271.
31. Larkin, K.T., & Zayfert, C. (1996). Anger management training with mild essential hypertensive patients. *Journal of Behavioral Medicine, 19,* 415–433.
32. Tafrate, R.C. (1995). Evaluation of treatment strategies for adult anger disorders. In H. Kassinove (Ed.), *Anger disorders: Definition, diagnosis, and treatment. Series in clinical and community psychology* (pp. 109–129). Philadelphia: Taylor & Francis.
33. Novaco, R.W. (1977). Stress inoculation: A cognitive therapy for anger and its application to a case of depression. *Journal of Consulting and Clinical Psychology, 45,* 600–608.
34. Linehan, M.M. (1993). *Cognitive-behavioral treatment of borderline personality disorder. Diagnosis and treatment of mental disorders.* New York: Guilford Press.
35. Feindler, E.L. (1995). Ideal treatment package for children and adolescents with anger disorders. In H. Kassinove (Ed.), *Anger disorders: Definition, diagnosis, and treatment. Series in clinical and community psychology* (pp. 173–195). Philadelphia: Taylor & Francis.
36. Del Vecchio, T., & O'Leary, K.D. (2004). Effectiveness of anger treatments for specific anger problems: A meta-analytic review. *Clinical Psychology Review, 24,* 15–34.
37. Elliott, F.A. (1976). Neurological factors in violent behavior (the dyscontrol syndrome). *Bulletin of the American Academy of Psychiatry and the Law, 4,* 297–315.
38. Macmillan, M. "The Phineas Gage Information Page," retrieved April 20, 2006 from www.degkin.edu.au/hbs/psychology/gagepage.
39. Fava, M., Anderson, K., & Rosenbaum, J.F. (1990). "Anger attacks": Possible variants of panic and major depressive disorders. *American Journal of Psychiatry, 147,* 867–870.

40. Fava, M., Anderson, K., & Rosenbaum, J. F (1993). Are thymoleptic-responsive "anger attacks" a discrete clinical syndrome? *Psychosomatics: Journal of Consultation Liaison Psychiatry, 34,* 350–355.
41. DiGiuseppe, R. (1995). Developing the therapeutic alliance with angry clients. In H. Kassinove (Ed.), *Anger disorders: Definition, diagnosis, and treatment. Series in clinical and community psychology* (pp. 131–149). Philadelphia: Taylor & Francis.
42. Deffenbacher, J.L. (1995). Ideal treatment package for adults with anger disorders. In H. Kassinove (Ed.), *Anger disorders: Definition, diagnosis, and treatment. Series in clinical and community psychology* (pp. 151–172). Philadelphia: Taylor & Francis.
43. Deutsch, C.J. (1984). Self-reported sources of stress among psychotherapists. *Professional Psychology: Research and Practice, 15,* 833–845.
44. Pope, K.S., & Tabachnick, B.G. (1993). Therapists' anger, hate, fear, and sexual feelings: National survey of therapist responses, client characteristics, critical events, formal complaints, and training. *Professional Psychology: Research and Practice, 24,* 142–152.

Chapter 4

An Overview of Pathological Gambling

Mark Griffiths

Gambling is one of the few activities that cuts across all barriers of race, class, and culture. Almost all surveys into gambling on a national level have concluded that there are more gamblers than non-gamblers but that most participants gamble infrequently.[1] Estimates based upon survey data from countries all over the world indicate that the majority of people have gambled at some time in their life.[2]

The introduction of national lotteries, the proliferation of gaming machines, the expansion of casinos, and the introduction of new media in which to gamble (e.g., Internet gambling, mobile phone gambling, interactive television gambling) have greatly increased the accessibility and popularity of gambling worldwide and, as a result, the number of people seeking assistance for gambling-related problems.[1] Commissions and official government reviews in a number of countries including the United States, the United Kingdom, Australia, and New Zealand have all concluded that increased gambling availability has led to an increase in problem gambling.

Despite token recognition of the complexity of gambling behavior, most research has been rigidly confined to narrow areas of specialization. Singular theoretical perspectives (e.g., behaviorism, cognitivism, addiction theory) have been assiduously pursued with few attempts to establish links or contrast them with other research programs. This assumes that a single explanation or theory is sufficient to explain every aspect of gambling behavior and that rival perspectives are thereby misguided. Yet, as a number of authors assert, this may not be so.[3–5]

Gambling is a multifaceted rather than unitary phenomenon.[4,5] Consequently, many factors may come into play in various ways and at different levels of analysis (e.g., biological, social, or psychological). Theories may be complementary rather than mutually exclusive, which suggests that limitations of individual theories might be overcome through the combination of ideas from different perspectives. This has often been discussed before in terms of recommendations for an "eclectic" approach to gambling[6] or a distinction between proximal and distal influences upon gambling.[7] However, for the most part, such discussions have been descriptive rather than analytical, and so far, few attempts have been made to explain why an adherence to singular perspectives is untenable. Accordingly, the aim of this chapter is to highlight limitations of existing theories of gambling at three increasingly specific levels of analysis: social, psychological, and biological.

Central to this view, no single level of analysis is considered sufficient to explain either the etiology or maintenance of gambling behavior. Moreover, this view asserts that all research is context-bound and should be analyzed from a combined, or biopsychosocial, perspective.[5] Variations in the motivations and characteristics of gamblers and in gambling activities themselves mean that findings obtained in one context are unlikely to be relevant or valid in another.[8] In each of the following sections, broad details of each level of analysis are provided, followed by discussions of the limitations and interdependence of each theoretical approach and the implications for research and clinical interventions.

PATHOLOGICAL GAMBLING: PREVALENCE AND HISTORY

Estimates of the number of probable adult pathological gamblers vary from just under 1 percent in the United Kingdom, 1.1–1.9 percent in the United States, and 2.3 percent in Australia.[2] These surveys have also indicated that pathological gambling is twice as common among males as it is among females, that nonwhites have higher rates than whites, and that those with poor education are more likely to be pathological gamblers.[1,2] In 1980, pathological gambling was recognized as a mental disorder in the third edition of the *Diagnostic and Statistical Manual of Mental Disorders (DSM–III)*[9] under the section "Disorders of Impulse Control" along with other illnesses such as kleptomania and pyromania. Adopting a medical model of pathological gambling in this way displaced the old image that the gambler was a sinner or a criminal.

Before the appearance of the *DSM–III* (1980), the subject of pathological gambling had produced an expanding body of literature by psychiatrists, psychologists, psychoanalysts, and social workers and had appeared under a variety of labels including "neurotic," "compulsive," "addictive," "excessive," and "pathological."[6] There now seems to be an increased preference among professionals for the term "pathological gambling" to describe individuals with severe gambling problems and this owes much to the consistent efforts of Moran, who argued that the phrase "pathological gambling" is descriptive as opposed to terms like "compulsive" or "addictive," which might suggest specific and homogenous etiologies.[10]

In diagnosing the pathological gambler, the *DSM–III* states that the individual is chronically and progressively unable to resist impulses to gamble and that gambling compromises, disrupts or damages family, personal, and vocational pursuits.[9] The behavior increases under times of stress, and associated features include lying to obtain money, committing crimes (e.g., forgery, embezzlement, fraud), and concealment from others of the extent of the individual's gambling activities. In addition, the *DSM–III* states that to be a pathological gambler, the gambling must not be due to antisocial personality disorder (see Table 4.1).

As Lesieur pointed out, these criteria were criticized for (1) a middle class bias, that is, the criminal offenses like embezzlement and income tax evasion were "middle class" offenses; (2) lack of recognition that many compulsive gamblers are self employed; and (3) exclusion of individuals with antisocial personality disorder.[11] Lesieur recommended that the same custom be followed for pathological gamblers as for substance abusers and alcoholics in the past, that is, allow for simultaneous diagnosis with no exclusions. In addition,

Table 4.1
***DSM–III* Diagnostic Criteria for Pathological Gambling**

The criteria state that maladaptive gambling is indicated by the following:

(A) The individual is chronically and progressively unable to resist impulses to gamble

(B) Gambling compromises, disrupts, or damages family, personal, and vocational pursuits, as indicated by at least three of the following:

    (1) Arrest for forgery, fraud, embezzlement, or income tax evasion due to attempts to obtain money for gambling

    (2) Default on debts or other financial responsibilities

    (3) Disrupted family or spouse relationships due to gambling

    (4) Borrowing money from illegal sources (loan sharks)

    (5) Inability to account for loss of money or to produce evidence of winning money if this is claimed

    (6) Loss of work due to absenteeism in order to pursue gambling activity

    (7) Necessity for another person to provide money to relieve a desperate financial situation

(C) The gambling is not due to Antisocial Personality Disorder

Source: American Psychiatric Association, *Diagnostic and Statistical Manual of Mental Disorders*, 3rd ed. (Washington, DC: American Psychiatric Association, 1980).

the criteria leave out the "problem gambler" who by self-admission, or by others' testimony, spends a disproportionate amount of time gambling but has yet to produce the serious consequences laid down in the *DSM–III*. The new criteria in the *DSM–III–R* (see Table 4.2) were subsequently changed, considering the criticisms and thus now modeled extensively on substance abuse disorders due to the growing acceptance of gambling as a bona fide addictive behavior.

However, in 1989, Rosenthal conducted an analysis of the use of the *DSM–III–R* criteria by treatment professionals.[12,13] It was reported that there was some dissatisfaction with the new criteria and that there was some preference for a compromise between the *DSM–III* and the *DSM–III–R*. As a consequence, the criteria were changed for *DSM–IV*[14] (see Table 4.3).

PHASES OF THE PATHOLOGICAL GAMBLER'S CAREER

The acquisition, development, and maintenance of pathological gambling is an area that is continually disputed. The exact causes and reasons for continuing gambling behavior seem to be dependent upon the individual, but there do seem to be some general underlying factors and re-occurring themes. Problem gambling generally begins in adolescence and may start following a major life stress, for example, the death of a parent or birth of a first child.[15] Such events may induce a need to escape from the problems of reality.

Lesieur and Custer have concluded that pathological gambling behavior consists of three stages—the winning phase, the losing phase, and the desperation phase.[16] The winning phase normally begins with small but

Table 4.2
***DSM–III–R* Diagnostic Criteria for Pathological Gambling**

The criteria state that maladaptive gambling is indicated by four of the following:

1. Frequent preoccupation with gambling or obtaining money to gamble
2. Person often gambles larger amounts of money or over a longer period than intended
3. Need to increase the size or frequency of bets to achieve the desired excitement
4. Restlessness or irritability if unable to gamble.
5. Repeatedly loses money gambling and returns another day to win back losses ("chasing")
6. is interpersonally exploitative, i.e., takes advantage of others to achieve his or her own ends
7. Person often gambles when expected to fulfill social, educational, or occupational obligations
8. Person has given up some important social, occupational, or recreational activity in order to gamble
9. Person continues to gamble despite inability to pay mounting debts or despite other significant social, occupational, or legal problems that the individual knows to be exacerbated by gambling

---

Source: American Psychiatric Association, *Diagnostic and Statistical Manual of Mental Disorders*, 3rd ed., rev. ed. (Washington, DC: American Psychiatric Association, 1987).

Table 4.3
***DSM–IV* Criteria for Pathological Gambling**

(A) Persistent and recurrent maladaptive gambling behavior is indicated by five (or more) of the following:

   (1) is preoccupied with gambling (e.g., preoccupied with reliving past gambling experiences, handicapping or planning the next venture, or thinking of ways to get money with which to gamble)

   (2) needs to gamble with increasing amounts of money in order to achieve the desired excitement

   (3) has repeated unsuccessful efforts to control, cut back, or stop gambling

   (4) is restless or irritable when attempting to cut down or stop gambling

   (5) gambles as a way of escaping from problems or of relieving a dysphoric mood (e.g., feelings of helplessness, guilt, anxiety, depression)

   (6) after losing money gambling, often returns another day to get even ("chasing" one's losses)

   (7) lies to family members, therapist, or others to conceal the extent of involvement with gambling

   (8) has committed illegal acts such as forgery, fraud, theft, or embezzlement to finance gambling

   (9) has jeopardized or lost a significant relationship, job, or educational or career opportunity because of gambling

   (10) relies on others to provide money to relieve a desperate financial situation caused by gambling

(B) The gambling behavior is not better accounted for by a Manic Episode.

Source: American Psychiatric Association, *Diagnostic and Statistical Manual of Mental Disorders*, 4th ed. (Washington, DC: American Psychiatric Association, 1994), 618.

successful bets in adolescence. Early wins prompt more skillful gambling, which usually leads to larger winnings. Most social gamblers stop at this stage. However, after a considerable big win maybe equaling or exceeding the individual's annual salary, the gambler accepts the thought that the occurrence can happen again.

The next stage—the losing phase—is characterized by unrealistic optimism on the gambler's part, and all bets are made in an effort to recoup their losses, which has been termed "the chase" by Lesieur.[17] The result is that instead of cutting their losses, gamblers get deeper into debt, preoccupying themselves with gambling, determined that a big win will repay their loans and solve all their problems. Family troubles begin (both marital and with relatives), and illegal borrowing and other criminal activities in an effort to get money usually start to occur.[18] At this point in the pathological gambler's career, family and friends may "bail out" the gambler.

Alienation from those closest to the pathological gambler characterizes the appearance of the final stage—the desperation phase. In a last-ditch, frenzied effort to repay his or her debts, illegal criminal behavior reaches its height, and when there are finally no more options left, the gambler may suffer from severe depression and have suicidal thoughts. It is then, usually at the insistence of the family (if not the courts), that the gambler must seek help. Because the pathological gambler is impatient, requiring immediate results, help should be aimed at priority areas, that is, legal and financial difficulties, counseling to resolve family and marital problems, and, most importantly, hospitalization for desperate patients who are depressed and suicidal.

More recently, Rosenthal has described a fourth phase called the "hopeless" or "giving up" phase.[12] This is where gamblers know they cannot possibly retrieve their losses and they do not care, leading to play for play's sake.

Explanations of Gambling Involvement

In general, research has consistently shown a positive relationship between the availability of gambling and both regular and problem gambling.[1,19] Whenever new forms of gambling are introduced, or existing forms become more readily available, there is an increase in gambling, suggesting that the demand for gambling products is closely linked to their supply. The more gambling industry infrastructure that is established (e.g., new venues), the larger the range of gambling products (e.g., through the application of new technologies), and the greater the industry's marketing efforts, the more likely people will be to gamble in the first place.

But why is gambling so popular? According to sociologists, gambling is an inherent component of human society,[20] and human beings have a natural penchant for play, risk, and competition. Gambling, they argue, fits easily with cultural values, virtues, and lifestyles,[21] so that when gambling becomes more accessible and socially acceptable, more people will gamble. As a form of social interaction, gambling provides a means by which people can escape the boredom of everyday life, adopt new roles, and enjoy the excitement of the "action," namely, the suspense, anticipation, and social reinforcement resulting from taking risks and being rewarded for one's daring.[22]

Almost all surveys of gambling have shown that these broad motivational factors are central to gambling and that attitudes toward gambling are positively related to availability and cultural acceptability. However, this perspective fails to take into account many key findings and observations in gambling research. Surveys have also shown that not everyone gambles and some people gamble more than others (e.g., pathological gamblers). Research has consistently shown that people often gamble for reasons other than broad social and economic reasons.[23] These other motivations may vary according to personal characteristics of the gambler and the type of gambling activity. Finally, broad social and economic theories fail to explain why certain gambling activities are more popular or "addictive" than others.

Demographic variations in gambling participation have been observed since surveys were first administered. Typically, gambling has been more popular in lower socioeconomic groups, in Catholics rather than Protestants, in unmarried people, in younger age groups, and in men.[24] Consistent with trends observed in overall participation rates, research has found that the incidence of gambling-related problems is considerably higher in lower socioeconomic groups and in younger people, and it is more likely to be associated with slot machine gambling, one of the few activities that attract similar numbers of men and women.[24] Accordingly, understanding demographic variations in overall participation is vital if one is to estimate the likely social effects of expansion or product changes in existing gambling markets.

Variations in gambling preferences are thought to result from differences in both accessibility and motivation. Older people tend to choose activities that minimize the need for complex decision making or concentration (e.g., bingo, slot machine gambling), whereas gender differences have been attributed to a number of factors, including variations in sex role socialization,[22] cultural differences,[7] and theories of motivation.[25]

Variations in motivation are also frequently observed among people who participate in the same gambling activity. For example, slot machine players may gamble to win money, for enjoyment and excitement, to socialize, and to escape negative feelings.[26] Some people gamble for one reason only, whereas others gamble for a variety of reasons. A further complexity is that people's motivations for gambling have a strong temporal dimension, that is, they do not remain stable over time.[15] As people progress from social to regular and finally to excessive gambling, there are often significant changes in their reasons for gambling. Whereas a person might have initially gambled to obtain enjoyment, excitement, and socialization, the progression to problem gambling is almost always accompanied by an increased preoccupation with winning money and chasing losses.

The Importance of the Structural Characteristics of Activities

Another factor central to understanding gambling behavior is the structure of gambling activities. Griffiths has consistently argued that gambling activities vary considerably in their structural characteristics, including the probability of winning, the amount of gambler involvement, the amount of skill that can be applied, the length of the interval between stake and outcome, and the magnitude of potential winnings.[5,27,28] Structural variations are also observed within certain classes of activities such as slot machines, where differences in reinforcement frequency, colors, sound effects, and machine features can influence the profitability and attractiveness of machines significantly.[26] Each of these structural features may (and almost certainly does) have implications for gamblers' motivations and the potential "addictiveness" of gambling activities.

For example, skillful activities that offer players the opportunity to use complex systems, study the odds, and apply skill and concentration appeal to many gamblers because their actions can influence the outcomes. Such characteristics attract people who enjoy a challenge when gambling. They may also contribute to excessive gambling if people overestimate the effectiveness of their gambling systems and strategies (see discussion of cognitive theories below). Chantal and Vallerand have argued that people who gamble on these activities (e.g., racing punters) tend to be more intrinsically motivated than lottery gamblers in that they gamble for self-determination (i.e., to display their competence and to improve their performance).[29]

People who gamble on chance activities, such as lotteries, usually do so for external reasons (i.e., to win money or escape from problems). This was confirmed by Loughnan, Pierce, and Sagris in a clinical survey of problem gamblers.[30] Here, racing punters emphasized the importance of skill and control considerably more than slot machine players. Although many slot machine players also overestimate the amount of skill involved in their gambling,[6] other motivational factors (such as the desire to escape worries or to relax) tend to predominate. Thus, excessive gambling on slot machines may be more likely to result from people becoming conditioned to the tranquilizing effect brought about by playing rather than just the pursuit of money.

Another vital structural characteristic of gambling is the continuity of the activity, namely, the length of the interval between stake and outcome. In nearly all studies, it has been found that continuous activities (e.g., racing, slot machines, casino games) with a more rapid play rate are more likely to be associated with gambling problems.[28] The ability to make repeated stakes in short time intervals increases the amount of money that can be lost and also increases the likelihood that gamblers will be unable to control spending.[31] Such problems are rarely observed in noncontinuous activities, such as weekly or biweekly lotteries, in which gambling is undertaken less frequently and where outcomes are often unknown for days. Consequently, it is important to recognize that the overall social and economic impact of expansion of the gambling industry will be considerably greater if the expanded activities are continuous rather than noncontinuous.

THEORIES OF GAMBLING BEHAVIOR

Although sociological, situational, and demographic factors can explain why some people are more likely to gamble than others, these theories cannot explain why some people gamble more than others or what factors contribute to behavior maintenance in gambling. Psychological theories become important at this level. Research in this area is remarkably diverse. Almost every major branch of psychology (e.g., cognitivism, behaviorism, Freudian theory, addiction theory) has been utilized in an attempt to understand gambling. Despite this, it is possible to distinguish two broad, general perspectives: first, theories that attribute ongoing behavior and excessive gambling to habitual processes that are the consequences of gambling; second, theories that state that variations in behavior result from variations in the characteristics, or makeup, of individual gamblers. In other words, whereas the first places a stronger emphasis upon psychological determinants of gambling, the second emphasizes biological differences between individuals.

Central to psychological explanations is the idea that every person who gambles has the potential to become a problem gambler. This is because gambling activities are difficult to resist by their very nature: they involve excitement, risk-taking, and the possibility of monetary gains. The more a person gambles, the more difficult it becomes to resist the temptation to commence a gambling session or stop once gambling has commenced.[32] Accordingly, it has been suggested that there is no neat distinction between problem gambling and normal gambling; rather there is a continuum from social gambling to regular gambling to problem gambling.

People who gamble regularly may display many of the same behaviors as people with gambling problems, although to a lesser degree. This view gives rise to conceptualizations of problem gambling that emphasize the developmental and habitual nature of problem gambling behavior rather than individual pathology. This perspective avoids terms such compulsive, addiction, or pathology in preference for terms such as impaired control.[31] Although researchers' views differ concerning the psychological mechanisms behind loss of control, three general classes of theory will be used to illustrate the limitations of psychological accounts. They are behaviorist theories that explain persistent gambling as a conditioned process; need state models that see gambling as a form of psychological or physiological dependence;

and cognitive theories that attribute excessive gambling to erroneous beliefs about the potential profitability of gambling.

Behaviorist Approaches

Both classical and operant conditioning principles have been applied to the study of gambling. In operant explanations for problem gambling,[33] persistent gambling is seen as a conditioned behavior maintained by intermittent schedules of reinforcement, most likely a variable-ratio schedule. This involves the provision of infrequent rewards after varying numbers of responses. On the other hand, proponents of classical conditioning models argue that people continue to gamble as a result of becoming conditioned to the excitement or arousal associated with gambling, so that they feel bored, unstimulated, and restless when they are not gambling. Both the classical and operant perspectives have been central to the development of measures of "impaired control" over gambling[34] and clinical interventions using desensitization, aversive conditioning, and satiation techniques.[2] In each of these examples, it is assumed that the more a person gambles, the more his or her behavior is dictated by factors beyond the person's control.

Despite evidence supporting both theories, neither is entirely satisfactory on its own. Classical conditioning theory seems useful to explain people's motivation to commence a gambling session but appears less useful to explain persistent gambling behavior. Conversely, while operant conditioning might explain ongoing behavior, it appears less useful in explaining why people commence gambling or recommence gambling after a prolonged period of abstinence.[6] Researchers have also raised questions about the extent to which gambling behavior adheres to operant theory at all, since gamblers lose more than they win and because reinforcement magnitudes are not independent of player responses, for example, stake sizes.[33,35] Nevertheless, the importance of subtle variations in machine characteristics upon behavior reinforces the role of operant conditioning in the maintenance of behavior, although perhaps in more subtle ways than was envisaged.[28]

It is important to recognize that these theories cannot stand in isolation. As with other psychological theories, conditioning theories cannot explain why people exposed to similar stimuli respond differently—why some gamble whereas others do not or why some people gamble more than others. In addition, the effectiveness or strength of the conditioning effect may be a function of motivational factors and type of activity. Some, but not all, people gamble for excitement or relaxation, and as discussed above, people satisfy these needs by different activities. Thus, it is unlikely that classical conditioning will affect all types of gambling or gamblers. Similar difficulties plague attempts to develop general operant theories of gambling. Some activities appear to suit this form of explanation more than others. Examples include slot machines and scratch tickets where there is a short time interval between stake and outcome and where outcomes are entirely determined by chance. It seems more difficult to apply these principles to skilled gambling games such as blackjack, poker, and sports betting, where player decisions can significantly influence outcomes.

Need-State Models and Theories of Addiction

Much of the discussion relating to classical conditioning also applies to need-state theories of gambling, which assume that people gamble to escape unpleasant feeling states such as anxiety, depression, and boredom. These perspectives have been applied to all facets of gambling, including involvement, ongoing behavior, and excessive gambling. They are incorporated into the *DSM–IV* classification for pathological gambling (i.e., gambling as a way of escaping from problems or intolerable feeling states). Although not all researchers agree that these motivations signify the existence of a physiological addiction,[36] most agree that people can become psychologically addicted to gambling.

The concept of arousal has been studied most extensively, but results have not been consistent.[35,37,38] Arousal increases have been observed in some studies but not in others, and most increases have been relatively small. Variations in arousal have neither covaried reliably with the persistence of behavior nor with the onset of gambling sessions. Walker has questioned the explanatory value of arousal theories arguing that the excitement of gambling is unlikely to be independent of people's desire to win money.[7]

Similar problems have plagued attempts to associate gambling with anxiety and depression. While a considerable number of studies have revealed that negative mood states commonly accompany gambling or predict the duration of gambling sessions,[39–43] most analyses have been confined to problem gamblers and high-frequency gamblers. For this reason, it is unclear whether these mood states are also associated with less frequent gambling. Moreover, it is not possible to determine whether mood states precede or arise as a consequence of gambling. Indeed, as Walker points out,[7] it may be that gamblers become depressed as a result of losing more money than they can afford.

Again, the temporal dimension suggests that the role of mood states is unlikely to be independent of the gambler's characteristics. As with arousal, it is unlikely that avoidance of negative feeling states will be common to all activities or all gamblers. For example, slot machines appear to reduce anxiety, whereas racing provides arousal and excitement. In addition, variations in gambling motivation among participants involved in the same activity suggest that not all people gamble to satisfy unfulfilled needs. It is also unclear why some people apparently have a greater need for arousal or relaxation than others and whether this would be sufficient to explain differences between normal and excessive gambling? It is important to place behavior in a social context to understand how gambling compensates for, or assuages, problems or deficits experienced in other areas of life. Alternatively, as will be suggested later in this chapter, it may be useful to look for dispositional or biological differences to explain the varying motivations and behaviors of individual gamblers.

Cognitive Theories

Despite the fact that the odds of almost all activities are weighted strongly in favor of the house, gamblers continue to believe they can win money from gambling. This observation leads to the conclusion that gambling may be maintained by irrational or erroneous beliefs. For example, people overestimate the extent to which they can predict or influence gambling outcomes and tend to misjudge how much money they have won or lost. This hypothesis has been confirmed in numerous studies showing that people overestimate the degree of skill or control which can be exerted in chance activities,[44,45] and also in studies using the "thinking aloud" method that reveal high levels of irrationality in verbalized statements made during gambling sessions.[46] These findings have been confirmed not only under laboratory conditions but also in ecologically valid gambling settings, using regular gamblers.[46,47]

Based upon these findings, it has been suggested that irrational thinking may be related to problematic gambling behavior,[48,49] with persistent behavior thought to be the result of people's overconfidence in their ability to win money.[7,46,49] Evidence suggests that problem gamblers frequently overestimate the amount of control and skill involved in gambling.[30] Unfortunately, some of these observations have also been made using students with no gambling experience[47] indicating that irrational beliefs are not positively related to level of gambling involvement. A further problem is that irrationality does not appear to covary with other observable facets of gambling, such as the level of risk taking or reinforcement frequency. Alternatively, where irrationality positively relates to involvement, few differences in behavior have been observed. Consequently, Dickerson and Baron have concluded that irrational thinking is probably more a reflection of demand characteristics than a rational underlying behavior.[50] A lot of what people say may only result from the difficulty of trying to come up with rational, meaningful statements in chance-determined situations.

In additional to these conceptual difficulties, it is also possible that contextual factors play a role in cognitive research. For example, Griffiths found that regular players had greater difficulty than occasional players in verbalizing their thoughts while they were gambling.[46] Regular players seemed capable of gambling without attending to what they were doing, suggesting (a) that cognitive processes did not play a major role in the maintenance of their behavior or (b) that the original justifications or rationales for behavior were less accessible. In either case, Griffiths's observations suggested that temporal factors (e.g., how long a person has been gambling) appear to be important. Therefore, all other things being equal, it appears that valid comparisons cannot be drawn between gamblers with differing levels of gambling experience; for what holds for infrequent gamblers might not hold for regular players, and vice versa.

Finally, it is again important to observe that cognitive theories need to take structural variations in activities into account. Many cognitive processes thought to underlie gambling behavior (e.g., overestimations of control, biased attributions) are more likely to be observed when activities are perceived as having some skill component.[6] With some activities, there is a genuine possibility for skillful play (e.g., racing, blackjack, table poker). The more people play or know about these activities, the greater their awareness of the skills involved. Thus, beliefs about control and skill are neither completely irrational nor consistent across players. Instead, in these situations, researchers must examine the quality of play—for example, to what extent the person adheres to optimal strategies—rather than look for evidence of irrational thinking.[51]

Even in activities where outcomes are chance-determined, there are likely to be variations in the extent to which gamblers' perceive that the outcomes are solely chance-determined (e.g., roulette and craps are probably more likely to be perceived as skillful than Australian slot machines because of the greater complexity of the rules and the possibility for variations in playing strategy). Therefore, it may be ineffective to compare results across studies using different chance activities without controlling for variations in perceived skill.

Biological and Dispositional Theories

Social and psychological explanations are insufficient to explain the full complexity of gambling behavior. Whether ongoing behavior is explained in terms of behaviorism, need-state models, or cognitive theories, it remains unclear why one person gambles more heavily than another. In other words, while it seems likely that increased involvement with gambling is likely to contribute to loss of control over behavior, development of irrational beliefs, and greater psychological dependence, it is important to determine what makes some gamblers more susceptible to these factors than others. It is here that research into biological and personality factors becomes important. Central to this research is to ascertain whether pathological gamblers possess qualities that would predispose them to excessive gambling. Much of this literature was summarized by Walker,[7] so this discussion is confined to three research areas: whether problem gamblers are particularly disposed toward developing an addiction; whether they have a greater need for arousal; and whether gamblers are naturally more impulsive than non-gamblers.

Studies into the first question have been undertaken by examining overlaps between potentially addictive and problematic behaviors with alcohol, illicit drugs, and gambling. This includes research into problem gamblers with psychoactive substance abuse problems or those who also have drug or alcohol use problems, or both.[43,52–57] The incidence of cross addictions in populations of pathological gamblers has been cited as evidence for the existence of an addictive personality type. In addition, research by Comings and colleagues, for example, has suggested a genetic basis for gambling in some people.[58] They reported that a variant of the dopamine D2 receptor gene (DRD2), which has been associated with other addictions, including alcoholism, was found in 51 percent of pathological gamblers compared with only 26 percent of controls. The effect of this gene was more closely associated with pathological gambling than any other addiction. This suggested that the genetic variants of the DRD2 gene may play a significant role in pathological gambling, which supports the concept that variants in this gene are an important risk factor for addictive behaviors. However, there are some genes that appear to be unique to problem gambling.[59]

Although intriguing, such data does not provide convincing evidence for the existence of a biological basis for gambling addiction. For a start, many pathological gamblers do not have other addictions.[60] Moreover, as Comings and colleagues show, only half of the problem gamblers possessed the so-called gambling gene, suggesting that this gene is not a necessary factor in the etiology of gambling addiction.[58] Finally, researchers have questioned the notion of physiological addiction altogether, arguing that there is very little evidence to support the applicability of traditional addiction models to gambling.[39,60] Not all gamblers experience cravings, withdrawal symptoms, or tolerance in the traditional addictions sense, suggesting that excessive gambling is more likely to arise as a result of other processes. If the term "addiction" is to be used at all, it is better used in a general sense to denote a condition broadly characterized as a repetitive and uncontrollable behavior that has undesirable consequences for individuals and those around them.[6]

Second, attempts have been made to associate gambling with an excessive desire for arousal or risk taking. For example, Brown hypothesized that pathological gamblers are habitually underaroused or understimulated and need gambling to reach an optimal level of arousal.[61] However, the available evidence offers little support for this notion. While studies by Wolfgang and Anderson and Brown have shown that regular gamblers tend to score higher on measures of sensation seeking than controls,[62,63] other studies have failed to find any associations at all,[64,65] or, paradoxically, studies have found that problem gamblers tend to score lower than population norms on the sensation-seeking scale.[40,66,67] This has been attributed to the fact that problem gamblers tend to engage in a very limited range of activities compared with other people, which limits the number of items endorsed (their scores) on the sensation-seeking scales. Consequently, it seems unlikely that this variable provides a reliable basis for distinguishing problem gamblers from other gamblers.

Thirdly, researchers have tried to associate excessive gambling with the inability to control impulses. This notion was central to the development of the first psychiatric definition of gambling in the *DSM–III*,[9] which classified pathological gambling as a form of impulse disorder, not unlike compulsive stealing (kleptomania) and hair-pulling (trichotillomania). Gamblers were hypothesized to have experiences characteristic of other recognized impulse disorders, such as physical and psychological tension prior to the commencement of gambling and the experience of a strong sense of pleasure or release once the activity had commenced.[68] Implicit in this explanation was the idea that gambling was unplanned, or involuntary, and highly repetitive.

Despite the inconsistency of psychometric evidence on this topic, clinical observations suggest that a loss of control is common to problem gambling.[69] Researchers have argued that there are similarities between problem gambling and children with attention deficit disorder (ADD),[70] in that both are characterized by limited attention spans, impulsive behavior, inability to delay gratification and insensitivity to punishment. Carlton ad colleagues confirmed this by administering a modified ADD scale to a sample of 16 problem gamblers and found that they scored significantly higher on ADD items than a control group.[71] This suggested the possibility that ADD during childhood may be an antecedent to the development of gambling problems in adulthood. Recent psychobiological evidence suggests that such traits can be directly linked to deficiencies in the production of certain neurotransmitters thought to be associated with impulse control. One of these substances is serotonin (5-hydroxtryptamine or 5-HT), which has an inhibitory effect upon the cortex and is associated with more controlled behavior.[68] Several studies of biological markers including the enzyme monoamine oxidase indicate that problem gamblers have deficits in the serotonin system.[72,73] This enzyme is also a marker for impulsivity and sensation-seeking traits. Findings from a variety of other biochemical and pharmacological studies are consistent with the view that problem gamblers are significantly more likely than non–problem gamblers to have impaired serotonergic function.[74]

The question that remains, however, is how researchers will ascertain the direction of causality, namely, whether decreased 5-HT levels are the result, or cause, of excessive gambling. This problem extends to all attempts to draw associations between dispositions and gambling behavior. This indicates the importance of a temporal dimension in gambling. Since gambling is likely to influence the characteristics of gamblers, it may be unwise to assume that observations of one sample can be generalized to other samples of gamblers with different levels of gambling experience.

Physiological accounts assume that such factors should override other environmental or contextual factors and allow for the development of a general theory of gambling addiction. However, this is clearly not so. Apart from the conceptual difficulties associated with determining a causal relationship between characteristics and behavior, these theories are unable to account for the full diversity of gambling patterns and behavior. They fail to explain demographic differences in the preference for activities and variations in motivation. Neither can they explain why some activities are more addictive than others and why the structural characteristics of specific activities (e.g., slot machines) can influence behavior. Therefore, it appears that excessive gambling is likely to result from both dispositional and psychological factors and the complex interaction between them. Psychological explanations must play a role because of the obvious importance of external factors (e.g., environmental and situational variables) in the development of gambling habits. However, it is also clear that internal factors influence how certain individuals respond to these situations. The implications of this observation for the study and treatment of problem gambling are discussed below.

CONCLUSIONS AND IMPLICATIONS FOR RESEARCH AND INTERVENTIONS

In summary, it seems that gamblers are first influenced by sociological factors, for example, the availability of gambling opportunities, attitudes and habits of parents, friends and peer groups, as well as a lack of alternative activities. During the middle stages of development, there are many factors that heavily influence the maintenance of gambling behavior. Three of these factors are schedules of reinforcement, the "escape" qualities of gambling, and cognitive biases, all of which have been summarized in this chapter. While it remains unclear exactly how some people come to gamble excessively, it is agreed that persistent gambling eventually leads to a desperate "spiral of options" where gambling is largely maintained by the desire to win money, recover losses, and pay back debts.[17] Gambling is thus a complex, multidimensional activity that is unlikely to be explained by any single theory. Instead, this research is best served by a biopsychosocial model that stresses the individual and idiosyncratic nature of the development of gambling problems and emphasizes the role of contextual factors internal and external to the process of gambling itself.[3,5]

Recognition of this complexity has important implications for gambling research both in terms of the selection of samples and data analysis. First, the existence of structural variations in activities suggests that results obtained using one activity cannot be generalized to other activities that are not structurally equivalent. Existing research suggests that continuity and the element of skill involved are two factors that must be similar in order for valid comparisons to be made. Second, studies of gambling motivation are unlikely to be valid unless both individual and situational factors are taken into account. Since motivations differ across demographic groups (e.g., different genders and ages), across activities, and over time, studies must ensure that these factors are controlled before drawing conclusions. Samples should contain equal numbers of men and women of a similar age with similar levels of gambling experience. Alternatively, in situations where this cannot be achieved, gender, age, and experience should be used as covariants, or as the first variables in regression analyses.

Third, in recognition that personality may influence the strength of experimental effects, it is important that researchers match comparison groups in terms of these variables. For example, cognitive experiments investigating the illusion of control should include measures of "desirability for control,"[75] whereas arousal experiments should include measures of gambling motivation. In addition, researchers should not assume that biological differences or psychological factors will explain all gambling behavior. Instead, it may be useful to explore the interaction between these different levels of analysis, for example, by examining whether variations in the structural characteristics of activities (e.g., reinforcement frequency) affect people with, or without, the characteristic under observation.

Implications for Prevention, Intervention, and Treatment

Since sociological factors appear to be critical in the acquisition of gambling behavior, prevention needs to be aimed at the social and situational antecedents. This can be approached from a number of levels (e.g., societal, school, family, individual), some of which may be more practical than others. Since problem gamblers start gambling at a significantly earlier age than non-pathological gamblers, an obvious step would be for governments to legislate against young people gambling (i.e., below 18 years of age). A "blanket ban" on gambling would, in most cases, reduce acquisition until at least late adolescence. Both parents and peers may model gambling; therefore, the family's role in maintaining gambling behavior should be addressed in therapy, and prevention plans should aim to increase the gambler's contact with non-gambling peers. Also, evidence or knowledge of a gambler's own negative thoughts or feelings about gambling behavior and a gambler's irrational biases may provide useful cues for behavior modification.[6]

These findings have led to suggestions to enhance educational awareness of the dangers of gambling not only among children and adolescents but also parents, guardians, and teachers. Although recommendations of this nature typically tend to focus upon the need for greater awareness of the true odds and the unprofitability of gambling, this approach needs to be applied with caution. It is quite possible for education to have the opposite effect, namely, to increase students' knowledge of how to gamble. In addition, it is questionable whether knowing the true odds has a significant effect upon dissuading people from gambling, given that many problem gamblers are well educated and have, in some cases, some knowledge of basic mathematics. For many, the belief that they are inherently lucky or different from others helps maintain their interest in gambling. Accordingly, educational campaigns that focus upon the negative consequences of gambling and alternatives to it may have greater success. While these sorts of campaigns are unlikely to prevent gambling in all young people, they might reduce (a) the total number of adolescents who start to gamble and (b) the amount of time adolescents spend gambling.

The fact that some gamblers are socially rewarded for gambling cannot be altered directly, but more adaptive personal and social skills can be taught as responses to stress (i.e., emotional antecedents), for example, relaxation, assertion, and social skills training.[6] Alternatively, where people seek the company of other gamblers as a way to escape from unpleasant feeling states or life stress, the development of alternative interests, hobbies, and social networks should be afforded priority during intervention. This approach could also be extended to people who gamble alone. An essential aspect of treatments should be to identify and address the factors that are antecedents to gambling, those that provide the underlying motivation and social and cultural context in which the behavior has developed. Only when these are addressed can treatments be extended to more specific psychological aspects of the behavior itself. This is because these broader social and structural factors influence a person's exposure to gambling, his or her opportunities to gamble, and his or her ability to recover. Detailed analysis of the person's daily schedule and the nature and extent of available social supports is essential during this phase of treatment.

Viewing problem gambling as a biopsychosocial process recognizes the diversity of psychological factors involved in maintaining the behavior as well as the fact that problem gamblers are not a homogeneous group;[5] in fact, there appear to be a number of subtypes. This has major treatment implications. For instance, Griffiths outlined two very different types of gamblers.[6] The first type appeared to be addicted to gambling itself and played to test skill, gain social rewards, and, mostly, for excitement (i.e., the buzz or high). This was termed a "primary addiction" and appears to be a mixture of Moran's "subcultural" and "impulsive" types of gamblers.[10] Identifying the environmental, situational, or emotional factors that precede a gambling session would be the next stage in the intervention. The use of imaginal desensitization, counterconditioning, and situational exposure are methods that have been used to teach people to resist the urge to gamble. Of course, therapists differ in their view concerning the factors underlying this urge. Whereas some emphasize the learned or conditional quality of the behavior and emphasize the role of stimulus control, others may emphasize irrational beliefs or the person's desire to obtain physiological stimulation from the activity.

Furthermore, as emphasized by Griffiths, a second type of gambler may gamble for the reasons described earlier, such as escape.[6] These gamblers are usually depressed and socially isolated and could be described as having a secondary addiction in that the player uses gambling as an escape from a primary problem (e.g., broken home, relationship crisis). It seems that this type of "escape gambler" is common. This type appears to be a mixture of Moran's "neurotic" and "symptomatic" types.[10] If the primary problem is resolved by excessive gambling, then playing should disappear. This distinction obviously has clinical usefulness and may also help explain conflicting research, some of which states that gambling is a social activity and some of which states that it is a solitary activity. As discussed above, such gamblers are likely to benefit from any intervention that tries to find alternative activities that take the place of gambling. Like Griffiths, more recent writings by Blaszczcynski and Nower suggest there are different subtypes of gamblers that follow different pathways.[76]

Conclusions

Examining gambling and problem gambling as a biopsychosocial behavior makes it evident that individual differences and broader contextual factors must be considered and not ignored.[5] This chapter provides evidence that a narrow focus upon one theoretical perspective in research and clinical interventions may, in many cases, not be justified. Such an approach fails to consider the interrelationships between different levels of analysis. It would be of limited value to many gamblers whose problems have a different etiology, which may be multifaceted. As Gambino and Shaffer pointed out nearly three decades ago, individuals are self-determining agents; therefore, a taxonomy of situations must be developed to describe the vast majority of contexts and conditions in which people use substances or engage in habitual behaviors to alter their perceived experience.[77]

Gambino and Shaffer also make the important point that these behaviors are not completely self-developed or understood by the people themselves and should be examined more broadly. This is because gambling becomes a habitual behavior. Since the perceived experience of the individual can change over time, it is possible that focusing upon the self-reported factors currently maintaining the behavior does not provide insights into the factors that led to the behavior developing. Thus, when one takes a biopsychosocial view, it becomes possible to perceive individual gambling in terms of its broader social and cultural context. This approach also suggests that different perspectives and approaches may be beneficial, so long as they appear to apply to the particular gambler concerned. Moreover, it indicates that a variety of treatments could be beneficial if experienced simultaneously.

APPENDIX 1: THUMBNAIL SKETCHES OF PROBLEM GAMBLERS (ADAPTED FROM GRIFFITHS[6])

Gary

Gary is 19 years old. He experienced an unsettled early life and had been in care and in youth custody for offenses committed to feed his addiction to slot machines. His gambling manifested itself in other forms, such as horse racing, and the consequences were debilitating socially, financially, and emotionally. He regularly followed the same pattern of spending. He would receive a payment of £80 benefits, buy a large breakfast in the local cafe and a small amount of tobacco, and then proceed to spend the remainder on a slot machine in the cafe. He would always play until such a time as his money was gone regardless of whether he had won anything or not. Although he experienced a high when playing on the machines, he was unable to understand his behavior. In addition, he would normally exhibit bouts of aggressive behavior followed by a period of depression that would continue until the receipt of his next benefits payment. To survive the interim period, Gary would sell his possessions and borrow heavily from other people.

Brian

Brian is 17 years old. He comes from a stable background but is now serving an 18-month prison sentence for burglary offenses to fund his gambling addiction. He began playing slot machines from a very early age, and even at nine years of age he was stealing £10 at a time from his parents to play the machines. Brian was always being suspended from school for bad behavior and was eventually taken into voluntary care. His parents blame themselves particularly because they knew about his playing of the machines from an early age and never tried to stop him. Brian says he plays the machines because he gets a buzz from the lights, music, and possible jackpot. During an average playing session he will spend between £50 and £80. On one occasion he stole £140 and then spent it in the course of one afternoon. He claims he just cannot stop playing.

Dave

Dave is 19 years old and is serving a youth custody sentence for theft. He is the second eldest son in a family of five, and there is no history of gambling in his family. As a child he played slot machines at the seaside with money given to him by his parents. His problem became evident at 16 years of age with constant arrests for stealing to play the machines. To stop him playing the machines, Dave's parents escorted him to and from his place of work until they thought he was out of the habit. As soon as they stopped meeting him his gambling started again, and he was then taken to Gamblers Anonymous (GA) by his mother. Although he enjoyed GA, his gambling did not stop, and on one occasion when his parents refused to lend Dave some money to gamble, he took a tranquillizer overdose. The shock of the attempted suicide renewed the family's efforts to help him. He got a job in a cinema but the foyer housed a fruit machine and he was soon stealing from the till to play it. He has now served a number of custodial sentences, but the pattern is always the same after release. He gets his check, cashes, it and then goes and spends it all at once down at the arcade in about two hours.

Jeremy

Jeremy is 18 years old and is an only child. He has been gambling on slot machines since childhood. No one knew he had a problem until he burgled his school and was caught. His parents noticed he had changed from a happy go lucky lad to a bad-tempered monster but did not know why. He had started to develop a problem and as a consequence began to steal small amounts of money from the home, used dinner money to play the machines, and began to be truant from school in order to go to the arcade. Over the years he repeatedly stole items from home—including various valuables and the television set. He is now serving a sentence for credit card fraud.

REFERENCES

1. Abbott, M.W., Volberg, R.A., Bellringer, M., & Reith, G. (2004). *A review of research aspects of problem gambling.* London: Responsibility in Gambling Trust.
2. Orford, J., Sproston, K., Erens, B., & Mitchell, L. (2003). *Gambling and problem gambling in Britain.* Hove, England: Brunner-Routledge.
3. Griffiths, M.D., & Larkin, M. (2004). Conceptualizing addiction: The case for a "complex systems" account. *Addiction Research and Theory, 12,* 99–102.
4. Shaffer, H.J., LaPlante, D.A., LaBrie, R.A., Kidman, R.C., Donato, A.N., & Stanton, M.V. (2004). Towards a syndrome model of addiction: Multiple expressions, common etiology. *Harvard Review of Psychiatry, 12,* 1–8.
5. Griffiths, M.D. (2005). A "components" model of addiction within a biopsychosocial framework. *Journal of Substance Use, 10,* 191–197.
6. Griffiths, M.D. (1995). *Adolescent gambling.* London: Routledge.
7. Walker, M.B. (1992). *The psychology of gambling.* Oxford: Pergamon Press.
8. Dickerson, M.G. (1995). Problem gambling: Future directions in research, treatment, prevention and policy initiatives. In J. O'Connor (Ed.), *High stakes in the nineties* (pp. 73–86). Sixth National Conference of the National Association for Gambling Studies, Fremantle, Western Australia.
9. American Psychiatric Association. (1980). *Diagnostic and statistical manual of mental disorders* (3rd ed.). Washington, DC: Author.
10. Moran, E. (1970). Varieties of pathological gambling. *British Journal of Psychiatry, 116,* 593–597.
11. Lesieur, H. (1988). Altering the DSM-III criteria for pathological gambling. *Journal of Gambling Behavior, 4,* 38–47.
12. Rosenthal, R.J. (1989, November). *Compulsive gambling.* Paper presented at the California Society for the Treatment of Alcoholism and Other Drug Dependencies, San Diego, CA.
13. American Psychiatric Association. (1987). *Diagnostic and statistical manual of mental disorders* (3rd ed., rev. ed.). Washington, DC: Author.
14. American Psychiatric Association. (1994). *Diagnostic and statistical manual of mental disorders* (4th ed.). Washington, DC: Author.
15. Griffiths, M.D. (2003). Adolescent gambling: Risk factors and implications for prevention, intervention, and treatment. In D. Romer (Ed.), *Reducing adolescent risk: Toward an integrated approach* (pp. 223–238). London: Sage.
16. Lesieur, H. R., & Custer, R.L. (1984). Pathological gambling: Roots, phases, and treatment. *Annals of the American Academy of Political and Social Sciences, 474,* 146–156.

17. Lesieur, H.R. (1984). *The chase: Career of the compulsive gambler* (2nd ed.). Rochester, VT: Schenkman Books.

18. Griffiths, M.D. (2004). Betting your life on it: Problem gambling has clear health related consequences. *British Medical Journal, 329,* 1055–1056.

19. Griffiths, M.D. (2003). Problem gambling. *The Psychologist : Bulletin of the British Psychological Society, 16,* 582–584.

20. Goffman, E. (1967). *Interaction ritual.* New York: Anchor.

21. Abt, V., Smith, J.F., & McGurrin, M.C. (1985). Ritual, risk, and reward: A role analysis of race track and casino encounters. *Journal of Gambling Behavior, 1,* 64–75.

22. Abt, V., & Smith, J.F. (1984). Gambling as play. *Annals of the American Academy of Political and Social Sciences, 474,* 122–132.

23. Griffiths, M.D. (1996). Pathological gambling: A review of the literature. *Journal of Psychiatric and Mental Health Nursing, 3,* 347–353.

24. Griffiths, M.D., & Delfabbro, P. (2001). The biopsychosocial approach to gambling: Contextual factors in research and clinical interventions. *Journal of Gambling Issues, 5,* 1–33. Retrieved April 20, 2006 from http://www.camh.net/egambling/issue5/feature/index.html

25. Delfabbro, P.H. (2000). Gender differences in Australian gambling: A critical summary of sociological and psychological research. *Australian Journal of Social Issues, 35,* 145–158.

26. Griffiths, M.D. (2002). *Gambling and gaming addictions in adolescence.* Leicester, England: British Psychological Society/Blackwells.

27. Griffiths, M.D. (1993). Fruit machine gambling: The importance of structural characteristics. *Journal of Gambling Studies, 9,* 101–120.

28. Griffiths, M.D. (1999). Gambling technologies: Prospects for problem gambling. *Journal of Gambling Studies, 15,* 265–283.

29. Chantal, Y., & Vallerand, R.J. (1996). Skill versus luck: A motivational analysis of gambling involvement. *Journal of Gambling Studies, 12,* 407–418.

30. Loughnan, T., Pierce, M., & Sagris, A. (1997, June). *The Maroondah Assessment Profile for Problem Gambling (G-Map™): A new direction in problem gambling counseling.* Paper presented at the Tenth International Conference on Gambling and Risk-Taking, Montreal, Canada.

31. O'Connor, J., Dickerson, M., & Phillips, M. (1995). Chasing and its relationship to impaired control over gambling. In J. O'Connor (Ed.), *High Stakes in the Nineties* (pp. 149–162). Sixth National Conference of the National Association for Gambling Studies, Fremantle, Western Australia.

32. Dickerson, M.G. (1989). Gambling: A dependence without a drug. *International Review of Psychiatry, 1,* 157–172.

33. Delfabbro, P.H., & Winefield, A.H. (1999). Poker machine gambling: An analysis of within session characteristics. *British Journal of Psychology, 90,* 425–439.

34. Baron, E., Dickerson, M., & Blaszczynski, A. (1995). The scale of gambling choices: Preliminary development of an instrument to measure impaired control of gambling

behavior. In J. O'Connor (Ed.), *High Stakes in the Nineties* (pp.153–167). Sixth National Conference of the National Association for Gambling Studies, Fremantle, Western Australia.

35. Griffiths, M.D. (1993). Tolerance in gambling: An objective measure using the psychophysiological analysis of male fruit machine gamblers. *Addictive Behaviors, 18*, 365–372.

36. Walker, M.B. (1989). Some problems with the concept of "gambling addiction": Should theories of addiction be generalized to include excessive gambling? *Journal of Gambling Behavior, 5*, 179–200.

37. Coventry, K.R., & Hudson, J. (2001). Gender differences, physiological arousal and the role of winning in fruit machine gamblers. *Addiction, 96*, 871–879.

38. Diskin, K.M., & Hodgins, D. (2003). Psychophysiological and subjective arousal during gambling in pathological and non-pathological video lottery gamblers. *International Gambling Studies, 3*, 37–51.

39. Blaszczynski, A., & McConaghy, N. (1989). Anxiety and/or depression in the pathogenesis of addictive gambling. *International Journal of the Addictions, 24*, 337–350.

40. Blaszczynski, A.P., McConaghy, N., & Frankova, A. (1990). Boredom proneness in pathological gamblers. *Psychological Reports, 67*, 35–42.

41. Dickerson, M.G., Cunningham, R., Legg England, S., & Hinchy, J. (1991). On the determinants of persistent gambling III: Personality, prior mood, and poker machine play. *International Journal of the Addictions, 26*, 531–548.

42. Dickerson, M.G., Hinchy, J., Legg England, S., Fabre, J., & Cunningham, R. (1992). On the determinants of persistent gambling behaviour I: High-frequency poker machine players. *British Journal of Psychology, 83*, 237–248.

43. Ramirez, L.F., McCormick, R.A., Russo, A.M., & Taber, J.I. (1984). Patterns of substance abuse in pathological gamblers undergoing treatment. *Addictive Behaviors, 8*, 425–428.

44. Langer, E.J. (1975). The illusion of control. *Journal of Personality and Social Psychology, 32*, 311–328.

45. Langer, E.J., & Roth, J. (1983). Heads you win, tails it's chance: The illusion of control as a function of the sequence of outcomes in a purely chance task. *Journal of Personality and Social Psychology, 32*, 951–955.

46. Griffiths, M.D. (1994). The role of cognitive bias and skill in fruit machine gambling. *British Journal of Psychology, 85*, 351–369.

47. Ladouceur, R., Gaboury, A., Bujold, A., Lachance, N., & Tremblay, S. (1991). Ecological validity of laboratory studies of videopoker gaming. *Journal of Gambling Studies, 7*, 109–116.

48. Ladouceur, R., & Walker, M.B. (1996). A cognitive perspective on gambling. In P.M. Salkovkis (Ed.), *Trends in Cognitive and Behavioural Therapies* (pp. 89–120). London: John Wiley & Sons.

49. Wagenaar, W.A. (1988). *Paradoxes of Gambling Behaviour*. London: Erlbaum.

50. Dickerson M.G., & Baron, E. (2000). Contemporary issues and future directions for research into pathological gambling. *Addiction, 95,* 1145–1159.
51. Keren, G., & Wagenaar, W.A. (1985). On the psychology of playing blackjack: Normative and descriptive considerations with implications for decision theory. *Journal of Experimental Psychology, 114,* 133–158.
52. Linden, R.D., Pope, M.G., & Jonas, J.M. (1986). Pathological gambling and major affective disorder: Preliminary findings. *Journal of Clinical Psychiatry, 47,* 202–203.
53. Ciarrocchi, J., & Richardson, R. (1989). Profile of compulsive gamblers in treatment: Update and comparisons. *Journal of Gambling Behavior, 5,* 53–65.
54. Lesieur, H.R., Blume, S.B., & Zoppa, R.M. (1986). Alcoholism, drug abuse and gambling. *Alcoholism: Clinical and Experimental Research, 10,* 33–38.
55. Lesieur, H.R., & Heineman, M. (1988). Pathological gambling among youthful substance abusers in a therapeutic community. *British Journal of Addictions, 83,* 765–771.
56. Griffiths, M.D. (1994). Co-existent fruit machine addiction and solvent abuse in adolescence: A cause for concern? *Journal of Adolescence, 17,* 491–498.
57. Griffiths, M.D. (1994). An exploratory study of gambling cross addictions. *Journal of Gambling Studies, 10,* 371–384.
58. Comings, D.E., Rosenthal, R.J., Lesieur, H.R., Rugle, L.J., Muhleman, D., Chie, C., et al. (1996). A study of dopamine D2 receptor gene in pathological gambling. *Pharmacogenetics, 6,* 223–234.
59. Slutske, W.S., Eisen, S., True, W.R., Lyons, M.J., Goldberg, J., & Tsuang, M. (2000). Common genetic vulnerability for pathological gambling and alcohol dependence in men. *Archives of General Psychiatry, 57,* 666–673.
60. Blaszczynski, A. (1996, November). *Is pathological gambling an impulse control, addictive or obsessive compulsive disorder?* Paper presented at the Seventh National Conference of the National Association for Gambling Studies, Melbourne, Australia.
61. Brown, R.I.F. (1986). Arousal and sensation-seeking components in the general explanation of gambling and gambling addictions. *International Journal of the Addictions, 21,* 1001–1016.
62. Wolfgang, A.K. (1988). Gambling as a function of gender and sensation seeking. *Journal of Gambling Behavior, 4,* 71–77.
63. Anderson, G., & Brown, R.I.F. (1984). Real and laboratory gambling, sensation-seeking and arousal. *British Journal of Psychology, 75,* 405–410.
64. Allcock, C.C., & Grace, D.M. (1988). Pathological gamblers are neither impulsive nor sensation-seekers. *Australian and New Zealand Journal of Psychiatry, 22,* 307–311.
65. Ladouceur, R., & Mayrand, M. (1986). Caractéristiques psychologiques de la prise de risque monétaire des joueurs et des non-joueurs à la roulette. *International Journal of Psychology, 21,* 433–443.

66. Blaszczynski, A., Wilson, A.C., & McConaghy, N. (1986). Sensation seeking in pathological gambling. *British Journal of Addiction, 81*, 113–117.
67. Dickerson, M.G., Hinchy, J., & Fabre, J. (1987). Chasing, arousal and sensation seeking in off-course gamblers. *British Journal of Addiction, 82*, 673–680.
68. McGurrin, M.C. (1992). *Pathological gambling: Conceptual, diagnostic, and treatment Issues.* Sarasota, FL: Professional Resource Press.
69. McCormick, R.A. (1994). The importance of coping skill enhancement in the treatment of the pathological gambler. *Journal of Gambling Studies, 10*, 77–86.
70. Goldstein, L., Manowitz, P., Nora, N., Swartzburg, M., & Carlton, P.L. (1985). Differential EEG activation and pathological gambling. *Biological Psychiatry, 20*, 1232–1234.
71. Carlton, P.L., Manowitz, P., McBride, H., Nora, R., Swartzburg, M., & Goldstein, L. (1988). Attention deficit disorder and pathological gambling. *Journal of Clinical Psychology, 48*, 487–488.
72. Blanco, C., Orensanz-Munoz, L., Blanco-Jerez, C., & Saiz-Ruiz, J. (1996). Pathological gambling and platelet MAO activity: A psychobiological study. *American Journal of Psychiatry, 153*, 119–121.
73. DeCaria, C., Hollander, M.E., Begaz, T., Schmeidler, J., Wong, C.M., Cartwright, C., et al. (1998). *Reliability and validity of a pathological gambling modification of the Yale-Brown Obsessive Compulsive Scale (PG-YBOCS): Preliminary findings.* Paper presented at the 12th National Conference on Problem Gambling. Las Vegas, NV.
74. Blanco, C., Ibanez, A., Saiz Ruiz, J., Blanco-Jerez, C., & Nunes, E.V. (2002). Epidemiology, pathophysiology, and treatment of pathological gambling. *CNS Drugs, 13*, 397–407.
75. Burger, J.M., & Cooper, H.M. (1979). The desirability of control. *Motivation and Emotion, 3*, 381–393.
76. Blaszczynski, A., & Nower, L. (2002). A pathways model of pathological gambling. *Addiction, 97*, 487–500.
77. Gambino, B., & Shaffer, H. (1979). The concept of paradigm and the treatment of addiction. *Professional Psychology, 10*, 207–223.

Chapter 5

Kleptomania

Jon Grant and Daniel Kim

THE HISTORY OF KLEPTOMANIA

Shoplifting appears to date back centuries. In fact, as long as there have been people selling merchandise, there have been people stealing it.[1,2] Although present for centuries, shoplifting seems to have become a serious problem in the 19th century with the rise of the department store (p. 4).[3] With easy access to a wide array of objects, there was an attendant increase in shoplifting. Newspapers in Europe and America ran daily articles about the rampant behavior of shoplifting.[2] When well-to-do middle-class women were caught stealing from department stores, however, the courts, the medical community, and society needed to explain this phenomenon.[2] It was from this context that the first scientific discussion of kleptomania emerged.

In 1816, Andre Matthey, a Swiss physician, used the word *klopemanie* (from the Greek words *kleptein* [to steal] and *mania* [insanity]) to describe the behavior of a distinct group of thieves that would impulsively or compulsively steal worthless or unneeded objects.[2,4] In 1838, two French physicians, Jean-Etienne Esquirol (Matthey's mentor) and C.C. Marc (Esquirol's pupil), changed the term to *kleptomanie* and included it among the *monomanias*, a group of disorders characterized by involuntary and irresistible actions that were mental diseases, not moral depravities (p. 183).[3] Thus, people suffering from kleptomania were seen as being forced to steal by this form of moral insanity (p. 184).[3]

Because most shoplifters appeared to be women, the discussion of kleptomania in the 19th and early 20th centuries became part of the ongoing medical debate about the relationship of insanity to the female reproductive system (pp. 186–187).[3] Kleptomania was discussed alongside female pelvic disorders, hysteria, and other diseases of uterine organs. This inclusion of kleptomania within an ongoing medical discussion of gender is clearly seen in one of the first well-publicized cases of possible kleptomania in the British legal system at the end of the 19th century. In 1896, Mr. and Mrs. Walter Castle, two American citizens, were arrested in London for shoplifting. Given their socially prominent status, the *New York Times* and the *San Francisco Chronicle* covered the story with almost daily articles for the month of the trial. Mrs. Castle was described as suffering from a "diseased condition of the moral nature." One physician characterized Mrs. Castle's behavior as a "disorder of the mind" due to a "long-neglected uterine and rectal disease" (p. 186).[3] In fact, several physicians agreed that disordered menstruation, hemorrhoids, and uterine irregularities resulted in various forms of mania (including kleptomania) in women (p. 186).[3] Although various stolen items were found among Mr. Castle's personal belongings, he was exonerated from all responsibility. Premenstrual tension, menstrual disturbance, and postpartum conditions were all proposed as prominent factors in female shoplifting.

Although shoplifting has continued unabated since the 19th century, the labeling of certain shoplifters as kleptomaniacs largely disappeared by 1920.[2] This may have occurred for several reasons: first, no one in the scientific community was able to offer proof that female reproductive issues caused shoplifting; second, greater numbers of men were being apprehended for shoplifting;[1] third, many stores began using house detectives to embarrass and frighten middle-class women without pressing charges; and fourth, society became intolerant of what was perceived as an excuse for middle-class and wealthy women.[2] Although episodic mention is made of kleptomania in the scientific literature of the early 20th century, it would not generate concentrated scientific interest again until the early 1990s. In 1952, the first *Diagnostic and Statistical Manual of Mental Disorders (DSM–I)* included kleptomania as a supplementary term rather than as a distinct diagnosis, but kleptomania was then left out altogether in the *DSM–II* (1968). Since its reappearance in the *DSM–III* (1980), it has been categorized as an impulse control disorder not elsewhere classified and remains this way in the current *DSM–IV–TR* (2000).

WHAT IS KLEPTOMANIA? CLINICAL CHARACTERISTICS OF COMPULSIVE SHOPLIFTING

According to the *DSM–IV–TR*, a diagnosis of kleptomania requires the following: (1) recurrent failure to resist impulses to steal objects that are not needed for personal use or for their monetary value; (2) increasing sense of tension immediately before committing the theft; (3) pleasure, gratification, or relief at the time of committing the theft; (4) stealing not committed to express anger or vengeance and not in response to a delusion or a hallucination; (5) stealing not better accounted for by conduct disorder, a manic episode, or antisocial personality disorder.[5] Furthermore, the objects stolen are usually of little value and affordable to the individual, who will then typically discard, hoard, secretly return, or give them away.[6] Individuals may avoid stealing when immediate arrest is likely, but the chances of apprehension are usually not fully taken into account. The impulse to steal is experienced as wrong, senseless, and incompatible with the individual's self-concept. Although a sense of pleasure, gratification, or relief is experienced at the time of the theft, individuals will describe a feeling of guilt, remorse, or depression soon afterwards.[7]

No national epidemiological study of kleptomania has been performed, but studies of kleptomania in various clinical samples suggest that the disorder is not uncommon. One study of depressed patients (n = 107) found that 4 (3.7%) suffered from kleptomania,[8] while a related study of patients with alcohol dependence (n = 79), found that 3 (3.8%) also reported symptoms consistent with kleptomania.[9] Studies of pathological gamblers have found rates of comorbid kleptomania ranging from 2.1 percent to 5 percent.[10,11] Interestingly, a study of bulimia patients found that 24 percent met *DSM–III–R* criteria for kleptomania.[12] A recent study of psychiatric inpatients with multiple disorders (n = 204) revealed that 7.8 percent (n = 16) endorsed current symptoms consistent with a diagnosis of kleptomania and 9.3 percent (n = 19) had a lifetime diagnosis of kleptomania.[13]

Of the four studies that have assembled large numbers of patients with kleptomania (n = 108), 68 (63.0%) were female.[4,14–16] Although the majority of reported cases of kleptomania indicate a female predominance, these findings may be biased, as women may be more likely than men to present for psychiatric evaluation. Also, the legal system may be more likely to send female shoplifters for psychiatric evaluation while sending male shoplifters to prison.[6]

The average age at onset of stealing behavior is typically during adolescence, although there are reports of new onset stealing behaviors occurring as early as 4 years of age[17] and as late as 77 years of age.[18] The mean age at time of evaluation is typically mid- to late thirties. Women usually present for evaluation at a younger age than men. For example, one study reported that the average age for women at time of evaluation was 35 years of age, while for men it was 50 years of age.[6] The length of time between age of onset and age at evaluation reinforces the guilt, shame, and secrecy involved in this disorder. The rates of marriage ranged from 35 percent[19] to 83 percent,[20] while university level education ranged from 19 percent[19] to 100 percent.[21] One study found that most of the patients were in the middle to lower economic brackets.[20]

According to *DSM–IV–TR*, three typical courses of this illness have been described: sporadic with brief episodes and long periods of remission; episodic with protracted periods of stealing and periods of remission; and chronic with some degree of fluctuation.[5] Most patients in the studies reported sudden onset with a chronic course.[16] A study of 22 kleptomaniacs revealed that they stole, on average, 2.3 times a week and had urges 3.7 days out of the week. Of those studied, 18.2 percent reported never having a day without symptoms and no one went longer than three weeks without stealing. Of those that were apprehended, 79 percent reported that urges to steal were virtually abolished, but only for an average of 3.5 days. Subjects reported that they stole mainly from stores (department, grocery, clothing, houseware), friends, relatives, and work. All stated they could afford what they stole but did not understand why they stole. Most reported that the value of stolen items increased over time and that most items were kept (or hoarded), although many were given away, returned, or discarded.[15] Examples of commonly stolen objects include sweets, newspapers, food, books, and clothes.[14]

ARE ALL SHOPLIFTERS KLEPTOMANIACS? A COMPARISON OF KLEPTOMANIA AND TYPICAL SHOPLIFTING

Kleptomaniacs differ from ordinary shoplifters in that they do not steal for personal gain but rather for symptomatic relief.[4] Apart from this, they may have many similarities, as the "profile of a typical shoplifter referred for psychiatric examination is a 37-year-old married female, employed at the professional end of the occupational spectrum, who is suffering from a depressive neurosis and who steals an item of insignificant value or use to herself."[22]

The exact prevalence of shoplifting is unknown (because many who steal are never caught), but one study found that 10 percent of randomly chosen customers followed while shopping were observed stealing.[23] In fact, it is estimated that more than $10 billion worth of goods are stolen from retailers each year, which translates into more than $25 million per day.[24] The vast majority of shoplifters are described as amateurs with sporadic activity, with no known history of criminal activity, and who steal for their own consumption rather than for resale.[25] One author has suggest that "the incidence of shoplifting is so widespread that one must give serious consideration to the possibility that it is a product of characteristics that are allied to or are part of the basic essence of human nature."[26] Studies involving apprehended, legally referred shoplifters indicate that shoplifting may be more common in women (ranging from 52 to 100%) than in men. But as with kleptomania, these rates may be falsely elevated because women may be more likely to be referred for psychiatric evaluation than are men. Male shoplifters are more likely to be apprehended during adolescence and early adulthood, whereas women are more likely to be apprehended during puberty/early adulthood and around the age of menopause.[4] Some of these same studies also revealed that shoplifting was not related to lower socioeconomic level and that most stole for personal gain.[4] Rates of kleptomania among people who are arrested for shoplifting have ranged from 0 percent to 8 percent.[4] According to the *DSM–IV–TR*, fewer than 5 percent of shoplifters are identified as kleptomaniacs.[5] Again, these rates may be falsely low due to incomplete psychiatric evaluations, lack of strict diagnostic criteria for kleptomania, and selection bias in these samples.[4]

A study that compared kleptomaniacs to shoplifters interviewed directly after apprehension found that 58 percent of the shoplifters were male compared to only 32.4 percent of kleptomania patients.[27] The mean age among shoplifters was 27 years and among kleptomaniacs, 41 years. Although none of the shoplifters met *DSM* criteria for kleptomania, approximately one-fifth had not stolen for personal use and had eventually discarded the object.[27] The study also found that both groups reported the same degree of impulsivity and a feeling of not being oneself. On the other hand, kleptomaniacs reported a relatively greater number of previous thefts compared to shoplifters, which supports the compulsive aspect of kleptomania. The course of shoplifting is not exactly known, but it appears that it can be chronic, as there are reports of middle-aged and elderly persons who continue to steal. Overall, this study found that many shoplifters, although they do not meet criteria for kleptomania, share characteristics with kleptomaniacs and therefore may benefit from treatment.[27]

Given that both typical shoplifting and kleptomania may start at a relatively early age, it is important to briefly examine childhood and adolescent stealing. A young child generally has little, if any, concept of stealing—for him or her, desiring or wanting means possession of the object. By the age of 6 or 7, children begin to realize they are doing something wrong when they take something that doesn't belong to them.[28] Children may steal because they are unhappy, lonesome, jealous, fearful, or craving attention.[29] For older children and adolescents, stealing can be used to gain acceptance from a group, but is also a strong predictor of future delinquency and a marker for families lacking in warmth and personal stimulation. A strong attachment to parents decreases involvement in shoplifting.[30]

Overall, studies have shown that roughly 40 percent of apprehended shoplifters are adolescents. A study involving almost 1,700 adolescents found that 37 percent reported shoplifting at least once in the prior 12 months.[25] The percentage of respondents peaked around the 10th grade and then declined, which is consistent with official crime statistics.[25] So why are so many adolescents stealing? The researchers hypothesized that this could be a function of immaturity during a stressful transition to adulthood, an inability to purchase certain items, and increased opportunity (the steepest gain of independence occurs around age 16 when most adolescents are allowed to drive and work).[25] On the other hand, the adolescents stated they shoplifted because of the novelty and risk involved, social reasons, and desire for the product. The majority of shoplifters in this study were male, which contrasts the popular view that shoplifting is a female crime but which supports U.S. government statistics that thievery is strongly male dominated during the teenage years.[25] Additionally, no relationship was found between family occupational status and adolescent shoplifting. How many of these adolescent shoplifters currently suffer from, or will develop a problem with kleptomania is not clear. Longitudinal studies of this nature are needed to help clinicians better assess who should receive treatment.

IS KLEPTOMANIA A SYMPTOM OF A LARGER PROBLEM?

The Relationship of Kleptomania to Other Psychiatric Ilnesses

Kleptomania has been classified as an impulse control disorder not elsewhere classified since its introduction to *DSM–III* in 1980. Other disorders included in this category include intermittent explosive disorder (discrete episodes of losing control of aggressive impulses), pyromania (recurrent, deliberate, and purposeful setting of fires), pathological gambling (persistent and recurrent maladaptive gambling that causes economic problems and significant social, personal, or occupational disturbances), and trichotillomania (recurrent pulling out of one's hair).[5] The essential feature of these disorders is the failure to resist an impulse, drive, or temptation to perform an act that is harmful to the person or to others. For most of these disorders, the individual feels an increasing sense of tension or arousal before committing the act and then experiences pleasure, gratification, or relief at the time of committing the act. Following the act there may or may not be regret, self-reproach, or guilt.

Symptoms may be one way of grouping disorders, but other ways include grouping by common etiologies and treatment. Some have proposed that kleptomania may be more appropriately placed among other disorders such as depression and obsessive-compulsive disorder (OCD). One way of examining this is to look at other illnesses that occur in patients with kleptomania (comorbidities), as well as illnesses in first-degree relatives of kleptomaniacs. High rates of comorbid psychiatric disorders have been found in patients with kleptomania. Rates of lifetime comorbid mood disorders have ranged from 59[15] to 100 percent[4] with lifetime comorbid bipolar disorder ranging from 9 percent[15] to 27[21] to 60 percent.[4] High lifetime rates of comorbid anxiety disorders (60%–80%),[4,30] impulse control disorders (20%–46%),[10] substance use disorders (23%–50%),[4,15] and eating disorders (60%)[4] have also been reported.

In terms of family history, 20–35 percent of first-degree relatives appear to suffer from mood disorders, while 15–20 percent suffer from substance use disorders.[16,31] One study has also found that obsessive-compulsive disorder may be elevated in first-degree relatives (25%),[16] but this finding has not been found consistently (7%).[31] And finally, one study found that although rates of individual psychiatric disorders in family members did not differ significantly between kleptomania patients and normal controls, patients with kleptomania were more likely to have a first-degree relative with a psychiatric disorder compared to normal controls.[32]

To explain these comorbidities and family histories, various suggestions have been proposed for kleptomania's classification. Some have suggested that kleptomania as well as a number of other disorders with impulsive features are related to either obsessive-compulsive disorder, forming an "obsessive-compulsive spectrum," or to mood disorders ("an affective spectrum disorder").[33] The grouping of impulse control disorders within either an obsessive-compulsive or an affective spectrum is based on symptom similarities, comorbidities, family history, and treatment responses. Like people who suffer from OCD, kleptomania patients report repetitive thoughts and behaviors and the high rates (63%) of hoarding.[15] Unlike OCD, however, the shoplifting of kleptomania is pleasurable and the behavior is often driven by cravings or urges. Given these descriptions, kleptomania may also share features of disorders characterized by impulsivity, such as bipolar disorder, substance use disorders, and attention deficit disorder.

Kleptomania has also been thought to be merely a symptom of an antisocial or borderline personality disorder. One study consisting of 28 individuals with kleptomania found that 10.7 percent met criteria for borderline personality disorder, while only 3.5 percent had antisocial personality disorder. Interestingly, the most frequently co-occurring disorder was paranoid personality disorder (17.9%) which is characterized by long-standing suspiciousness and mistrust of people. The results of this study suggested that kleptomania occurs independently of any particular personality disorder.[34] On the other hand, another study of 37 kleptomaniacs found that many displayed antisocial traits (not personality disorder), suggesting a lack of a clear boundary between kleptomaniacs and ordinary thieves.[14] Grant also found that kleptomaniacs have personality dimensions that are suggestive of borderline temperament, but this is not specific to kleptomania and there was not enough evidence to suggest kleptomania as a symptom of borderline personality disorder.[34]

Despite multiple suggestions as to where kleptomania should be classified, there is evidence to suggest that it should remain where it is. One study found that kleptomaniacs were no more likely than comparison subjects to endorse symptoms of depression, bipolar disorder, or OCD, but they did have a higher prevalence of impulse control disorders. The findings of this study support kleptomania in its current category of "impulse control disorders not elsewhere classified" and may suggest a common etiology among them.[32]

The Personal, Family, Social, and Economic Impacts of Kleptomania

One of the criteria for kleptomania is "pleasure, gratification, or relief at the time of committing the theft,"[5] How much pleasure and gratification does a kleptomaniac experience from this disorder? From various studies attempting to answer this question, it seems as though there is more suffering than pleasure or gratification. In a study of 22 kleptomaniacs, 100 percent reported trying unsuccessfully to stop stealing, and 100 percent had increased urges to steal when trying to stop.[15] Attempts to control urges to steal involved not leaving the house, shopping with friends and family, shopping when stores are busy, and thinking about getting caught. In addition, 64 percent reported being apprehended and 23 percent had been jailed. The vast majority (77.3%) experienced guilt and shame, with 27.3 percent reporting psychiatric hospitalization and 18.2 percent considering suicide because of their behavior. Only 41.7 percent told their spouses due to shame and guilt.[15]

A study of 40 kleptomaniacs revealed 77.5 percent had been arrested for shoplifting and 17.5 percent served jail time. Of those studied, 97.5 percent actively lied to loved ones about their behavior, and 47.5 percent felt this directly led to deterioration of these relationships. Among this group, 42.5 percent also reported significant work impairment through time wasted dealing with urges, guilt, and personal/legal consequences of behavior.[35] Those who suffer from kleptomania also report high levels of perceived stress (i.e., the degree to which people find their lives to be unpredictable, uncontrollable, and stressful), which appears to be associated with the severity of kleptomania symptoms.[36] Individuals with kleptomania also have significantly poorer life satisfaction compared to the general population, which may highlight the moral and legal repercussions of this disorder.[37]

Little is known about how much kleptomania contributes to economic losses, so most of the figures are extrapolated from shoplifting. The incidence of shoplifting has substantially increased in the past 40 years, partly because of the increase in supermarket and display merchandising.[38] Some suggest that

kleptomania is a consequence of consumerism and the abundance of com-
modities in modern society.[39] As previously mentioned, over $10 billion worth
of goods are stolen from retailers each year (over $25 million a day) and there
are 23 million shoplifters (or 1 in 11 people) in the United States. If the prevalence of kleptomania is 6 per 1,000 persons,[6] then there are approximately
1.2 million individuals with kleptomania (of the 200 million American adults)
responsible for the loss of $500 million a year.[35] Shoplifting results in increased
prices to cover anticipated losses, as well as delays and intrusions from locks,
tags, and surveillance.[25]

"Tell Me about Your Childhood" . . . Proposed Psychodynamic Hypotheses

The past two centuries of kleptomania's history are littered with various theories and hypotheses that attempt to explain this baffling disorder but achieve
no consensus on causation. The early to mid-1900s saw an increase in the popularity of psychodynamic and psychoanalytic theories of kleptomania, although
many of these writings assumed that kleptomania and stealing had the same
meanings and causes.[40] Kleptomania has been interpreted as a reflection of
unconscious defenses against anxiety, forbidden instincts or wishes, unresolved
conflicts, prohibited sexual drives, fear of castration, and sexual arousal, sexual
gratification, and orgasm during the act of thievery.[41] The association of stealing
and sexuality has appeared in various writings and has been described as being
"an ungratified sexual instinct," as well as a forbidden secret such as masturba-
tion.[42] This was reported in a case of a 57-year-old white female kleptomaniac
who "claims that although frigid, afraid of sex, and never able to attain orgasm, she
experienced her first orgasm when apprehended for the first time."[42] Symbolic
meaning has also been attributed to the act of stealing, the stolen object, and the
victim of the theft.[41] Stealing by a woman was viewed as symbolic of stealing
a penis, while objects stolen represented anal fixation.[43] Cupchik felt thievery
among upstanding citizens was an effort to obtain symbolic compensation for
an actual or anticipated loss.[38] Some object relationists have seen stealing as a
way of controlling a frightening and dangerous object by reinstating a sense of
omnipotence, while some self psychologists have interpreted stealing as a way to
prevent fragmentation of the self and as a response to narcissistic injury.[6] There
has also been focus on kleptomania's relationship with anxiety and depression.
The act of stealing has been interpreted as a risk-taking behavior performed by
a depressed subject with an antidepressant significance, as a symptom of stress,
or as a way of relief from stressful conditions.[44] In children who report feeling
injured or neglected, kleptomania may gratify two needs: the actions themselves

may be gratifying and the stolen objects might dispel feelings of deprivation.[43] Analogously, some reported that the need for stimulation results in artificial methods (such as shoplifting) to increase psychological tension. There are no data, however, to confirm or refute any of these theories.[6]

WHAT ABOUT BRAIN CHEMISTRY? PROPOSED NEUROBIOLOGICAL HYPOTHESES OF KLEPTOMANIA

Multiple case reports discuss neurological and medical conditions as well as medications that have induced kleptomania-like behavior, but the findings of these studies should be interpreted with caution, as they may or may not have direct relevance to kleptomania occurring in the absence of these factors. Thomas Nyffeler described a 32-year-old male with a brain tumor (craniopharyngioma with right-sided extension) who developed kleptomania symptoms within weeks after surgery. These findings suggest that disruption of specific neuronal pathways in the brain (especially of the prefrontal cortex) could result in impairments of response suppression and development of disorders of the compulsive-addictive spectrum. Furthermore, compulsive-addictive behaviors may be more common after right-sided brain damage than after left-sided brain damage.[45]

Anat Aizer described two cases of head trauma resulting in new onset kleptomania-like symptoms.[46] A 43-year-old male with blunt trauma to the front/side (frontotemporal region) of the head resulted in 5–10 minutes of unconsciousness and normal neurological imaging and examination. Soon afterwards he developed personality changes and kleptomania-like symptoms, which remitted with citalopram (antidepressant) and therapy. Although brain imaging showed no abnormalities, it was hypothesized that damage to this patient's frontal lobe resulted in his clinical condition, as lesions to this region commonly induce personality changes and are associated with poor planning and faulty decision making. The second case involved a 34-year-old male who fell from first-floor level, resulting in a three-day coma. Imaging revealed a bruise on the left side of the brain (left temporal lobe). Soon afterwards he began to develop kleptomania-like symptoms, which fully remitted with venlafaxine (antidepressant) and naltrexone (medication for opiate addiction and other addictive behaviors).

The underlying biological mechanism of urge-based disorders may involve the processing of incoming reward inputs by the ventral tegmental area-nucleus accumbens-orbital frontal cortex (VTA-NA-OFC) circuit.[47,48] This circuit influences behavior by modulating animal and human motivation (e.g., urges, cravings). Dopamine may also play a major role in the regulation of this region's functioning.[49] One hypothesis is that differences in these regions may result in craving behavior seen in kleptomania and other impulse control disorders. The efficacy of naltrexone (see below) lends further support to this hypothesis. Naltrexone is a medication that is used to treat opiate and alcohol addiction and is thought to modulate dopamine neurons in this area.[50]

Because serotonergic systems have been implicated in impaired impulse regulation, serotonin dysregulation may also be a clue to the pathophysiology of kleptomania (as well as other impulse control disorders). Given the evidence of serotonin dysregulation in trichotillomania, pathological gambling, and other obsessive-compulsive spectrum disorders, pharmacologic intervention for kleptomania has focused on the use of selective serotonin reuptake inhibitors (SSRIs).[51] The use of SSRIs is based on the hypothesis that the etiology of these disorders stems from low levels of serotonin in brain synapses.[41] On the other hand, there are reported cases of kleptomania emerging during treatment of depression with SSRIs. Three cases involve a 54-year-old female, 45-year-old male, and 65-year-old male with new onset of kleptomania-like symptoms during treatment of depression with SSRIs such as fluvoxamine and fluoxetine. It is not entirely clear what the causative agent in each case was or if these patients represent a particular subgroup.[52]

WHAT CAN BE DONE ABOUT KLEPTOMANIA? A MULTIDISCIPLINARY APPROACH TO TREATMENT

At this time, the available treatments for kleptomania offered by mental health professionals include various forms of psychotherapy and pharmacotherapy, but studies exploring the efficacy of these treatments are extremely limited. The majority of findings are based on case reports, small case series, and small numbers of individuals with kleptomania who have been willing to participate in research studies. Treatments are typically selected on a case-by-case basis and involve patient preference and appropriateness to the respective modality. Typically a patient will either take medications alone or take medications in conjunction with therapy. One study found that 68 percent sought medication treatment, but 0 percent told their physician about kleptomania symptoms. Instead, these patients presented with symptoms of anxiety and depression. Furthermore, no treating physician screened for kleptomania symptoms.[15]

As discussed in an earlier section, psychoanalytic and psychodynamic theories were used to try to understand kleptomania, and thus psychoanalytic and psychodynamic psychotherapy were the treatment of choice for many decades.[41] The efficacy of this treatment modality, however, is unknown due to lack of controlled studies. Case reports reveal that some patients responded well to this type of therapy, sometimes in conjunction with medications, while others showed no improvement despite years of therapy.[41] No improvements in kleptomania symptoms were reported in a group of 11 patients (out of 20) undergoing psychodynamic psychotherapy.[4]

With regards to therapy, cognitive-behavioral therapy (CBT) has largely replaced psychoanalytic and psychodynamic psychotherapies in the treatment of kleptomania. Several strategies used in kleptomania include the following: covert sensitization (i.e., the patient is instructed to imagine herself stealing and then to imagine a negative outcome such as being caught or feeling nauseous or short of breath), aversion therapy (i.e., aversive breath holding until mildly painful whenever an urge to steal or an image of it is experienced), and systematic desensitization (i.e., helping the patient achieve a relaxed state through progressive muscle relaxation and asking the patient to imagine the different steps of the stealing episode, meanwhile suggesting that he or she could better control the urge to steal by controlling the anxiety).[51] CBT suffers from a lack of controlled studies, but case reports reveal that some patients respond well to this, especially in conjunction with medication. One case described a 77-year-old female with onset of kleptomania at age 73 who responded well to covert sensitization, in conjunction with medication and a self-imposed ban on shopping.[18] Another case described a 43-year-old male with new onset kleptomania and personality changes after head trauma and loss of consciousness during an automobile accident. He achieved full remission with citalopram 40mg/d and CBT.[46] One case study reported a 39-year-old male with kleptomania who responded well to CBT (including covert sensitization).[53]

Typically medications are used in conjunction with therapy (CBT or psychodynamic/psychoanalytic psychotherapy). Currently there are no medications approved by the Food and Drug Administration to treat kleptomania. As with the therapies, current knowledge about the pharmacotherapy of kleptomania is based on case reports, case series, and an open-label studies and is also guided by etiological and neurobiological hypotheses.

Selective serotonin reuptake inhibitors (SSRIs) are medications commonly used to treat depression and a variety of anxiety disorders including obsessive-compulsive disorder and panic disorder. One case series reported that 2 patients achieved remission of kleptomania with fluoxetine while 7 did not.[4] A combination of fluoxetine 40mg/d and lithium 600mg/d resulted in minimal or no chronic urges to steal in a 40-year-old female.[54] A case series of 5 patients reported success with fluoxetine up to 40mg/d (4 patients) and paroxetine up to 20mg/d (1 patient).[55] An 11-year-old girl with kleptomania and attention deficit hyperactivity disorder achieved symptom remission with sertraline and methylphenidate (stimulant).[56] A 38-year-old Chinese male with kleptomania and OCD was successfully treated with fluvoxamine 300mg/d.[57] A 29-year-old male with kleptomania achieved almost complete symptom remission with paroxetine 30mg/d.[58] A 48-year-old female with kleptomania and premenstrual dysphoric disorder (PMDD) experienced marked intensification of kleptomania prior to menses. Symptoms from both disorders abated with escitalopram 10mg/d.[59] As discussed in a prior section, the emergence of new onset kleptomania during use of SSRIs for depression was reported in 3 patients.

Other non-SSRI antidepressants that have been used to treat kleptomania include trazodone, imipramine, desipramine, and monoamine oxidase inhibitors (MAO-Is). A 23-year-old female with bulimia nervosa and kleptomania experienced remission of bulimic symptoms with tranylcypromine 60mg/d (an MAO-I) and remission of kleptomania with trazodone 300mg/d, whereas a 19-year-old female with bulimia, depression, and kleptomania experienced no symptom relief with trazodone 400mg/d. Instead, a trial of fluoxetine 80mg/d achieved virtual remission of depression and kleptomania and 80% reduction of bulimia.[4] Imipramine alone (3 cases) and desipramine alone (1 case) were not found effective, but nortriptyline achieved remission in 1 patient. Imipramine in combination with fluoxetine was beneficial for another patient.[41] Overall, findings do not support use of MAO-Is, which were ineffective for 5 patients except for 1 (who was also on trazodone).[4]

Mood stabilizers, including lithium, valproic acid, carbamazepine, topiramate, and lamotrigine, have been used "off label" to treat kleptomania. Lithium with fluoxetine achieved a substantial decrease in stealing urges in a 40-year-old female.[54] Of 4 trials where lithium was administered alone, only 1 patient experienced good remission.[41] A 37-year-old female with bipolar disorder and kleptomania achieved full remission of kleptomania and manageable mood swings with valproic acid 2,000 mg/d.[60] Carbamazepine with clomipramine failed to improve kleptomania symptoms.[41] Topiramate has been used successfully either alone or in conjunction with an SSRI.[61]

Naltrexone is classified as an opioid receptor antagonist and is used to curb urges in opiate and alcohol addiction. In addition, naltrexone has shown some promise in the treatment for kleptomania, based on case reports and an open-label study. In an outcome study of 17 patients with kleptomania treated with naltrexone for up to three years, 76.5 percent reported reduction in urges to steal, 41.1 percent reported no stealing behavior, and 52.9 percent were rated "not ill at all" or having "very mild" kleptomania symptoms.[62] Another study conducted by Grant involving 10 kleptomaniacs on naltrexone showed that 20 percent reported complete remission, while 80 percent reported significant reduction in urges.[50] Three additional case reports revealed complete remission of kleptomania on naltrexone 50–150 mg/d.[63–65]

Other medications that have been used include benzodiazepines (sedatives), including clonazepam and alprazolam (in conjunction with other treatment modalities), which are especially effective in tension relief.[41] There are some reports of electroconvulsive therapy (ECT) being used to treat kleptomania, but typically in the presence of depressive symptoms as well. Three case reports revealed ECT being effective for depressive and possibly for kleptomania symptoms.[4] ECT should probably be used only for patients who suffer from co-occurring depression.[41]

Despite the increasing use of medications to treat kleptomania, perhaps a self-imposed ban on shopping by the patient is still the most common method of treatment. This way people suffering from kleptomania can impose such treatment without having to seek help.[6] But with increasing understanding awareness, and education about this illness, perhaps fewer people will have to suffer in shame and secrecy, as we are finding that kleptomania is a potentially treatable illness.

REFERENCES

1. Murphy, D.J. (1986). *Customers and thieves: An ethnography of shoplifting.* Brookfield, VT: Gower Press.
2. Segrave, K. (2001). *Shoplifting: A social history.* Jefferson, NC: McFarland & Company.
3. Abelson, E.S. (1989). *When ladies go a-thieving: Middle-class shoplifters in the Victorian department store.* New York: Oxford University Press.
4. McElroy, S.L., Pope, H.G., & Hudson, J.I. (1991). Kleptomania: A report of 20 cases. *American Journal of Psychiatry, 148,* 652–657.
5. American Psychiatric Association. (2000). *Diagnostic and statistical manual of mental disorders* (4th ed., text revision). Washington, DC: Author.
6. Goldman, M. (1991). Kleptomania: Making sense of the nonsensical. *American Journal of Psychiatry, 148,* 986–996.
7. Grant, J.E., & Kim, S.W. (2002). Temperament and early environmental influences in kleptomania. *Comprehensive Psychiatry, 43,* 223–228.
8. Lejoyeux, M., Arbaretaz, M., McLoughlin, M., & Ades, L. (2002). Impulse control disorders and depression. *Journal of Nervous and Mental Disorders, 190,* 310–314.
9. Lejoyeux, M., Feuche, N., Loi, S., Solomon, J., & Ades, L. (1999). Study of impulse-control disorders among alcohol-dependent patients. *Journal of Clinical Psychiatry, 60,* 302–305.
10. Grant, J.E., & Kim, S.W. (2003). Comorbidity of impulse control disorders in pathological gamblers. *Acta Psychiatric Scandanavia, 108,* 207–213.
11. Specker, S.M., Carlson, G.A., Christenson, G.A., & Marcotte, M. (1995). Impulse control disorders and attention deficit disorder in pathological gamblers. *Annuals of Clinical Psychiatry, 7,* 175–179.

12. Hudson, J.I., & Pope, H.G. (1990). Affective spectrum disorder: Does antidepressant response identify a family of disorders with a common pathophysiology? *American Journal of Psychiatry, 147,* 552–564.

13. Grant, J.E., Potenza, M.N., Levine, L., & Kim, D. (in press). Prevalence of impulse control disorders in adult psychiatric inpatients. *American Journal of Psychiatry.*

14. Sarasalo, E., Bergman, B., & Toth, J. (1996). Personality traits and psychiatric and somatic morbidity among kleptomaniacs. *Acta Psychiatric Scandanavia, 94,* 358–364.

15. Grant, J.E., & Kim, S.W. (2002). Clinical characteristics and associated psychopathology of 22 patients with kleptomania. *Comprehensive Psychiatry, 43,* 378–384.

16. Presta, S., Marazziti, D., Dell'Osso, L., Pfanner, C., Pallanti, S., & Cassano, G.B. (2002). Kleptomania: Clinical features and comorbidity in an Italian sample. *Comprehensive Psychiatry, 43,* 7–12.

17. Phelan, J. (2002). Childhood kleptomania: Two clinical case studies with implications for further research. *Psychology and Education—An Interdisciplinary Journal, 39,* 19–21.

18. McNeilly, D., & Burke, W. (1998). Stealing lately: A case of late-onset kleptomania. *International Journal of Geriatric Psychiatry, 13,* 116–121.

19. Dannon, P., Lowengrub, K., Iancu, I., & Kotler, M. (2004). Kleptomania: Comorbid psychiatric diagnosis in patients and their families. *Psychopathology, 37,* 76–80.

20. Wiedemann, G. (1998). Kleptomania: Characteristics of 12 cases. *European Psychiatry, 13,* 67–77.

21. Bayle, F., Caci, H., Millet, B., Richa, S., & Olié, J.P. (2003). Psychopathology and comorbidity of psychiatric disorders in patients with kleptomania. *American Journal of Psychiatry, 160,* 1509–1513.

22. Bradford, J., & Balmaceda, R. (1983). Shoplifting: Is there a specific psychiatric syndrome? *Canadian Journal of Psychiatry, 28,* 248–253.

23. Astor, S.D. (1969). Shoplifting: Far greater than we know? *Security World, 6,* 12–13.

24. Retrieved April 20, 2006 from http://shopliftingprevention.org/main.asp

25. Cox, D., Cox, A., & Moschis, G. (1990). When consumer behavior goes bad: An investigation of adolescent shoplifting. *Journal of Consumer Research, 17,* 149–159.

26. Meyers, T.J. (1970). A contribution to the psychopathology of shoplifting. *Journal of Forensic Science, 15,* 295–310.

27. Sarasalo, E., Bergman, B., & Toth, J. (1997). Theft behavior and its consequences among kleptomaniacs and shoplifters: A comparative study. *Forensic Science International, 86,* 193–205.

28. Castiglia, P. (1999). Stealing/Shoplifting. *Journal of Pediatric Health Care, 13,* 248–249.

29. Spock, B., & Parker, S.J. (1998). *Dr. Spock's baby and child care* (7th ed.). New York: Pocket Books.

30. McElroy, S. L., Hudson, J. I., Pope, H. G., Keck, P., & White, K. (1992). The DSM-III-R impulse control disorders not elsewhere classified: Clinical characteristics and relationship to other psychiatric disorders. *American Journal of Psychiatry*, *149*, 318–327.

31. McElroy, S. L., Hudson, J. I., Pope, H. G., Keck, P., & White, K. (1991). Kleptomania: Clinical characteristics and associated psychopathology. *Psychological Medicine*, *21*, 93–108.

32. Grant, J. E. (2003). Family history and psychiatric comorbidity in persons with kleptomania. *Comprehensive Psychiatry*, *44*, 437–441.

33. McElroy, S. L., Phillips, K. A., & Keck, P. E. (1994). Obsessive compulsive spectrum disorder. *Journal of Clinical Psychiatry*, *55*(Suppl. 10), 33–51.

34. Grant, J. E. (2004). Co-occurrence of personality disorders in persons with kleptomania: A preliminary investigation. *Journal of American Academy of Psychiatry Law*, *32*, 395–398.

35. Aboujaoude, E., Gamel, N., & Koran, L. (2004). Overview of kleptomania and phenomenological description of 40 patients: Primary care companion. *Journal of Clinical Psychiatry*, *6*, 244–247.

36. Grant, J. E., Kim, S. W., & Grosz, R. (2003). Perceived stress in kleptomania. *Psychiatric Quarterly*, *74*, 251–258.

37. Grant, J. E., & Kim, S. W. (2005). Quality of life in kleptomania and pathological gambling. *Comprehensive Psychiatry*, *46*, 34–37.

38. Cupchik, W., & Atcheson, J. (1983). Shoplifting: An occasional crime of the moral majority. *Bulletin of the American Academy of Psychiatry Law*, *11*, 343–354.

39. Dannon, P. (2002). Kleptomania: An impulse control disorder? *International Journal of Psychiatric Clinical Practice*, *6*, 3–7.

40. Goldman, M. (1992). Kleptomania: An overview. *Psychiatric Annuals*, *22*, 68–71.

41. Durst, R., Katz, G., Teitelbaum, A., Zislin, J., & Dannon, P. N. (2001). Kleptomania: Diagnosis and treatment options. *CNS Drugs*, *15*, 185–195.

42. Fishbain, D. (1987). Kleptomania as risk-taking behavior in response to depression. *American Journal of Psychotherapy*, *41*, 598–603.

43. Murray, J. (1991) Kleptomania: A review of the research. *The Journal of Psychology*, *126*, 131–138.

44. Marazziti, D., Mungai, F., Giannotti, D., Pfanner, C., & Presta, S. (2003). Kleptomania in impulse control disorders, obsessive-compulsive disorder, and bipolar spectrum disorder: Clinical and therapeutic implications. *Current Psychiatry Reports*, *5*, 36–40.

45. Nyffeler, T., & Regard, M. (2001). Kleptomania in a patient with a right fronto-limbic lesion. *Neuropsychiatric Neuropsychological Behavioral Neurology*, *14*, 73–76.

46. Aizer, A., Lowengrub, K., & Dannon, P. (2004). Kleptomania after head trauma: Two case reports and combination treatment strategies. *Clinical Neuropharmacology*, *27*, 211–215.

47. Mogenson, G.J., Jones, D.J., Yim, C.Y. (1980). From motivation to action: Functional interface between the limbic system and motor system. *Progress in Neurobiology, 14*, 69–97.

48. Koob, G.F., & Bloom, F.E. (1988). Cellular and molecular mechanisms of drug dependence. *Science, 242*, 715–723.

49. Kuhar, M.J., Ritz, M.C., & Boja, J.W. (1991). The dopamine hypothesis of the reinforcing properties of cocaine. *Trends in Neuroscience, 14*, 299–302.

50. Grant, J.E., & Kim, S.W. (2002). An open-label study of naltrexone in the treatment of kleptomania. *Journal of Clinical Psychiatry, 63*, 349–355.

51. Grant, J.E., & Potenza, M.N. (2004). Impulse control disorders: Clinical characteristics and pharmacological management. *Annuals of Clinical Psychiatry, 16*, 27–34.

52. Kindler, S., Dannon, P., Iancu, I., Sasson, Y., & Zohar, J. (1997). Emergence of kleptomania during treatment for depression with serotonin selective reuptake inhibitors. *Clinical Neuropharmacology, 20*, 126–129.

53. Kohn, C., & Antonuccio, D. (2002). Treatment of kleptomania using cognitive and behavioral strategies. *Clinical Case Studies, 1*, 25–38.

54. Burstein, A. (1992). Fluoxetine-lithium treatment for kleptomania. *Journal of Clinical Psychiatry, 53*(1), 28–29.

55. Lepkifker, E., Dannon, P., Ziv, R., Iancu, I., Horesh, N., & Kotler, M. (1999). The treatment of kleptomania with serotonin reuptake inhibitors. *Clinical Neuropharmacology, 22*, 40–43.

56. Feeney, D., & Klykylo, W. (1997). Treatment for kleptomania. *Journal of the American Academy of Child and Adolescent Psychiatry, 36*, 723–724.

57. Chong, S., & Low, B. (1996). Treatment of kleptomania with fluvoxamine. *Acta Psychiatric Scandanavia, 93*, 314–315.

58. Kraus, J. (1999). Treatment of kleptomania with paroxetine. *Journal of Clinical Psychiatry, 60*, 793.

59. Aboujaoude, E., Gamel, N., & Koran, L. (2004). A case of kleptomania correlating with premenstrual dysphoria. *Journal of Clinical Psychiatry, 65*, 725–726.

60. Kmetz, G., McElroy, S., & Collins, D. (1997). Response of kleptomania and mixed mania to valproate. *American Journal of Psychiatry, 154*, 580–581.

61. Dannon, P. (2003). Topiramate for the treatment of kleptomania: A case series and review of the literature. *Clinical Neuropharmacology, 26*, 1–4.

62. Grant, J.E. (2005). Outcome study of kleptomania patients treated with naltrexone: A chart review. *Clinical Neuropharmacology, 28*, 11–14.

63. Kim, S.W. (1998). Opioid antagonists in the treatment of impulse-control disorders. *Journal of Clinical Psychiatry, 59*, 159–162.

64. Dannon, P., Iancu, I., & Grunhaus, L. (1999). Naltrexone treatment in kleptomanic patients. *Human Psychopharmacology Clinical and Experimental, 14*, 583–585.

65. Grant, J.E., & Kim, S.W. (2001). A case of kleptomania and compulsive sexual behavior treated with naltrexone. *Annuals of Clinical Psychiatry, 13*, 229–231.

Chapter 6

Mood Disorders in Children and Adolescents

Jarrod M. Leffler and Mary A. Fristad

Mood disorders occur in approximately 5 percent of children and adolescents at any point in time. Awareness of mood disorders among the general public is increasing, as evidenced by an explosion of magazine and newspaper stories, television features, popular press books, and Web sites coving the topic as well as television and print article advertisements for pharmacologic interventions. However, there are many controversies in the field, over both how to diagnose depression and bipolar disorder in youth and how to treat these conditions once they are recognized. In this chapter, we briefly reflect on contemporary portrayals of mood disorders in the media, then we present clinical vignettes representative of mood disorders in children and adolescents. Next, we outline a history of diagnosing and treating depressive and bipolar disorders in youth, ending with an overview of current diagnostic controversies. Then we review how to assess depression and mania in youth, providing developmentally appropriate examples of how symptoms appear in youth and discussing possible differential diagnoses. We summarize what is known about biological treatments (e.g., pharmacotherapy, light therapy, and electroconvulsive therapy) and psychotherapy treatments for depressive and bipolar disorders in youth, and we discuss current treatment issues in the news (e.g., antidepressants linked to increased suicidality in youth). Finally, we conclude with a summary of resources families can use to educate themselves about mood disorders.

IN THE MEDIA

You are likely, at some point in your life, to meet or know someone with depression or bipolar disorder. Additionally, you are increasingly likely to hear mood disorders described as relatively common conditions afflicting celebrities and other public figures. The *New York Times* recently published an article titled "Hypomanic? Absolutely. But Oh So Productive!"[1] This article not only brought bipolar disorder to the nation's attention by being published in one of the largest print media sources in the world, but it joined numerous other professional, scientific, and lay publications in the discussion of bipolar disorder (see Resources).[2,3] There have also been books written for children in an attempt to help them better understand the illness (see Resources).

A recent Google Internet search identified 517,000 sites for "childhood mood disorders" and 577,000 for "adolescent mood disorders." Numbers for more specific searches were similarly high. The search phrase "childhood depression" resulted in 3,100,000 identified sites, while "childhood bipolar disorder" and "childhood mania" resulted in 483,000 and 248,000 sites, respectively. Similarly, when searching for "adolescent depression," 3,630,000 sites were found, while the terms "adolescent bipolar disorder" and "adolescent mania" resulted in 757,000 and 645,000 sites, respectively. The public's attention also has been raised regarding mental illness via new government-sponsored implementation of national screening days for depression and anxiety.

Although mood disorders can be quite debilitating, some individuals who have suffered from them have been highly successful in their professional lives. A partial list of famous persons who have battled mood disorders includes John Quincy Adams (former U.S. president); Buzz Aldrin (astronaut); Ludwig van Beethoven (composer); Ray Charles (musician); Winston Churchill (former British prime minister); Kurt Cobain (musician); Rodney Dangerfield (comedian); F. Scott Fitzgerald (writer); Ernest Hemingway (writer); Audrey Hepburn (actress); Abraham Lincoln (former U.S. president): Georgia O'Keeffe (painter); Sylvia Plath (poet); and Boris Yeltsin (former Russian president). Given the frequency with which adults with mood disorders report their onset in childhood and adolescence,[4] it is important to understand the history of recognizing mood disorders in youth.

CLINICAL VIGNETTES*

Samuel

Upon meeting with Samuel, a 10-year-old male, he reported becoming easily irritated and annoyed by his friends and family members, and he has had homicidal thoughts about these individuals. When irritated, Samuel often slammed doors,

---

* In the vignettes, all names have been changed and identifying information concealed to protect the privacy of the individuals.

destroyed property, and yelled excessively. Samuel also reported that he experienced suicidal ideation, and he had a significant history of engaging in self-harming behaviors by cutting himself with a knife. Samuel reported ongoing negative views about his social and physical abilities, significant discomfort from daily stomachaches, and frequent periods of tearfulness. Samuel's mother, Mrs. Jones, reported that Samuel displayed a loss of energy and appeared unmotivated. Additionally, Samuel experienced difficulty falling asleep for two to three hours almost every night and experienced waking up in the middle of the night once or twice a week. Given the number, duration, frequency, and severity of his symptoms, Samuel was diagnosed with and treated for major depressive disorder (MDD).

Amy

Amy, a 15-year-old female, abruptly began to display significant hypersexual behaviors. For example, she frequently attempted to kiss her mother with an open mouth while sticking out her tongue; opened her mother's blouse, exposing her chest; touched the genital areas of male and female peers at school; and against her parents' wishes wore provocative and revealing clothing that was often too small for her. Around the same time, Amy began to laugh without provocation, and when she tried to talk, her speech was sometimes so rapid that she stuttered. Additionally, her laughter and giggling interfered with what she was saying. When she did speak, others had difficulty following her line of thought. Amy began to sleep two to four hours a night, waking with a high level of energy. She described her mood as "very excited all the time." After a week of this unusual behavior, Amy became very sad and tearful, and she yelled at her family to "Just leave me alone." She began to sleep 12–14 hours a day and still would fall asleep in class. Her grades began to suffer and she complained school was boring. Upon repeated questioning, both she and her mother denied she had ever been sexually abused or exposed to inappropriate sexual content (e.g., X-rated movies, pornography). Because of the frequency, intensity, number, and duration of her symptoms, Amy was diagnosed with and treated for bipolar I disorder.

HISTORY OF DIAGNOSING MOOD DISORDERS

Depression

We have learned much about youth mood disorders in the past two decades. Prior to the 1980s, many mental health professionals believed that children, due to their underdeveloped psyches, were unable to experience affective disturbances. According to psychodynamic theory, the immature superego and lack of stable self-concept in childhood prevented depression from occurring in this age group.[5]

Others postulated that depression could not exist in children because the behaviors described as features of the illness are transiently prevalent in all children and can therefore not be described as deviant.[6] However, further work has validated the presence of depression in children.[7] Epidemiological studies suggest the prevalence rate of child and adolescent depressive disorders ranges from 1.6 to 8.9 percent.[8] Rates of depression for preschoolers have been reported to range between 1 and 4 percent.[9] In youth aged 9 to 17 rates of 5 percent have been reported.[8] Prevalence rates in the general population of clinically significant depression have been found between 0.4 and 2.5 percent and 0.4 and 8.3 percent for children and adolescents, respectively, with lifetime rates of depression in school-age children at about 3 percent.[8] Lifetime prevalence rates of major depression in adolescents are reported to be between 9 and 14 percent.[10] Prevalence rates of dysthymic disorder range from 0.6 to 1.7 percent for children and 1.6 to 8.0 percent for adolescents.[10]

Bipolar Disorder

In the 1920s, Emil Kraepelin discussed the clinical presentation of manic depression, an illness that presented with the switching between elevated and depressed emotions, cognitions, and behaviors. These symptoms consisted of flight of ideas, elevated and expansive mood, pressured speech, depressed mood, and cognitive stupor.[11] Others more specifically reported cases of manic depression in children and adolescents.[12,13] Within the past decade, bipolar disorder in youth has received increased public and professional interest.[14,15] Research has found lifetime prevalence rates for bipolar disorder to be about 1 percent with an additional 5.7 percent reporting subthreshold symptoms quite possibly related to bipolar II disorder or cyclothymia.[16] Sixty percent of adults diagnosed with bipolar disorder retrospectively reported onset of the illness in childhood or adolescence.[4] A perceived increase in childhood bipolar disorder can be related to the increased knowledge professionals and the public have about the disorder. Additionally, increased media coverage in the past decade has added to the public's awareness and outcry regarding the illness. Other possible reasons childhood bipolar disorder is diagnosed more frequently include (1) an increasing number of children at a younger age being prescribed psychotropic medications that may exacerbate manic symptoms and episodes and (2) the successful treatment of many adults who then go on to have families of their own and ultimately have children with similar mood disorders. These topics are discussed in more detail later in the chapter.

CURRENT DIAGNOSTIC CONVENTIONS

Youth depressive and bipolar disorders can have a chronic and morbid course with significant costs to individuals, families, peers, and society due to suicidality, dropping out of school, health care costs (i.e., medical and psychiatric), teen/early pregnancies, substance use, and legal issues.[16] Diagnosis for these illnesses is based on the criteria set forth by the American Psychiatric Association (APA) and described in the fourth edition, text revision, of the *Diagnostic and Statistical Manual of Mental Disorders (DSM–IV–TR)*.[17]

Depression

A mental or medical health care provider (i.e., a medical doctor, psychologist, social worker, or counselor) who applies the guidelines set forth in the *DSM–IV–TR* can make the diagnosis of major depressive disorder (MDD), dysthymia, or depressive disorder-not otherwise specified (NOS). Criteria to diagnose depressive disorders in youth are the same as for adults and include the presence of depressed mood or irritable mood and/or loss of pleasure for at least two weeks, a decline from previous functioning, significant distress or impairment in areas of functioning, and four additional symptoms from the following list: significantly increased or decreased appetite; sleeping too much or too little; too much or too little energy; fatigue; feelings of worthlessness and guilt; decreased ability to concentrate; and morbid or suicidal ideation or attempt.[17] Dysthymic disorder is more chronic and persistent than MDD. Dysthymia requires depressed or irritable mood for one year (two years in adults), with at least two symptoms similar to those of MDD. Additionally, medical illnesses should be ruled out as a reason for symptoms being present (e.g., thyroid difficulties can cause changes in energy levels, eating, and sleeping patterns). Depressive disorder-NOS is diagnosed when an individual experiences symptoms of MDD or dysthymia but the severity, intensity, and number or frequency of symptoms fall short of meeting the diagnostic criteria of MDD or dysthymia.[17]

During childhood, boys and girls experience similar rates of depression. However, gender differences emerge by ages 12 to 13.[18] The onset of MDD is more likely to occur between the ages of 11 and 14, with dysthymia occurring even earlier.[19] Currently, we know little about ethnic and cultural differences in rates of youth depression. Youth of parents with mood disorders have a higher chance of developing mood disorders than youth of non-mood-impaired parents.[20]

Bipolar Disorder

There are various types of bipolar disorders based on the types and severity of moods experienced. Their cardinal feature is mania. In bipolar I disorder, mania presents as a distinct period of excessively elevated, expansive, or irritable mood persisting for at least one week. In bipolar II disorder, the level of elevated mood is less, or hypomanic, and usually only lasts four days. In bipolar I and bipolar II, three or more of the following symptoms accompany the elevated mood (four symptoms if the mood change is irritability): increased self-esteem; decreased need for sleep; increased amount or pace of speech; distractibility; racing thoughts; increased goal-directed behavior; and over-involvement in pleasurable activities.[17] Mania may alternate or co-occur with depression. In cyclothymia, multiple periods of hypomania and mini-depressions occur without a break for more than two months at any one time. Bipolar disorder-not otherwise specified (BP-NOS) refers to manic and depressive symptoms that do not meet criteria for any other bipolar disorder. For example, youth whose symptoms are intense but brief (lasting two to three days at a time two to three times a month) or whose symptoms are low in number would receive the diagnosis of BP-NOS. Another diagnosis to consider is mood disorder due to a general medical condition. This diagnosis requires that a significantly prominent mood disturbance, either depressed or elevated, is present as the result of a medical condition (e.g., hypothyroid condition, brain tumor, seizure disorder).

Bipolar disorder that starts in childhood differs in several ways from bipolar disorder in adults. Adults often experience longer mood cycles than youth.[21] Additionally, youth are more likely to experience rapid cycling or mixed episodes (manic and depressive symptoms occurring at the same time).[22]

Family history is associated with increased risk for bipolar disorder.[23] The rates of mood disorders in youth of parents with bipolar disorder range from 5 percent to 67 percent whereas 0 percent to 38 percent of youth born of parents without bipolar disorder developed mood disorders.[23] Rates of other psychological disorders range from 5 percent to 52 percent for youth with parents diagnosed with bipolar disorder and from 0 percent to 25 percent for youth of parents without bipolar disorder.[23]

Many adolescents with major depression (6% to 49%) develop manic symptoms.[24] Risk factors for "switching" from depression to mania include hypersomnolence, psychotic symptoms, early age of onset, and family history of bipolar disorder.[25] Youth with bipolar disorder are at high risk for suicidality.[16]

DIAGNOSTIC ISSUES

In the process of determining whether a mood disorder exists, two key concerns must be addressed. They are differential diagnosis, meaning there are other possible disorders that may better account for the youth's disturbance, and comorbidity, meaning that more than one disorder is present at the same time. Both are reviewed below.

Differential Diagnosis

Accurate diagnosis, which directs appropriate psychopharmacology, psychotherapy, and other necessary services, is difficult, and if not done correctly it can lead to negative outcomes. For instance, if a youth has mania but is misdiagnosed with attention deficit hyperactivity disorder (ADHD) and prescribed a stimulant, this medication could trigger a manic or psychotic episode. Additionally, if the youth was medicated for a depressive episode but actually had bipolar disorder, the antidepressant could trigger a manic episode.

Disorders that are sometimes confused with mood disorders include ADHD, anxiety, schizophrenia, oppositional defiant disorder, conduct disorder, post-traumatic stress disorder, and others to be discussed in this section. Although many childhood psychiatric disorders share similar symptoms and symptoms of mania and depression are present in other psychiatric disorders, the collection of symptoms and their frequency, intensity, number, and duration as well as the level of impairment and disruption they cause the individual and those around him or her assist in identifying the most accurate explanation of distress.

Depression

Conditions that may mimic depression include bereavement, adjustment disorder with depressed mood, anorexia nervosa, ADHD, anxiety disorders, somatization disorder, and possibly schizophrenia, if psychotic symptoms are present. Bereavement is in response to the death of a loved one (e.g., a family member, friend, or pet). Usually the individual's sad mood does not last beyond two months, and if it does, a diagnosis of MDD might be considered. Additionally, bereavement does not include symptoms such as excessive guilt about the event, suicidal ideation, excessive feelings of worthlessness, chronic and significant deficits in functioning, or hallucinations.[17] Adjustment disorders are the result of a stressor; they begin within three months of the event, dissipate within six months, and do not meet diagnostic criteria for MDD.

Anorexia nervosa shares with MDD the symptoms of weight loss, worthlessness, guilt, and decreased self-esteem. However, weight loss in anorexia is driven by a fear of being fat, whereas weight loss in MDD is due to a loss of appetite. Weight loss, guilt, and decreased self-esteem in anorexia are related to body image distortions, whereas in depression these symptoms tend to be more global. Because lack of nutrition can produce symptoms of fatigue and cognitive slowing in anorexia, weight stabilization is necessary before clearly determining what other symptoms are present. Additionally, a youth who continues to lose weight while on a calorie-enhanced program and being monitored by a physician or dietician is more likely experiencing an eating disorder or other medical condition rather than MDD.

Attention problems and restlessness are hallmark features of ADHD. For these disturbances to "count" as symptoms of depression, they need to change markedly from their baseline for the youth. While anxiety and mood disorders share several symptoms (e.g., restlessness, irritability, difficulty concentrating, sleep disturbance, fatigue), MDD requires loss of pleasure or dysphoric mood as a cardinal symptom. Somatization disorder requires physical pain, which is not a required symptom of MDD, and the severity of physical complaints exceeds that typically experienced by individuals suffering from MDD. Finally, while psychosis is a central feature of schizophrenia, it can also occur when MDD is severe. In the case of MDD with psychotic features, the psychosis resolves as the mood disorder improves. This is not true in schizophrenia.

Bipolar Disorder

Some possible differential diagnoses for bipolar disorder in youth include conduct disorder, ADHD, schizophrenia, schizoaffective disorder, intermittent explosive disorder, and post-traumatic stress disorder.

Youth with both conduct disorder and mania can appear surly and irritable, and on the surface their diagnoses can be difficult to differentiate. However, the level of irritability that a youth with bipolar disorder displays can become significantly more violent with less provocation. Further, the progression of conduct disorder is more prolonged. One can also differentiate mania form conduct disorder by noting that the former but not the latter includes flight of ideas, rapid speech, sleep disturbance, altered mood states, grandiosity, and may include psychotic features.

Mania and ADHD share similar symptoms including excessive energy, quick speech, irritability, distractibility, and lack of forethought in planning. However, when youth with bipolar disorder display an increase in behavior levels, they demonstrate an increase in goal-directed behavior whereas youth with ADHD do not.[26] Further, although youth with ADHD may become irritable, youth with bipolar disorder display mood cycles that include elation, depression, and irritability. Clinicians can distinguish more readily between ADHD and mania by identifying the duration, frequency, and intensity of elation, grandiosity, racing thoughts, hypersexuality, and decreased need for sleep.[26]

Bipolar disorder in youth may be inappropriately identified as schizophrenia. Therefore, schizophrenia should be considered as a differential diagnosis, especially in late-teens.[27] This may occur because manic symptoms can mimic psychosis due to rapid and tangential speech, flight of ideas, auditory and visual hallucinations, and paranoia.[26] However, individuals with schizophrenia may present as socially withdrawn and display more bizarre behaviors. Further, the course of developing schizophrenia is more disturbed and chronic compared to an acute onset in mania. Also, the presentation of prior depressive episodes may distinguish bipolar disorder from schizophrenia. Schizoaffective disorder and bipolar disorder both require the occurrence of a depressive, manic, or mixed mood episode. However, schizoaffective disorder also requires the presentation of two of the following: hallucinations; delusions; disorganized language and thought process; severely disturbed behavior; and symptoms suggestive of a loss of normal functioning (i.e., decrease in goal-directed behavior, loss of emotional range, and poverty or decline in thought and speech).

While intermittent explosive disorder carries with it severe episodes of aggressive behaviors, it lacks the inclusion of manic and depressive mood states, sleep disturbances, and thought and speech disturbances. Adjustment disorder with mixed disturbance of emotion and conduct requires the identification of a stressor within the past three months that prompted an emotional and behavioral response in excess of what would be expected. Post-traumatic stress disorder involves experiencing, witnessing, or being confronted with a physically or emotionally threatening event that invoked feelings of fear, helplessness, or horror. The individual may then experience a decrease in sleep, hyperarousal, rapid speech, and irritability. However, these symptoms differ from those of bipolar in that there usually is not the presence of elevated and silly mood, increase in goal-directed behavior, and grandiosity. Additionally, experiencing a life-threatening event is not usually a precipitant to bipolar disorder.

Medical illness should also be considered in the different diagnosis. Medical problems that may mimic or cause symptoms of mania include encephalitis, multiple sclerosis, Wilson's disease, acquired immune deficiency states, hyperthyroidism, seizures, complications in autoimmune disorders, right-sided cerebrovascular accident, closed and open head injuries, and brain tumors.[28] Medications such as corticosteroids, which are used to reduce various types of inflammation related to illnesses (e.g., asthma, inflammatory bowel disease), aminophyline, pseudoephedrine, and antibiotics such as clarithromycin, erythromycin, and amoxicillin may incite episodes of mania.[28] As previously mentioned, stimulant and antidepressant medications may elicit symptoms of mania. Additionally, illicit substances such as marijuana, cocaine, and Ecstasy can contribute to elevated moods.

Comorbidity

Depression

Comorbidity is common in youth with MDD.[10] The most likely disorder to co-occur with MDD is anxiety. Between 18 and 75 percent of youth with depressive disorders also have one or more anxiety disorders.[29,30] Other comorbid disorders include conduct disorder, 33 percent; oppositional defiant disorder, 13 percent in children and 7 percent in adolescents, but rates as high as 50 percent have been found as well; ADHD, 15 percent in children and 6 percent in adolescents; substance use disorders, 1 percent in children and 11 percent in adolescents; and eating disorders.[10,29,30]

Bipolar Disorder

Similarly, comorbidity is high in youth with bipolar disorder, with a majority of youth with bipolar I and II disorders meeting diagnostic criteria for at least one other psychiatric disorder.[31] Some of the more common disorders include oppositional defiant disorder, 47 to 79 percent; conduct disorder, 12 to 17 percent; ADHD, 63 to 87 percent; anxiety disorders, 14 to 23 percent; and substance abuse in adolescents, 18 percent.[22,31]

TREATMENT

This section reviews various types of biological and psychotherapeutic interventions used to treat mood disorders. Some are less conventional but have been found to be effective (e.g., light therapy and electroconvulsive treatment), whereas others are more traditional and familiar to professionals and lay persons (e.g., medications and talk therapy).

Biological Treatments

Biological treatments include different types of interventions (e.g., oral or external) that in some way, once delivered to the individual, alter physiological events in the body. These events include increasing or decreasing chemicals in the brain by sending signals to certain parts of the brain or by delivering specific chemicals to targeted locations in the brain.

Pharmacotherapy

Pharmacotherapy (i.e., medication) is a common treatment component for mood disorders. While we know a considerable amount about pharmacotherapy in adults with mood disorders, our knowledge of youth psychopharmacology is, unfortunately, scanty. Psychotropic medications have been found to help reduce mood symptoms in adults. More specifically, antidepressants such as Prozac, Celexa, Zoloft, and Paxil have been found to improve depressive mood states, while mood stabilizers such as lithium, Lamictal, and Depakote[32] and atypical antipsychotics such as Zyprexa, Seroquel, Risperdal, Geodon, and Abilify[33] have successfully managed elevated mood and disruptive behaviors related to bipolar disorder. This success has prompted controlled medication trials with youth, and some studies have found similar success. For example, some antidepressant medications have been found to effectively treat depressive symptoms in youth, and some mood stabilizers have been found to successfully treat manic episodes. Other studies have found that antidepressants for youth are no more effective than placebo treatments.[34] While there are no controlled studies in youth evaluating the effectiveness of atypical antipsychotic medications, case studies have demonstrated their positive impact on managing manic episodes and related symptoms.[28] In summary, many more studies are needed to thoroughly understand the potential risks and benefits of medications for mood disorders in children and adolescents.

Trends in prescribing psychotropic medications to youth have fluctuated. More specifically, rates of prescriptions for these classes of medications in youth have increased dramatically in the past decade.[35] Between 1994 and 2003, prescriptions for selective serotonin reuptake inhibitors (SSRIs), a type of antidepressant, more than tripled from 4.6 per 1,000 to 14.5 per 1,000 children ages 5 to 17 years old, whereas prescriptions for tricyclic antidepressants decreased from 6.5 per 1,000 to 1.3 per 1,000.[35] During this time period there was no change in the prescription of lithium. However, anticonvulsants had a twofold increase from 3.5 per 1,000 to 6.9 per 1,000 children. More specifically, the increase in anticonvulsants was noted among individuals diagnosed with bipolar disorder.[35]

The increasing amount of psychotropic medication prescription and use in youth has alarmed and gained the attention of parents, professionals, and youth advocates. One only needs turn on the television or open newspapers and magazines to find this out. For example, the *Today Show* covered this topic on June 22, 2005. *Time, Newsweek,* and the *New York Times* have also recently addressed this topic.[14,36,37] These concerns relate to the positive and negative acute- and long-term effects these medications have on youth. Although many medications improve mood symptoms, many carry with them significant potential risks.

Side effects, or unwanted reactions to medications, do occur. There are documented cases in which youth have been prescribed an SSRI for depression and then displayed manic symptoms (e.g., excessively elevated mood and irritability).[28] Predictors that best identified if a youth would experience disinhibition related to medications included younger age (less than eight); if disinhibited behaviors were present before the administration of the medication trial; and if the youth experienced clinically diagnosed ADHD.[38] However, others suggest that there is no evidence that antidepressants promote manic symptoms in youth. Results are mixed on the possibility of stimulant medications inducing manic episodes. Some studies have found no effects of stimulant use exacerbating manic symptoms, whereas other outcomes suggest an association between the administration of stimulant medication and the onset of manic symptoms.[39] Overall, the most significant current concern regarding the safety of youth being treated with psychotropic medications is the potential of suicidal ideation and attempts related to antidepressant medications in the treatment of mood disorders. Controlled studies have found mixed results regarding the increase of such thoughts and actions in youth being treated with these medications.[40]

Recently the pharmaceutical companies who develop and sell these medications have been scrutinized for lack of consumer protection. More specifically, outcomes have suggested that SSRIs are linked to suicidal ideation and attempts in youth. These results prompted the U.S. Food and Drug Administration (FDA) in June 2003 to alert medical professionals about the possibility of danger these medications pose to their younger clients. Further, the FDA began to propose and initiate more stringent guidelines and consumer information regarding the use of antidepressant medication in the treatment of youth diagnosed with mood disorders. These guidelines, which were voted on by the FDA in September 2004, called for black-box warnings stating the potentially dangerous side effects of taking antidepressant medications. The following month the FDA directed all manufacturers of antidepressant medications to add a black-box warning to these medications. More recently, practice parameters in the United Kingdom suggest that psychotherapy should be the first line of treatment for youth with depression.[41] Thus, as with any potentially potent intervention, benefits must be weighed against risks when deciding whether or not to use medications.

Light Therapy

Light therapy is used to increase the level of neurochemicals produced in the brain by exposing the individual to specially designed artificial light sources. In the 1980s researchers began to consider how the effects of bright light exposure to suppress and release melatonin impacted seasonal changes in mood.[42] The Society for Light Treatment and Biological Rhythms spawned from this research. Light therapy is effective at improving symptoms of seasonal and nonseasonal depression,[43] as well as treating depressed mood in a pediatric population.[44]

Electroconvulsive Therapy

Electroconvulsive therapy (ECT), another type of biological treatment, was first used in the 1940s. Since its introduction, it has been employed to treat various psychiatric illnesses in youth and adults, including severe depression, schizophrenia, and dementia. Historically, ECT has been criticized for its severe side effects (e.g., short-term memory impairment, broken bones due to convulsions). However, with the inception of newer medications (e.g., muscle relaxants and anesthetics) the patient is less likely to harm himself or herself during the procedure, and recent studies have documented less memory impairment than had previously occurred.[45] Despite ECT's effectiveness at treating severe pathology in youth,[46] it continues to be a last resort treatment for chronic and treatment-resistant mood disorders. Newer and potentially more effective treatments with fewer side effects are being developed. These include transcranial magnetic stimulation (TMS) and vagus nerve stimulation (VNS).

Summary

The overarching goal of biological treatments is to treat, rather than ameliorate, psychological distress. This distinction is important to make. For example, in treating acute medical illnesses such as the flu, the illness runs its course but medication helps ease suffering from the symptoms. Chronic illnesses such as diabetes and cancer are managed by adhering to a medication regimen. Biological treatments for mood disorders share similar ties with both acute and chronic illness treatment. More specifically, psychotropic medications do not cure the illness but instead ease and improve some symptoms. Curing the illness, in the medical sense of the phrase, does not occur. Maintenance on a medication regimen may bring the illness into remission, just as judicious insulin management can keep diabetes under control. Thus, while medications may improve mood symptoms, they will not completely ameliorate the illness. Therefore, other methods of treatment must be considered in conjunction with medications.

Psychotherapeutic Treatments

Psychotherapy, or talk therapy, is another form of intervention for youth with mood disorders. As with medications, psychotherapy does not cure a mood disorder but instead provides strategies for the youth to manage his or her symptoms. Overall, psychotherapy has been found to be an effective intervention for ameliorating emotional and behavioral distress in youth.[47]

Depression

Various types of psychotherapy have been studied to determine their effectiveness in improving depressive symptoms in youth. Those with significant research support are discussed below.

Social skills training addresses deficits in interpersonal socialization. Depressed youth have social problem-solving, social information-processing, and conflict-negotiation skills deficits.[48] Social skills training assists depressed youth in improving their problem-solving and interpersonal skills deficits and in maintaining these gains over time.[48,49]

Cognitive behavioral therapy (CBT) attempts to ameliorate depressive symptoms by changing an individual's cognitive distortions and increasing positive mood states and interpersonal interactions. The goal is to teach youth alternative problem-solving skills and hypothesis testing, increasing interpersonal social skills and confronting and challenging negative cognitions. CBT is clinically effective at decreasing levels of depression, negative cognitive distortions, and suicidality.[50] Individual CBT produces larger treatment gains for youth between the ages of 9 and 18 with depression than family therapy, relaxation training, self-modeling, or supportive therapy.[51] These results were consistent across ethnic groups. Individual CBT and CBT with parental involvement appear superior to other forms of treatment for youth with depression.[51]

Interpersonal Family Therapy (IFT) focuses on patterns of family interactions that impact the youth's depression and as deals with the effects of depression on the family system. Pilot studies indicate that IFT is beneficial at decreasing levels of emotional disturbance in youth.[52]

Interpersonal Psychotherapy for Adolescents (IPT-A) takes into account not only the youth's cognitions and behaviors but also interpersonal interactions and the associated patterns of communication.[52] By identifying and altering dysfunctional interactions, an individual should experience more positive interactions and, therefore, lower levels of depressive symptoms.[52] IPT-A has a large psychoeducational element, which focuses on increasing interpersonal skills in the individual. Although developed as an individual therapy, youth treated with IPT-A may also have their caregivers involved in the sessions.

Psychoeducation combines CBT and family therapy components to increase the youth's and caregiver's awareness of mood disorders and symptoms, identify family patterns and interactions that may exacerbate mood symptoms, and develop strategies to better manage mood disorders. Psychoeducation programs have been successful at alleviating emotional distress and improving family interactions.[53,54] Psychoeducation treatment with older youth has increased caregivers' knowledge of mood disorders.[54]

Bipolar Disorder

There is less research on psychotherapy for youth with bipolar disorder. However, it is agreed that pharmacotherapy is standard treatment for bipolar disorder, with psychosocial interventions serving as an important adjunctive treatment.[28] Given the degree of impairment that results from mood disorders, as previously discussed, effective treatments are necessary. The U.S. Surgeon General's *Report on Mental Health* also identified and outlined the need for such interventions.[55] One type of intervention, psychoeducation, has been studied by three groups of researchers and is reviewed below.

Multi Family Psychoeducation Group (MFPG) and *Individual Family Psychoeducation (IFP)* are manual driven treatments for youth with mood disorders and their caregivers.[54] MFPG is provided in a group format (e.g., parent group and child group), allowing for both youth and caregiver to experience similar treatment interventions simultaneously and then collaborate on weekly projects to practice treatment topics outside of group. IFP is provided in an individual therapy format with some sessions dedicated to either the youth or caregiver and some dedicated to working collaboratively with both the youth and caregiver. IFP also employs weekly projects for the youth and caregiver to practice skills outside of treatment. Both MFPG and IFP assist to increase caregivers' knowledge of mood disorders; positive communication with their children; knowledge about medications, mental health services, and educational interventions for their children; and coping and problem-solving skills. Simultaneously, MFPG and IFP assist youth to increase their knowledge of mood disorders; increase their communication skills; and develop coping and problem-solving skills.

Child- and Family-Focused Cognitive Behavioral Therapy (CFF-CBT) implements CBT tenets in an individual and family setting.[56] CFF-CBT uses the acronym RAINBOW to identify treatment topics that focus on symptom education and management as well as coping and problem-solving skills development. Additionally, the rainbow of colors is used to identify mood disturbance severity and baseline functioning.

Family-Focused Treatment for Adolescents (FFT-A) originated from a similar treatment for adults with bipolar disorder.[57] This treatment involves educating the youth and family regarding mood cycling and factors that influence these changes; symptom management; medication education; identifying the strengths of the youth; and addressing ways to increase mood stability in the family environment.

Preliminary results suggest that MFPG, IFP, CFF-CBT, and FFT-A are promising treatments that warrant further research.[54–57] However, given the limited number of these empirically supported outcome studies for the treatment of youth with bipolar disorder, more research development and implementation of treatments for this population is necessary.

Summary

Psychotherapeutic/psychosocial interventions are effective treatments for youth experiencing mild to moderate mood disorders. However, when the level of distress is severe, the combination of psychosocial treatment and medications is often necessary. Combination therapy is more often the choice for youth with bipolar disorder, given that medications and adjunctive psychosocial treatments provide the most effective treatment results.

CONCLUSION

Depression and bipolar disorder presenting prior to adulthood is a real phenomenon that has received growing awareness among parents, professionals, the government, and youth advocates. The stories of youth and their illnesses as well as their treatments have been covered by every large media source and can be readily found with the click of a mouse on any major Internet search engine. Throughout history, mood disorders have impacted countless individuals. Today we know more than ever about how to diagnose and treat mood disorders. However, treatments carry with them risk as well as potential benefit. Hopefully, increased public awareness will accelerate the drive to obtain new, safe, and effective treatments for depression and bipolar disorder in youth.

RESOURCES

Books for Children with Mood Disorders

Brandon and the Bipolar Bear by T. Anglada
The Storm in My Brain by Child and Adolescent Bipolar Foundation (CABF)
Kid Power Tactics for Dealing with Depression by N. and S. Dubuque
Matt, the Moody Hermit Crab by C. McGee
My Bipolar, Roller Coaster, Feelings Book by B. Hebert
Anger Mountain by Bryna Hebert

Books for Adolescents with Mood Disorders

When Nothing Matters Anymore: A Survival Guide for Depressed Teens by B. Cobain
Recovering from Depression: A Workbook for Teens by M.E. Copeland and S. Copans

Conquering the Beast Within: How I Fought Depression & Won ... and How You Can, Too by C. Irwin

Everything You Need to Know about Bipolar Disorder & Manic Depressive Illness by M.A. Sommers

Books for Parents of Children/Adolescents with Mood Disorders

A Parent's Survival Guide to Childhood Depression by S. Dubuque

Raising a Moody Child: How to Cope with Depression and Bipolar Disorder by M.A. Fristad and J. Goldberg Arnold

New Hope for Children and Teens with Bipolar Disorder by B. Birmaher

The Bipolar Child by D. Papolos and J. Papolos

The Ups and Downs of Raising a Bipolar Child by J. Lederman and C. Fink

If Your Child is Bipolar: The Parent-to-Parent Guide to Living with and Loving a Bipolar Child by C. Singer and S. Gurrentz

Organization, Support Groups, and Web Sites

National Alliance for the Mentally Ill (NAMI): www.nami.org

National Mental Health Association (NMHA): www.nmha.org

Depression and Bipolar Support Alliance (DBSA): www.dbsalliance.org

Child & Adolescent Bipolar Foundation (CABF): www.bpkids.org or www.cabf.org

Juvenile Bipolar Research Foundation (JBRF): www.bpchildresearch.org

Parenting Bipolars: A Survival Guide for Parents: www.parentingbipolars.com

Bipolar Children Newsletter: www.bipolarchild.com

REFERENCES

1. Carey, B. (2005, March 22). Hypomanic? Absolutely. But oh so productive! *The New York Times*, p. F1.

2. Gartner, J. (2005). *The hypomanic edge, the link between (a little) craziness and (a lot of) success in America*. New York: Simon & Schuster.

3. Steele, D. (1998). *His bright light: The story of Nick Traina*. New York: Delta.

4. Lish, J.D., Dime-Meehan, S., Whybrow, P.C., Price, R.A., & Hirschfeld, R.M.A. (1994). The National Depressive and Manic-Depressive Association (DMDA) survey of bipolar members. *Journal of Affective Disorders, 31,* 281–294.

5. Rie, H.E. (1966). Depression in childhood: A survey of some pertinent contributors. *Journal of the American Academy of Child Psychiatry, 5,* 653–685.

6. Lefkowitz, M.M., & Burton, N. (1978). Childhood depression: A critique of the concept. *Psychological Bulletin, 85,* 716–726.

7. Fleming, J.E., & Offord, D.R. (1990). Epidemiology of childhood depressive disorders: A critical review. *Journal of American Academy of Child and Adolescent Psychiatry, 29,* 571–580.

8. Angold, A., & Costello, E.J. (2001). The epidemiology of depression in children and adolescents. In I.M. Goodyer (Ed.), *The depressed child and adolescent* (2nd ed., pp. 143–178). New York: Cambridge University Press.

9. Kashani, J.H., Holcomb, W.R., & Orvaschel, H. (1986). Depression and depressive symptoms in preschool children from the general population. *American Journal of Psychiatry, 143,* 1138–1143.

10. Lewinsohn, P.M., Hops, H., Roberts, R.E., Seeley, J.R., & Andrews, J.A. (1993). Adolescent psychopathology: I. prevalence and incidence of depression and other DSM-III-R disorders in high school students. *Journal of Abnormal Psychology, 102,* 133–144.

11. Kraepelin, E. (1921). *Manic depressive insanity and paranoia.* Edinburgh, Scotland: E & S Livingstone.

12. Barrett, A.M. (1931). Manic depressive psychosis in childhood. *International Clinics, 3,* 205–217.

13. Strecker, E.A. (1921). The prognosis in manic-depressive psychosis. *New York Medical Journal, 114,* 209–211.

14. Kalb, C. (2003, September 22). Troubled souls. *Newsweek, 142,* 68–70.

15. Kluger, J., Song, S., & Simon, L. (2002, August 19). Young and bipolar. *Time, 160,* 38–48.

16. Lewinsohn, P.M., Klein, J.R., & Seeley, J.R. (1995). Bipolar disorder in a community sample of older adolescents: Prevalence, phenomenology, comorbidity, and course. *Journal of the American Academy of Child and Adolescent Psychiatry, 34,* 454–463.

17. American Psychiatric Association. (2000). *Diagnostic and statistical manual of mental disorders* (4th ed., text revision). Washington, DC: Author.

18. Cohen, P., Cohen, J., Kasen, S., Velez, C.N., Hartmark, C., Johnson, J., et al. (1993). An epidemiological study of disorders in late childhood and adolescence: I. Age- and gender-specific prevalence. *Journal of Child Psychology and Psychiatry, 34,* 851–867.

19. Kovacs, M., Feinberg, T.L., Crouse-Novak, M.A., Paulauskas, S.L., Pollock, M., & Finkelstein, R. (1984). Depressive disorders in childhood: II. A longitudinal study of the risk for a subsequent major depression. *Archives of General Psychiatry, 41,* 229–237.

20. Radke-Yarrow, M., Nottelmann, E., Martinez, P., Fox, M.B., & Belmont, B. (1992). Young children of affectively ill parents: A longitudinal study of psychosocial development. *Journal of the American Academy of Child and Adolescent Psychiatry, 31,* 68–77.

21. Goodwin, F.K., & Jamison, K.R. (Eds.). (1990). *Manic-depressive illness.* New York: Oxford University Press.

22. Findling, R.L., Gracious, B.L., McNamara, N.K., Youngstrom, E.A., Demeter, C.A., & Branicky, L.A. (2001). Rapid, continuous cycling and psychiatric co-morbidity in pediatric bipolar I disorder. *Bipolar Disorders, 3,* 202–210.

23. DelBello, M.P., & Geller, B. (2001). Review of studies of child and adolescent offspring of bipolar parents. *Bipolar Disorder, 3,* 325–334.

24. Geller, B., Zimerman, B., Williams, M., Bolhofner, K., & Craney, J.L. (2001). Bipolar disorder at prospective follow-up of adults who had prepubertal major depressive disorder. *American Journal of Psychiatry, 158,* 125–127.

25. Akiskal, H.S., Downs, J., Jordan, P., Watson, S., Daugherty, D., & Pruitt, D.B. (1985). Affective disorders in referred children and younger siblings of manic depressives: Mode of onset and prospective course. *Archives of General Psychiatry, 42,* 996–1003.

26. Geller, B., Zimerman, B., Williams, M., DelBello, M.P., Bolhofner, K., Craney, J.L., et al. (2002). DSM-IV mania symptoms in a prepubertal and early adolescent bipolar disorder phenotype compared to attention-deficit hyperactive and normal controls. *Journal of Child and Adolescent Psychopharmacology, 12,* 11–25.

27. Werry, J.S., McClellan, J.M., & Chard, L. (1991). Childhood and adolescent schizophrenic, bipolar, and schizoaffective disorders: A clinical and outcome study. *Journal of the American Academy of Child and Adolescent Psychiatry, 30,* 457–465.

28. Kowatch, R.A., Fristad, M., Birmaher, B., Dineen Wagner, K., Findling, R.L., Hellander, M., et al. (2005). Treatment guidelines for children and adolescents with bipolar disorder: Child psychiatric workgroup on bipolar disorder. *Journal of the American Academy of Child and Adolescent Psychiatry, 44,* 213–235.

29. Yorbik, O., Birmaher, B., Axelson, D., Williamson, D.E., & Ryan, N.D. (2004). Clinical characteristics of depressive symptoms in children and adolescents with major depressive disorder. *Journal of Clinical Psychiatry, 65,* 1654–1659.

30. Kashani, J.H., Carlson, G.A., Beck, N.C., Hoeper, E.W., Corcoran, C.M., McAllister, J.A., et al. (1987). Depression, depressive symptoms, and depressed mood among a community sample of adolescents. *American Journal of Psychiatry, 144,* 931–934.

31. Tillman, R., Geller, B., Bolhofner, K., Craney, J.L., Williams, M., & Zimerman, B. (2003). Ages of onset and rates of syndromal and subsyndromal comorbid DSM-IV diagnoses in a prepubertal and early adolescent bipolar disorder phenotype. *Journal of the American Academy of Child and Adolescent Psychiatry, 42,* 1486–1493.

32. McElroy, S.L., & Keck, P.E., Jr. (2000). Pharmacologic agents for the treatment of acute bipolar mania. *Biological Psychiatry, 48,* 539–557.

33. Glick, I.D., Murray, S.R., Vasudevan, P., Marder, S.R., & Hu, R.J. (2001). Treatment with atypical antipsychotics: New indications and new populations. *Journal of Psychiatric Research, 35,* 187–191.

34. Wagner, K.D., & Ambrosini, P.J. (2001). Childhood depression: Pharmacological therapy/treatment (Pharmacotherapy of childhood depression). *Journal of Clinical Child Psychology, 30,* 88–97.

35. Hunkeler, E.M., Fireman, B., Lee, J., Diamond, R, Hamilton, J., He, C.X., et al. (2005). Trends in use of antidepressants, lithium, and anticonvulsants in Kaiser Permanente-insured youths, 1994–2003. *Journal of Child and Adolescent Psychopharmacology, 15,* 26–37.

36. Cowell, A. (2004, September 21). Second thoughts on restricting drugs to treat depression in adolescents. *New York Times,* p. C6.

37. Harris, G. (2004, September 21). Study finds less youth antidepressant use. *New York Times*, pp. C1, C6.
38. Carlson, G.A., & Mick, E. (2003). Drug-induced disinhibition in psychiatrically hospitalized children. *Journal of Child and Adolescent Psychopharmacology, 13,* 153–164.
39. Soutullo, C.A., DelBello, M.P., Ochsner, J.E., McElroy, S.L., Taylor, S.A., Strakowski, S.M., et al. (2002). Severity of bipolarity in hospitalized manic adolescents with history of stimulant or antidepressant treatment. *Journal of Affective Disorders, 70,* 323–327.
40. Olfson, M., Shaffer, D., Marcus, S.C., & Greenberg, T. (2003). Relationship between antidepressant medication treatment and suicide in adolescents. *Archives of General Psychiatry, 60,* 978–982.
41. National Institute for Health and Clinical Excellences. (2005). *Depression in children and young people: Identification and management in primary, community and secondary care.* London: Author.
42. Rosenthal, N.E., Sack, D.A., Gillina, J.C., Lewy, A.J., Goodwin, F.K., Davenport, Y., et al. (1984). Seasonal affective disorder: A description of the syndrome and preliminary findings with light therapy. *Archives of General Psychiatry, 41,* 72–80.
43. Golden, R.N., Gaynes, B.N., Ekstrom, R.D., Hamer, R.M., Jacobsen, F.M., Suppes, T., et al. (2005). The efficacy of light therapy in the treatment of mood disorders: A review and meta-analysis of the evidence. *American Journal of Psychiatry, 162,* 656–662.
44. Swedo, S.E., Allen, A.J., Glod, C.A., Clark, C.H., Teicher, M.H., Richter, D., et al. (1997). A controlled trial of light therapy for the treatment of pediatric seasonal affective disorder. *Journal of the American Academy of Child and Adolescent Psychiatry, 36,* 816–821.
45. Taieb, O., Flament, M.F., Chevret, S., Jeammet, P., Allilaire, J.F., Mazet, P., et al. (2002). Clinical relevance of electroconvulsive therapy (ECT) in adolescents with severe mood disorders: Evidence from a follow-up study. *European Psychiatry, 17,* 206–212.
46. Rey, J.M., & Walter, G. (1997). Half a century of ECT use in young people. *American Journal of Psychiatry, 154,* 595–602.
47. Weisz, J.R., Weiss, B., Han, S.S., Granger, D.A., & Morton, T. (1995). Effects of psychotherapy with children and adolescents revisited: A meta-analysis of treatment outcome studies. *Psychological Bulletin, 117,* 450–468.
48. Sergin, C. (2000). Social skills deficits associated with depression. *Clinical Psychology Review, 20,* 379–403.
49. Stark, K.D., Rouse, L.W., & Livingston, R. (1991). Treatment of depression during childhood and adolescence: Cognitive-behavioral procedures for the individual and family. In P. Kendall (Ed.), *Child and adolescent therapy: Cognitive-behavioral procedures* (pp. 165–206). New York: Guilford Press.
50. Reinecke, M.A., Ryan, N.E., & DuBois, D.L. (1998). Cognitive-behavioral therapy of depression and depressive symptoms during adolescence: A review and

meta-analysis. *Journal of the American Academy of Child and Adolescent Psychiatry, 37,* 26–34.

51. Chorpita, B.F., Yim, L.M., Donkervoet, J.C., Arensdorf, A., Amundsen, M.J., McGee, C., et al. (2002). Toward large-scale implementation of empirically supported treatments for children: A review and observation by the Hawaii Empirical Basis to Services Task Force. *Clinical Psychology: Science and Practice, 9,* 165–190.

52. Mufson, L., Weissman, M.M., Moreau, D., & Garfinkel, R. (1999). Efficacy of interpersonal psychotherapy for depressed adolescents. *Archives of General Psychiatry, 56,* 573–579.

53. Asarnow, J.R., Jaycox, L.H., & Tompson, M.C. (2001). Depression in youth: Psychosocial interventions. *Journal of Clinical Child Psychology, 30,* 33–47.

54. Lofthouse, N., & Fristad, M.A. (2004). Psychosocial interventions for children with early-onset bipolar spectrum disorder. *Clinical Child and Family Psychology Review, 7,* 71–88.

55. U.S. Public Health Services. (2000). *Report of the Surgeon General's Conference of children's mental health: A national action agenda.* Washington, DC: Author.

56. Pavuluri, M.A., Graczyk, P.A., Henry, D.B., Carbray, J.A., Heidenreich, J., & Miklowitz, D.J. (2004). Child- and family-focused cognitive-behavioral therapy for pediatric bipolar disorder: Development and preliminary results. *Journal of the American Academy of Child and Adolescent Psychiatry, 43,* 528–537.

57. Miklowitz, D.J., George, E.L., Axelson, D.A., Kim, E.Y., Birmaher, B., Schneck, C., et al. (2004). Family-focused treatment for adolescents with bipolar disorder. *Journal of Affective Disorders, 82S,* S113–S128.

Chapter 7

Adult Depression: Features, Burdens, Models, and Interventions

Michael J. Constantino, Anna Lembke, Candice Fischer, and Bruce A. Arnow

Generally characterized by sad mood and associated cognitive, behavioral, and physical symptoms, depression is one of the most widespread psychiatric conditions. It has been estimated that over 18 million Americans will suffer from some type of depression each year[1] and that approximately 20 percent of the U.S. population will experience a significant depressive episode in their lifetime.[2] In addition to its high prevalence, depression has been associated with remarkably high rates of impairment across psychological, interpersonal, health, and occupational realms.[3,4] Furthermore, depression incurs considerable personal and societal costs,[5] including an extremely high economic burden.[1,6] In fact, unipolar major depression is projected to become the leading source of disease burden in established economies by 2020.[7] It is no wonder that Seligman argued that the public faces a depression "epidemic."[8]

Heightened recognition of its prevalence and appreciation of its damaging personal and societal effects have stimulated strong basic and applied research agendas aimed at better understanding depression, as well as how to prevent and treat it. A number of effective treatments, resting on different theoretical models of depression's etiology, have been developed for people suffering from depression. However, these treatments do not work for everyone, nor do they always prevent relapse or recurrence. Thus, research examining basic processes involved in depression onset and maintenance, as well as developing more effective treatments, continues. Focusing on the adult population, the present chapter presents a contemporary look at the clinical features, epidemiology, burdens, theoretical models, and associated treatments related to adult depression.

CLINICAL FEATURES

Classification, Symptomatology, and Differential Diagnosis

The current edition of the *Diagnostic and Statistical Manual of Mental Disorders (DSM–IV–TR)*[9] defines depression as a mood disorder. With its categorical approach to classifying mental illness, the *DSM–IV–TR* divides multiple mood disorders into four categories: (1) depressive disorders, (2) bipolar disorders, (3) substance-induced mood disorders, and (4) mood disorders due to a general medical condition. Our main focus is on the depressive conditions, and even more specifically on major depressive disorder in adults. The *DSM–IV–TR* diagnosis of major depressive disorder requires the presence of one or more depressive episodes that last for at least two weeks and cause marked distress or impairment in the person's life. A depressive episode is characterized by the individual experiencing a significantly dysphoric mood or loss of interest or pleasure in nearly all activities and at least four other symptoms, including appetite or weight changes, sleep difficulties, psychomotor agitation or retardation, loss of energy, feelings of worthlessness or excessive guilt, difficulty concentrating, and suicidal ideation. In addition to the time course and symptomatic picture, the diagnosis requires that the difficulties are not directly related to the physiological effects of a substance or a general medical condition (which would fall respectively into mood disorder categories 3 and 4 above). Moreover, the symptoms should not be better accounted for by a normal period (i.e., less than two months) of bereavement following a significant loss.

Also under the depressive disorders category, the *DSM–IV–TR* defines dysthymic disorder as a long-standing (at least two continuous years), low-grade depression. Generally speaking, the same symptoms as a major depressive episode apply. However, the diagnosis reflects fewer and less severe symptomatology, with less intense distress or impairment in the person's life. In a way, dysthymic symptoms become integrated into a person's baseline, normative functioning. Dysthymic individuals can also be diagnosed with major depressive disorder if full criteria for a depressive episode are met. When major depressive disorder occurs during an episode of dysthymia, it is referred to as "double depression."

Both major depression and dysthymia imply the absence of manic or hypomanic symptoms. Mania is characterized by abnormally expansive or irritable mood lasting for at least a week in addition to other symptoms such as grandiosity, decreased need for sleep, pressured speech, racing thoughts, distractibility, marked increase in goal-directed activity, and excessive involvement in activities that are pleasurable but have a high likelihood of negative consequences (e.g., spending large amounts of money, risky sexual behavior). Manic episodes are severe enough to cause marked impairment in social or occupational functioning or to require hospitalization. In contrast, hypomanic episodes, while involving similar symptoms, are less severe than full manic episodes and are associated with lower levels of social and occupational impairment. If someone does exhibit clinically significant expansive or irritable mood, the diagnosis would fall under category 2 above as a bipolar I disorder (which requires the presence of a full manic episode) or a bipolar II disorder (which requires the presence of a hypomanic episode and the absence of any history of full-blown mania). In the case of an individual having both low-grade depressive symptoms and hypomanic symptoms over an extended period of time, a diagnosis of cyclothymic disorder may be applicable.

When an individual has clinically significant mood symptoms (not directly related to substance use or a general medical condition) but otherwise fails to meet full criteria for a depressive or bipolar condition, he or she could be diagnosed with depressive (or bipolar) disorder not otherwise specified. Again, the main focus of this chapter is on relevant features of major depressive disorder.

Diagnostic Subtypes

In addition to the overarching mood disorder categories discussed above, the *DSM–IV–TR* includes multiple subtypes and specifiers to add further descriptive detail to an individual's condition. For major depressive disorder, a multitude of such specifiers exist. For example, an episode of depression can be qualified as having "melancholic" features, which include a specific cluster of symptoms including significant loss of pleasure, failure of mood to improve even when something good happens, early morning worsening of mood, marked psychomotor retardation, significant weight loss, and excessive and inappropriate guilt. "Atypical" features of major depression include mood reactivity, significant weight gain or increased appetite, excessive sleeping, leaden paralysis, and heightened sensitivity to interpersonal rejection. Postpartum onset in women reflects a rather severe depressive episode that occurs within four weeks after giving birth. The "seasonal pattern" specifier reflects a regular temporal relationship between the depressive episodes and the time of the year (e.g., consistently feeling depressed in the winter but not in the summer).

As mentioned previously, "double depression" reflects the combination of dysthymic disorder and major depressive disorder. "Chronic" major depression applies when the full criteria for a major depressive episode are met continuously for at least two years. This chronic subgroup has several distinctive features including high rates of recurrence, comorbid personality disorders, elevated rates of psychiatric hospitalizations, and, for women, low educational achievement, which may contribute to underemployment and lower income.[10]

Phenomenological Subtypes

Although the above *DSM–IV–TR* categories and subtypes capture some of the heterogeneity within depressive disorders, it is important to highlight several limitations of the categorical approach to classification. First, *DSM* categories may oversimplify the complex nature of depression, as well as other mental disorders, by focusing on symptom presentation rather than on the biological, psychological, and social etiological factors.[11] Second, the current criteria suggest that depression is an illness that either does or does not exist. Such a dichotomized perspective ignores the likelihood that depression manifests itself on a continuous scale and, thus, is better assessed in terms of degrees and clinical significance as opposed to numbers of symptoms and static temporal anchors.[11] Moreover, the categorical approach to diagnosis deflects attention from those with sub-syndromal symptoms, who suffer nonetheless.[2] And finally, although diagnostic and descriptive subtypes have been advanced, they may not accurately capture individual differences in one's phenomenological experience of depression. Without a better understanding of such differences in phenomenology, it is possible that treatment decisions could be misguided.

McWilliams, for example, presented a clinical vignette of how two individuals may be clinically depressed with essentially identical symptomatic profiles and yet have markedly different subjective experiences.[12] In her description, one man feels badly because he views himself as morally deficient, whereas the other man feels empty and views himself as defective (but not morally reprehensible). Both men are contemplating suicide, but for very different reasons. The former believes that his evilness is poisoning the world and that the world would be a better place without him. The latter feels no investment in improving the world but, rather, simply sees no reason to live. As discussed by McWilliams, the first person likely received messages from important others that he was bad, which led to a predominant feeling of guilt. The second person may have received little attention or few messages from important others, lacks a clear sense of self, and feels inconsequential, prompting a profound sense of shame. From a treatment perspective, if a psychotherapist were to respond to the first person with a supportive and overly sympathetic tone, the patient may feel that his negative self-view is being invalidated. This lack of verification and understanding on the part of the therapist may lead to even greater depression. With the second person, however, such warm and supportive interventions may instill a sense of hope and provide at least a temporary relief from his emptiness. The above vignettes speak to the limitations of a simple categorical perspective on depression and to the importance of including a self dimension in clinical diagnosis, subtyping, and treatment planning.[13] A fuller discussion of depression treatment occurs later.

In addition, several theorists have articulated phenomenological subtypes of depression based theoretically on one's early experiences, personality style, and self-schemas. Freud, for example, articulated two fundamental and relatively independent experiences of depression. One experience was predominantly interpersonal in nature with issues related to dependency, helplessness, and fear of loss and abandonment. The second experience was more intrapsychic and was characterized by self-criticism, concerns about self-worth and competence, and feelings of guilt and failure.[14]

Consistent with Freud's subtypes, Blatt argued that depressed individuals can be either anaclitic or introjective.[15] According to Blatt, anaclitic individuals' sense of self and well-being is closely tied to getting their dependency needs met from others (i.e., receiving a steady dose of love, support, and assurance). Thus, these individuals tend to value others only for their instrumental capacity to provide immediate gratification of these rather primitive attachment needs. When the other person is unable to meet these strong dependency demands, it provokes the anaclitic individual to feel unloved, unwanted, and abandoned, and, in turn, sad. The anaclitic individual is conceptually similar to Beck's sociotropic depressive subtype.[16] Introjective individuals, on the other hand, have much more of a self-preoccupation surrounding issues of perceived failure or personal inadequacy. Thus, these individuals view others not so much as a source of attachment gratification but more as an opportunity to provide approval, acceptance, and validation. The acceptance and positive impact of such feedback, however, is often short-lived, as introjective individuals' high self-criticism and self-loathing tend to predominate. Furthermore, the introjective individual's quest for approval and acceptance often precludes any fully present enjoyment of the moment. Intense feelings of guilt, shame, and self-doubt not surprisingly give rise to a dysphoric mood. The introjective individual is conceptually similar to Beck's autonomous depressive subtype.

The above discussion of diagnostic and theoretical subtypes of depression is by no means exhaustive. Rather, it is meant to highlight some of the more common types of depression, which despite having a similar symptom assemblage may nonetheless reflect significantly different causes, courses, and subjective experiences. Although there is not perfect agreement on the exact types and nature of depression or whether it is best to use a categorical or dimensional classification system, there is a consensus that depression can mean very different things for different people. Nonetheless, the *DSM–IV–TR* remains the most widely used diagnostic system, with its own merits. Most notably, this taxonomic system provides a common language that can facilitate clear communication among clinicians and researchers. Such research includes large-scale epidemiological studies, which allow us to estimate the prevalence and nature of clinical conditions. The epidemiological features of depression are discussed next.

EPIDEMIOLOGY

Prevalence and Course

Drawing on data from community samples in the United States, it has been estimated that 10 to 25 percent of women and 5 to 12 percent of men will experience depression at some point in their lifetime.[9] Point prevalence rates (i.e., the number of people at a given point in time who are experiencing the disorder) have been estimated at 5 to 9 percent for women and 2 to 3 percent for men. Greenberg et al. found that 8.7 percent of adults experienced depression in 2000 (i.e., 12-month prevalence),[1] which reflected a small decline from the 10.1 percent in 1990.[6] In addition to major depression, it has been estimated that 6 percent of the population will experience dysthymia or "double depression."[9] With the exception of the significant gender difference, depression rates tend to cut evenly across demographic domains, that is, ethnicity (although conceptions of depression can vary in other cultures), education, socioeconomic status, and marital status.[5] Within specific contexts, however, depression can be particularly common. For example, the 12-month prevalence rate for major depression is 2–3 times higher for medical patients than for community samples.[17] In addition, individuals suffering from chronic illnesses such as diabetes and asthma have a higher likelihood of having significant depressive symptoms than general community samples.[18, 19]

The onset of depression may occur at any point from childhood to old age. Considerable evidence has suggested that the average age of onset is in the early to mid-twenties.[2, 9] However, more recent epidemiological data suggest that depression is a disorder of younger onset for those born more recently.[2, 9]

Some studies have demonstrated that initial episodes of depression often occur in adolescence[20] and that there is a high likelihood that depressive episodes will recur in adulthood.[21, 22]

Full major depressive episodes typically develop over the course of days to weeks, often following a period of anxiety or mild depression. The length of each episode can vary, with untreated episodes often lasting at least six months.[9] According the *DSM–IV–TR*, naturalistic studies have revealed that one year following the diagnosis of a major depressive episode, 40 percent of individuals still meet full criteria, 20 percent continue to have subclinical depressive symptoms (i.e., partial remission), and 40 percent are no longer depressed (i.e., full remission). Although many individuals will completely recover from a major depressive episode, depression is a highly recurrent condition. In some estimates, over 75 percent of individuals have more than one episode.[23] The course of recurrent major depression varies from person to person. Some individuals have episodes that are separated by long periods of full remission. Others may have similar time between full episodes but only achieve partial remission. Still others may have clusters of episodes or may have an increasing number of episodes as they get older. And finally, some individuals with major depression (approximately 20%) will experience the full impact of depressive episodes lasting two or more years. What does seem consistent is that the number of previous episodes is a reliable predictor of future episodes. This point is underscored in community samples where people who have had two depressive episodes have a 70 percent chance of having another, and individuals having had three episodes have a 90 percent chance of having a fourth.[9] Other data suggest that without treatment, recurrence rates after two to three episodes range from 60–85 percent.[24, 25] Furthermore, periods of remission tend to shorten with each passing episode.[23, 26]

Gender Differences

There is a substantial gender difference in the prevalence of depression. It has been estimated in large-scale community epidemiological studies that women are 1.5 to 3 times more likely to experience clinical depression than men.[27, 28] Women also tend to report subclinical depression at a higher rate than men.[29] This gender difference is consistent across most demographic and cultural groups, as well as in different countries.[30] Furthermore, the gender difference appears to surface around the age of 12 to 13.[31] Prior to this, boys and girls have similar rates of depression. The 1.5–3 to 1 (female to male) ratio exists by late adolescence and remains through adulthood.[30] Data also suggest that the gender difference in depression is attributable to a greater number of index episodes in women than men, as opposed to differences in duration, recurrence, or speed of recovery from the illness.[28, 32]

Multiple explanations for the gender difference in depression have been advanced. For example, biological explanations have focused on hormonal changes in women during puberty, premenstruation, postpartum, and menopause, as well as possible gender differences in biological reactivity to stress.[30] Psychological explanations have included women's interpersonal orientation and the related emotional costs of being, compared to men, more emotionally tied to others and to the outcome of interpersonal events. Another psychological explanation focuses on the tendency for women to ruminate about their distress more than men.[33] Such rumination, it is argued, hinders one's ability to cope with and to overcome depression because it maintains negative thinking, decreases motivation, and interferes with concentration and problem-solving abilities. Social explanations have focused on chronic stressors that women face based on their social standing and traditional gender role obstacles.[34]

Although all of the above gender difference hypotheses have received theoretical and empirical attention, few have received unequivocal support. Furthermore, as argued by Kessler, many such theories are flawed in their focus on explaining gender differences in the chronicity of depression (for which a gender difference does not exist).[27] According to Kessler, there is ample reason to question all of the explanations presented above. The most plausible explanations for the gender difference, he argued, include sex hormones, genes, subtle socialization experiences in adolescence, and gender experiences that may lead to depression vulnerability. Recent work has also focused on the role of personality in explaining gender differences in depression. For example, Goodwin and Gotlib found that levels of neuroticism may moderate the association between gender and depression among adults.[34] Clearly, the gender difference issue is a complex one that will require future research with a clearly defined focus and appropriate methodology to address the seemingly primary question, why do women have more first episodes of depression than men?[27]

Comorbidity

Epidemiological studies reveal substantial comorbidity between depression and other disorders. For example, data from the World Health Organization Collaborative Study and the National Comorbidity Study showed that 62 percent and 74 percent, respectively, of patients with major depressive disorder also met criteria for one or more concurrent psychiatric disorders.[35,36] The most frequent co-occurring psychological conditions are anxiety disorders (especially generalized anxiety disorder, panic disorder, and post-traumatic stress disorder). In addition to psychological comorbidity, depression also tends to co-occur with medical conditions. For example, approximately 40 percent of people who suffer a stroke or myocardial infarction will develop some symptoms of depression afterward.[37, 38] There is also evidence that depression and chronic pain often coexist,[39] with a recent large primary care study showing that approximately two-thirds of patients with major depression also reported chronic pain.[40]

In addition to epidemiological comorbidity, there is some evidence that the co-occurrence of depression and medical conditions has an interactive effect on outcomes. For example, depression in diabetic patients is associated with poor glycemic control and increased risk for medical complications.[41] The mortality rate for persons recovering from myocardial infarctions is three times higher if the person is depressed versus nondepressed.[42] Depressed stroke patients are also at higher mortality risk than nondepressed stroke patients.[43] The combination of major depression plus disabling chronic pain is associated with significantly poorer health-related quality of life and more instances of panic disorder than among those with depression and non-disabling pain or without chronic pain.[40] While this list of comorbid conditions is by no means complete, it reveals that comorbid conditions are the norm rather than the exception among depressed individuals.

BURDENS

Personal, Familial, and Societal

Depression has a substantial functional impact on all aspects of the sufferer's life, including home, family, work, and school.[5, 44] Furthermore, depression produces adverse social outcomes, including some that may be irreversible—for example, decreased educational attainment and increased teenage parenting.[45, 46] In the Medical Outcomes Study, the functional impairment associated with depression was comparable to or greater than the impairment associated with other common and chronic medical conditions (e.g., hypertension, diabetes, arthritis).[47] Moreover, in the Global Burden of Disease Study, unipolar depression was second only to ischemic heart disease in disease burden in established economies.[7] Thus, depression produces more burden than problems like cardiovascular disease, alcohol use, and even injuries associated with road traffic accidents. As previously mentioned, depression is projected to supplant ischemic heart diseases as the leading cause of disease burden by 2020. And when focusing specifically on the middle years of life, depression is already—and by far—the single most burdensome illness in both developing and developed nations.[48]

In addition to personal emotional costs, depression has been shown to affect an individual's work functioning. Depressed individuals are more likely to experience work loss than those with any other mental illness.[48] Furthermore, depression leads to greater work loss than impairing nonpsychiatric conditions such as neurological problems, diabetes, and history of heart disease and cancer.[49] Another obvious personal and human cost is that of suicide, which accounts for over 30,000 deaths per year in the United States. Depression is a major risk factor for completed suicide. In fact, suicide rates for people experiencing a current depressive episode represent a 50-fold increase over the population base rate.[50] Depression also has a highly negative impact on family functioning. For example, maternal depression is associated with disruptions in children's emotional and cognitive development.[51] In addition, children of depressed parents are three times more likely than children of nondepressed parents to experience depression themselves.[52] Depression has also been associated with martial instability,[53] as well as marital dissatisfaction in women.[54]

Financial

The financial costs associated with depression include those related to direct care (e.g., psychiatric/medical services), mortality (e.g., suicide), and morbidity (e.g., reduced work productivity). In 1990, the financial burden of depression was estimated between 43.7 and 52.9 billion dollars.[6, 55] In 2000, the figure was 83.1 billion dollars.[1] The 2000 figure actually represents just a 7 percent increase over the inflation-adjusted figure of 77.4 billion for 1990, indicating that the financial burden of depression has remained rather stable, despite a significant increase from 1990 to 2000 in people seeking treatment.[1] For the 2000 overall cost figure, $26.1 billion (31%) was attributed to direct treatment costs, $5.4 billion (7%) to suicide-related costs, and $51.5 billion to work costs associated with absenteeism and reduced productivity due to depression. With respect to direct service costs, even after controlling for chronic medical illness, the medical costs of depressed individuals are approximately 1.5 to 2 times greater than those of individuals who are not depressed. In one study, depressed individuals visited the emergency room seven times more frequently than nondepressed individuals.[56] Clearly, depression is associated with large decrements in daily social and emotional functioning as well as overall quality of life. Furthermore, there is a huge cost to the individual and to the society at large in dealing with this prevalent and often chronic condition. Thus, there is a pressing need to improve our understanding of the etiology of depression. Contemporary theoretical models regarding the nature and causes of depression as well as associated treatment approaches are discussed next.

THEORETICAL MODELS AND ASSOCIATED TREATMENTS

The cause of depression is still poorly understood. The limited understanding that we do have can be likened to the parable of "The Blind Men and the Elephant"; different scientists deduce different explanations for its cause, depending upon the branch of science that they are studying. What we can say with some degree of certainty is that the cause of depression is multifactorial, with contributing elements from both nature and nurture.

Biological Models and Treatments

Heritability studies, in which scientists trace the patterns of inheritance of a given disease through multiple generations of one family, provide strong evidence that depression is at least in part genetic.[57] If a parent has depression, his or her child is at increased risk for developing depression but will not *necessarily* develop the disorder. Twin studies demonstrate that 40–50 percent of the risk of depression is genetic.[58] In other words, if one twin has depression, the other is at increased risk for developing depression, despite different environments and life experiences. Although the evidence is strong for a genetic contribution to depression, no specific gene has been identified.

Potential nongenetic causes of depression are also important. Emotional or physical traumas (e.g., childhood abuse, war, and isolation) are often associated with depression. Even a minor stressor can cause depression in individuals who are genetically predisposed.[59] The delicate balance between genetic vulnerability and environmental factors is different for each person. Physical illness can also be a trigger for depression, and some illnesses are more commonly associated with depression than others; for example, hypothyroidism, stroke, or Parkinson's disease.[60]

In addition to genetic and environmental factors, some scientists speculate that depression itself can lead to depression, in a process known as "kindling." Broadly speaking, the kindling hypothesis states that depression itself is traumatic to the brain, making depressed individuals more vulnerable to future depression.[61] This hypothesis is based in part on studies of seizure activity in rodents, where the amount of electrical stimulation needed to trigger a seizure is less and less with each subsequent seizure.[62] The kindling hypothesis is also consistent with the natural history of depression. As mentioned previously, the more episodes of depression the individual has experienced, the greater the likelihood of additional recurrences in the future.[26]

It can be confidently asserted that depression is associated with biochemical brain changes. Our understanding of such depression-related changes has advanced greatly in the last half century. Using special brain imaging techniques to compare depressed and nondepressed individuals, it is clear that many parts of the brain are involved in this disease process. It appears that some parts are too active during depression, and some parts too quiescent.[63] Three theories seek to explain what is happening on a biochemical level: the monoamine theory, the hypothalamic-pituitary-adrenal (HPA) axis dysregulation theory, and the neurotrophic damage theory. Each theory, as well as the evidence to support it, is discussed in turn. It is important to keep in mind that the validity of one theory does not necessarily refute the validity of another, and that all three may play some role in the pathophysiology of depression.

The monoamine theory of depression emerged from treatment response rather than systematic investigation into brain changes during depression. Neurons in the brain communicate with one another by sending signals. Molecules are released from the end (dendrite) of one neuron to receptors at the beginning (axon) of the next neuron. The space between neurons traversed by the molecule is called the synaptic cleft, and the molecule itself is called a neurotransmitter. Monoamine neurotransmitters include serotonin, norepinephrine, and dopamine. Antidepressant medications typically increase the amount of monoamine neurotransmitters in the synaptic cleft. Scientists postulated after the fact that monoamine neurotransmitters play a central role in the biochemistry of depression and that low levels of serotonin, norepinephrine, and/or dopamine in the cleft are responsible for the symptoms of depression. There is some evidence that supports this theory, in the form of low serotonin levels in the cerebrospinal fluid and brain parenchyma of depressed individuals.[64] The evidence, however, is generally quite sparse. Also, antidepressant medications typically take four to six weeks to take effect, but the levels of monoamines in the cleft rise immediately with medication, implying that antidepressant efficacy works by some other mechanism. Nonetheless, it is generally accepted that serotonin, norepinephrine, and dopamine play an important role in depression. That role, however, has yet to be fully determined.

The hypothalamic-pituitary-adrenal (HPA) axis dysregulation theory is a well-supported theory of how depression disrupts normal brain function. The HPA axis, under normal circumstances, mediates the stress response. Neurons in the hypothalamus (located in the brain itself) secrete corticotrophin releasing factor (CRF), which acts on the pituitary (located at the base of the brain) to release adrenocorticotrophin (ACTH). ACTH then travels through the bloodstream down to the adrenal glands (located above the kidneys in the abdominal cavity). The adrenal gland is then stimulated to make and release glucocorticoids, or cortisol. Cortisol, sometimes referred to as adrenaline, is the natural steroid made by the human body. Cortisol in turn circulates through the body and has profound effects on metabolism and brain function. It also has an inhibitory effect on the hypothalamus, called a negative feedback loop. The release of cortisol, under normal conditions, should lead to a decrease in CRF and a decrease in ACTH and ultimately cortisol.

However, under conditions of prolonged or severe stress, cortisol remains elevated at high levels, which in turn may damage key parts of the brain, such as the hippocampus. Damage to the brain may include dysfunction of the inhibitory feedback loop, thereby further prolonging elevated cortisol levels. This process may contribute to depression. Evidence for this theory includes the following: (a) animals exposed to early life stress show persistent HPA-axis abnormalities, which can be normalized with antidepressant treatment;[65] (b) increased activation of HPA axis is seen in about 50 percent of people with depression and can be corrected with antidepressant treatment;[66] and (c) increased activation measured by increased urinary cortisol, increased CRF in cerebrospinal fluid, or decreased ability of the exogenous synthetic glucocorticoid, dexamethasone, to suppress blood levels of cortisol and ACTH.

The neurotrophic damage theory posits that a more diffuse process causes depression, rather than a problem localized to any one brain region. This theory identifies lack of brain-derived neurotrophic factor (BDNF) as contributing to depression. BDNF is a chemical in the brain that regulates growth and differentiation of neurons. Support for this theory includes data showing that stress leads to decreased levels of BDNF in the hippocampus of rodents[67] and that long-term administration of antidepressants increases BDNF.[68]

Other theories regarding the pathophysiology of depression are more speculative.[69] One involves impairment in the brain reward pathways, the same area of the brain that mediates addiction to substances of abuse. Impairment of this region might affect an individual's ability to experience pleasure from everyday emotions and activities. The depressed person might be unable to take joy in food or sex or a good movie, because damage to the reward pathway prevents dopamine and endogenous opioids from contributing to a "natural high." Another theory implicates the hypothalamus, a region of the brain involved in the regulation of sleep, appetite, and circadian rhythms, which are often abnormal in depressed persons. And yet another theory involves the amygdala. The amygdala plays an important role in the conditioned fear response and is likely integral to emotional memory.

Despite our still limited understanding of what causes depression, we have come a long way in the treatment of depression. Depression today is treated with antidepressant medications, psychotherapy, or a combination thereof. More severe and treatment-resistant forms of depression are targeted with electroconvulsive shock therapy (ECT). In this section, we focus on the bio-logically based treatments.

Antidepressant medications were discovered serendipitously about 50 years ago, when it was found that medications to treat tuberculosis actually helped with mood. As scientists began studying how these medications worked, they discovered that the modulation of neurotransmitters such as serotonin and dopamine seemed to be the key to antidepressant efficacy. The acute mechanism of most antidepressants in existence today is the enhancement of serotonin, norepinephrine, or dopamine in the synaptic cleft. However, mood-elevating effects take weeks to months, suggesting that enhanced monoamine neuro-transmission per se is not the mechanism of the antidepressant effect. Some gradual downstream adaptation to the acute effects of the drugs is the likely mechanism; however, its exact nature remains a mystery. No one antidepres-sant has been shown to be superior to another, and the choice of antidepressant for a given individual usually depends on the treatment history of that person, as well as the side effect profile of the drug.

Patients who do not respond to the initial antidepressant trial are tried on another, and if that fails, yet another. Trial and error is important given that response is variable between individuals, and whereas one antidepres-sant might not be effective for a given patient, another may result in com-plete remission of symptoms. According to a recent study, up to 65 percent of patients ingesting up to three antidepressants consecutively show total or near-total remission of their symptoms of depression.[70] However, even these good response rates demonstrate that a large minority of patients with depression continue to have some or all of their symptoms, even after phar-macologic treatment.[71]

Other medications used to target symptoms of depression include antianxi-ety medications, antipsychotic medications, mood stabilizers, and sleep aids. A detailed discussion of how these medications are used alone or in combina-tion with other medications to treat depression is beyond the scope of this chapter. Suffice it to say that there continues to be as much art as science in finding the right medication to treat mood in any given individual.

Electroconvulsive shock therapy (ECT) is also an effective treatment for those depressed patients who fail to respond to more conventional treatments. Reported response rates are as high as 90 percent in some studies.[72] However, limitations associated with ECT include high relapse rates as well as memory impairment.[73] It is also still associated with significant stigma, in part related to film depictions of this kind of treatment. ECT serves the important pur-pose of providing relief of suffering in cases where no other treatment type has been effective.

The future holds promise for other new and exciting treatments for depression, from new medications to novel somatic interventions. A medication that works as a glucocorticoid receptor antagonist, RU486 mifepristone, may be useful in psychotic depression.[74] CRF receptor antagonists are also being explored.[66] In addition, truly experimental treatments that bypass medication and attempt to target the brain directly are also being studied, from transcranial magnetic stimulation to vagal nerve stimulation.[75]

Psychosocial Models and Treatments

In addition to the biological models discussed above, multiple psychosocial models have been advanced to explain the causes of depression. In this section, we discuss the general role of stress as a contributor to depression as well as cognitive, interpersonal, and psychodynamic theories and their related psychosocial treatments.

Stress and Depression

One of the more consistent findings in the literature is that there is a strong association between stressful life events and depression.[76] That said, the relationship is likely complex and inconsistent with a simple causal model.[11] Furthermore, the concept of stress is in and of itself complex. For example, with respect to depression, do a series of minor but unrelenting stressors have the same impact on one's mood as one circumscribed but intense stressor? Some data have revealed that approximately 50 percent of depressed individuals experienced a severe stressor prior to onset.[77] While these data suggest that stress may be an important risk factor for depression, they also allow for other explanatory factors. Many current theorists have dealt with the complexity of the stress-depression relationship by at least partially adopting a diathesis-stress perspective. From this perspective, individuals have varying degrees of vulnerability (diathesis) to an illness. When coupled with a certain level of stress, this vulnerability may give rise to the actual illness. This relationship is also likely quite nuanced. For example, is a high degree of vulnerability plus a severe stressor required to produce depression, or is one significant component sufficient?

Furthermore, individual differences on other psychological levels may interact with stress and depressive response. For example, in a recent prospective study, Constantino, Wilson, Horowitz, and Pinel found that stressful life events predicted depression in college students.[78] However, this relationship was moderated by a type of self-organization. That is, people who perceived strong distinctions between their different self-aspects were less likely to develop depression in response to stress when compared to people who had a lot of overlap in their self-representations. These findings were discussed in terms of Linville's notion of spillover.[79] That is, for people who have more distinctive self-aspects, it is less likely that any negative affect associated with one aspect (in response to a specific stressor) will spread, or spill over, to another. For example, a man may have representations of himself as a father, an employee, a little league coach, and a choir member. If this man perceives himself differently in each of these roles, then there would be less likelihood that a stressful event in one domain (e.g., getting fired) would spill over to his functioning as a father, coach, and choir member, thereby protecting him against a significant depressive response. If, however, this person tended to see himself very similarly across all domains and all of these self-representations were closely associated in memory, his getting fired may be more likely to permeate all domains. In this case, he may see himself as a general failure as an employee, father, coach, and choir member, thereby increasing the risk of a significant depressive response. Thus, a specific type of self-organization (i.e., low overlap among self-aspects) may be a protective factor for depression.

Cognitive Theories and Treatment

Since Beck first articulated his pioneer cognitive model of depression, there has been an expanded (and in many cases predominant) focus on cognitive processes as they relate to the onset, course, and treatment of depressive experiences.[80, 81] According to Beck's landmark theory, negative thinking lies at the core of depression, with the rationale that a person's behavior and affect are determined mainly by the way in which they structure, perceive, and understand the world.[81] From this perspective, it is not the external situation that determines how a person feels but the manner in which the situation is construed or appraised. More specifically, depressed individuals tend to have negative and pessimistic interpretations of themselves, their world, and their future—what Beck refers to as the *cognitive triad*.

Also according to cognitive theory, negative thinking has multiple levels. The first level involves *automatic thoughts*, which are posited to color negatively a person's perceptions of many or most situations or stressors, thereby enhancing or maintaining a depressed mood. People's thinking at this level is often characterized by *cognitive distortions*, or faulty information-processing. For example, depressed individuals tend to exhibit *black and white thinking*, for example, failing a test and deducing that you are a horrible student across all subjects or a failure across many other domains. A second level of thinking reflects *intermediate beliefs*, which reflect a deeper level of attitudes, assumptions, and rules that people apply to their self-perception. For example, a depressed person may assume that the only way that he or she will be liked by others is to work extremely hard in order to perform perfectly. Thus, when this individual does not live up to this impossible rule, resulting negative emotions are likely to occur. And finally, the deepest level of thinking reflects an individual's most central or *core beliefs* about the self. These beliefs, which often stem from previous experiences, are at the most fundamental level and tend to be global, rigid, and overgeneralized. Such organizing self-schemas are often regarded by the person as absolute truths, though they may be so fundamental that the person rarely articulates them—even to himself or herself. For example, a depressed man who had rejecting or invalidating parents may have developed a defectiveness schema characterized by a strong belief that he is bad, unwanted, or inferior and that he would be completely unlovable to significant others. As a result, this individual may be prone to interpreting the behavior of others as being consistent with this belief. In other words, he may be hypersensitive to perceived criticisms, rejections, or blame. In turn, these perceptions are likely to strengthen the organizing self-schema of being unlovable, thereby reinforcing the depressogenic state. Given people's inherent drive for consistency, early maladaptive schemas or core beliefs tend to fight for survival by way of these persistent feedback loops.[82]

Another variation on cognitive approaches to depression is Seligman's learned helplessness theory.[83] Seligman postulated that at the center of depression lies a learned feeling that our actions to change a given stressful situation are out of our control. Thus, depressed people believe that there is nothing that they can do to relieve their suffering or to bring gratification to their life. In short, these individuals believe that they are "helpless," and that there is nothing that can soothe their pain. Such individuals will subsequently adopt this passive and helpless stance across most or all life circumstances.

The learned helplessness understanding of depression has been revised in order to better account for why some people become helpless and depressed when they experience negative events while others do not. This revision takes into account the role of *attributions*, or ways in which a person explains what happens to them.[84] It is an example of a diathesis-stress model, where the diathesis is a pronounced tendency toward negative explanations for events and the stress is the experience of negative life events. According to this perspective, a depressed person will attribute the occurrence of negative life events to personal deficiencies that are internal, stable, and global. Consider two individuals who apply for a job, receive an interview, and are not offered the position. Individual A attributes not receiving the offer to his own (internal) unworthiness ("I did not receive the job offer because I am incompetent") and views the absence of a job offer as due to factors that are stable ("I'll never have the skills to get a good job") and global, that is, affecting many areas in his life ("I am a failure as a person and will not succeed in any area"). This individual will assume that negative outcomes will continue to occur in the future, that he will be powerless to prevent them, and that the pattern signifies general personal unworthiness, leading to depression. Individual B attributes not getting the job to situational factors, specifically, a lack of fit between his particular set of skills and the job requirements ("I did not get the job because it required knowing a computer language that I have not had the opportunity to learn yet"), views the problem as correctible, that is, temporary ("I am going to take a course to learn the specific skills that I need so that the next time this comes up I will be prepared"), and does not view the lack of a job offer as a reflection on his sense of self-worth. Individual B would not necessarily expect negative events to continue unabated, would feel a greater sense of control over his future, would not feel a pervasive sense of unworthiness, and would be far less vulnerable to depression than individual A.

Although other cognitive models exist, all models assume that negative cognitive processes play a significant role in the etiology of depression. Thus, cognitive approaches to treatment have developed from this assumption.

Over the past few decades, the emergence of cognitive therapy (CT) has been one of the major developments in the treatment of depression.[4] In fact, CT is a well-established, empirically supported treatment for depression that is widely recognized as one of the most effective psychosocial treatments available.[86] CT is at least as effective as other psychosocial or pharmacological approaches[87] and may be superior in reducing the rate of relapse and recurrence.[88]

The hallmark of the cognitive therapy (CT) approach is to explore how people's ways of thinking may be contributing to their difficulties. A primary goal of the cognitive therapist is to work collaboratively with his or her patients to assist them in developing new—and more accurate and adaptive—perspectives of self, other, world, and future. While there is a multitude of techniques,[85] the main principle is that events and experiences can be interpreted in many ways. Thus, CT therapists help patients to identify irrational and maladaptive automatic thoughts, cognitive distortions, intermediate beliefs, and eventually core views of self. Therapists also help patients to link their thoughts with their emotions and then help patients to challenge their distorted thoughts and to consider new ways of thinking. Cognitive therapists encourage patients to become scientists who treat their thoughts as hypotheses rather than as established facts and to learn to see that perception can change mood. In many cases, behavioral strategies complement the core cognitive strategies. For example, therapists will encourage patients to gather evidence concerning their beliefs, to test alternative viewpoints about a situation, and to try new methods of coping with situations. CT is a time-limited, structured, problem-oriented, and educational approach, in which the therapist is often active and directive. The approach is intended to have a here-and-now focus, though such a focus is certainly informed by one's history.

Interpersonal Theory and Treatment

Departing from cognitive approaches, interpersonal models of depression view relational difficulties as the core problem in depression. This model rests on many of the assumptions originally advanced by Sullivan[89] and Meyer[90]— the founders of the Interpersonal School of Psychology. From this framework, depression is understood as the result of three intertwined processes: neurovegatative symptoms and depressive affect, social and interpersonal relations, and personality and character problems.[91] On the one hand, interpersonal stressors are purported to play a crucial role in the onset of depression, and on the other hand, depression negatively impacts interpersonal relationships. The belief in this reciprocal interaction between mood and life events is at the core of the interpersonal theory of depression. Following from this model, Klerman and colleagues[92] developed interpersonal psychotherapy (IPT) specifically for the treatment of depression. IPT highlights the psychosocial and interpersonal underpinnings of depression and focuses mainly on current relationships and relational patterns. Within the IPT framework, improving interpersonal relationships is viewed as the vehicle for resolving depressive symptoms. One or several of four main areas of interpersonal difficulties can be the focus of IPT. These areas include grief, interpersonal role disputes, role transitions, and interpersonal deficits.[91] IPT proposes specific goals and strategies for the treatment of depressed patients with respect to each of these interpersonal problems.

Grief is the focus of treatment among patients for whom the onset of the depressive episode is connected to the death of a loved one. The goal of the therapy with these patients is to assist the healthy mourning process and to help them reestablish activities and relationships to replace what has been lost. For interpersonal role dispute, depression is related to a relationship in which the individuals have nonreciprocal or conflicting expectations of each other. In this case, the main goal of treatment is to identify the dispute (which may be covert), to develop a plan for change, and to modify expectations or faulty communication to resolve the interpersonal problem. In some cases, dissolution of the relationship may reflect the most adaptive outcome. The third problem area, called "role transition," applies to patients who are going through a major life change, such as retiring or starting a new job, moving to a new city, or being diagnosed with a medical illness. It is presumed that these patients become depressed because of difficulties meeting the demands of the new role or their inability to relinquish the old role. The goals for therapy with patients going through a "role transition" include mourning and accepting of the loss of the old role, developing a more positive evaluation of the new role, and restoring self-esteem by developing a sense of mastery in the demands of the new role. The last problem area is referred to as "interpersonal deficits." It is a reserved for patients who do not fit into any of the other three areas, show no evidence of an acute precipitant of depression, or have a long history of impoverished or unsuccessful interpersonal relationships. The goals for the treatment of patients with "interpersonal deficits" are to reduce the patient's social isolation and to encourage the formation of new relationships. Similar to CT, considerable research supports the effectiveness of IPT to the point that it is also considered a well-established, empirically supported treatment for depression that produces outcomes comparable to other psychosocial and psychopharmacological approaches.[93]

Psychodynamic Theories and Treatment

Since the beginning of the 20th century, a variety of psychoanalytic writers have attempted to explain and to understand the challenging concept of depression. Psychodynamic models of depression have typically focused on the emotional impact of childhood experiences on a person's perception of self and significant others. Freud described the onset of depression as triggered by the loss (either in reality or fantasy) of someone important in the person's life.[15] Different from normal grief or mourning, Freud suggested that the melancholic or depressed person undergoes an important loss of self-esteem. Abraham viewed the state of adult melancholia as stemming from a current disillusionment in love, which is perceived by the depressed person as a repetition of an early traumatic experience in which the person had a severe injury to his or her self-esteem.[94] Bibring emphasized the difficulty in self-esteem regulation as a key issue in depression.[95] According to this model, low self-esteem stems from the existing gap between the person's current self view and his or her aspirations as to whom they would like to be (ego ideal).

The primary focus of psychodynamic psychotherapy is on the gradual understanding of the person's depressive symptoms with respect to an underlying core depressive dynamic. The main treatment goal is for the person to gain insight into the ways in which these dynamics have become embedded in the person's perception of himself or herself as well as in relationships with others. As summarized by Busch, Rudden, and Shapiro, "Gradually, the patient begins to recognize the contexts that tend to elicit depression, to understand what is happening internally during those times, and to feel more in control of the depressed feelings" (p. 31).[96] While many traditional psychoanalytic treatments are lengthy (possibly lasting years), briefer psychodynamic treatments have also been developed (ranging anywhere from 5–40 sessions) that emphasize increased therapist activity during sessions and a limited central focus.[97] Although widely used with depression, psychodynamic treatments continue to have a limited evidence base relative to CBT or IPT. This lack of evidence does not necessarily imply that psychodynamic treatment is ineffective for depression but rather that the number of rigorous effectiveness studies remain limited at the current time.[93]

In conclusion, several psychosocial treatments have been shown to be at least as effective as psychopharmacological approaches to depressions, with CBT and IPT having the most impressive empirical support. In the case of preventing relapse or recurrence, there is some evidence that CBT may have an edge over other approaches. Furthermore, when it comes to chronic depressions, there is growing evidence that the combination of antidepressant medication and psychotherapy is the most effective strategy.[10]

SUMMARY

In this chapter, we have summarized contemporary information and perspectives regarding the clinical features, burdens, theoretical models, and treatments associated with adult depression. Categorically defined as a mood disorder within our current psychiatric nomenclature (though not without controversy), depression is a highly prevalent and often recurrent psychiatric condition that affects about twice as many women as men. Furthermore, there is substantial comorbidity among depression and other psychiatric and medical conditions. Whether on its own or in connection with other problems, depression gives rise to significant personal, societal, and economic costs and is expected to soon become the leading source of disease burden in established economies (it already ranks second).

With respect to understanding depression, multiple theoretical models have been advanced. The models all have corresponding research literatures, and many have treatments that stem from the particular theories. In the current chapter, we reviewed prominent biological models (e.g., genetics, biochemical change) and treatments (e.g., antidepressant medications, ECT) as well as psychosocial models (e.g., cognitive, interpersonal) and treatments (CBT, IPT). While significant progress has been made in understanding the mechanisms involved in the onset and course of depression, many questions remain.

Depression is a heterogeneous illness, which leaves much to be discovered regarding the essential features and explanatory mechanisms for different subtypes. What can be said with a fair degree of certainty is that the cause of depression is multifactorial, with many researchers accepting some semblance of a biopsychosocial (nature-nurture) perspective.

Despite our still rather limited understanding of depression and its causes, we have actually come a long way with regard to treatment. Episodes of depression can be treated fairly effectively (and comparably) with antidepressant medications or psychosocial therapies. In some cases (e.g., chronic depression), a combination of medication and psychotherapy seems most efficacious. For severe and treatment resistant depressions, ECT can often be effective, at least in terms of providing immediate relief from previously intractable symptoms. While there is an abundance of data speaking to the general effectiveness of psychopharmacological and certain psychosocial interventions (CBT and IPT) for depression, the fact remains that improvement rates in some studies remain fairly modest, with some patients dropping out prematurely, some achieving only partial response, and others not responding at all. Furthermore, even when patients do respond to a course of treatment, they remain vulnerable to future depression. As we have highlighted in this chapter, depression is a chronic condition that often requires long-term or at least episodic care. Thus, even though depression is one of the most studied psychological conditions, much work remains to be done to improve our understanding of its basic processes and to improve our interventions. And as argued by Arnow and Constantino, it is not enough to think simply about improving our ability to affect short-term symptom reduction.[10] Rather, it is imperative to take into account the chronicity of depression as well as its considerable functional impact on work and social function. Thus, effective treatments need to target long-term gain, relapse prevention, and areas of functioning beyond symptom-reduction. Fortunately, and appropriately, depression remains a high basic and applied research priority.

REFERENCES

1. Greenberg, P.E., Kessler, R.C., Birnbaum, H.G., Leong, S.A., Lowe, S.W., Berglund, P.A., et al. (2003). The economic burden of depression in the United States: How did it change between 1990 and 2000? *Journal of Clinical Psychiatry, 64,* 1465–1475.
2. Gotlib, I.H., & Hammen, C.L. (2002). Introduction. In I.H. Gotlib & C.L. Hammen (Eds.), *Handbook of depression* (3rd ed., pp. 1–20). New York: Guilford.
3. Klerman, G.L., & Weissman, M.M. (1992). The course, morbidity, and costs of depression. *Archives of General Psychiatry, 49,* 831–834.

4. Young, J.E., Weinberger, A.D., & Beck, A.T. (2001). Cognitive therapy for depression. In D.H. Barlow (Ed.), *Clinical handbook of psychological disorders* (3rd ed., pp. 264–308). New York: Guilford.

5. Pincus, H.A., & Pettit, A.R. (2001). The societal costs of chronic major depression. *Journal of Clinical Psychiatry, 62*(Suppl. 6), 5–9.

6. Greenberg, P.E., Stiglin, L.E., Finkelstein, S.N., & Berndt, E.R. (1993). The economic burden of depression in 1990. *Journal of Clinical Psychiatry, 54,* 405–418.

7. Murray, C.J.L., & Lopez, A.D. (Eds.). (1996). *The global burden of disease: A comprehensive assessment of mortality and disability from diseases, injuries, and risk factors in 1990 and projected to 2020.* Cambridge, MA: Harvard University Press.

8. Seligman, M.E.P. (1990). Why is there so much depression today?: The waxing of the individual and the waning of the commons. In R.E. Ingram (Ed.), *Contemporary psychological approaches to depression: Theory, research, and treatment* (pp. 1–9). New York: Plenum Press.

9. American Psychiatric Association. (2000). *Diagnostic and statistical manual of mental disorders* (4th ed., text revision). Washington, DC: Author.

10. Arnow, B.A., & Constantino, M.J. (2003). Effectiveness of psychotherapy and combination treatment for chronic depression. *Journal of Clinical Psychology/In Session, 59,* 893–905.

11. Ingram, R., & Trenary, L. (2004). Mood disorders. In J.E. Maddux & B.A. Win-stead (Eds.), *Psychopathology: Foundations for a contemporary understanding* (pp. 155–177). Mahwah, NJ: Lawrence Erlbaum Associates.

12. McWilliams, N. (1994). *Psychoanalytic diagnosis: Understanding personality structure in the clinical process.* New York: Guilford.

13. Constantino, M.J., & Castonguay, L.G. (2003). Learning from the basics: Clinical implications of social, developmental, and cross-cultural study of the self. *Journal of Psychotherapy Integration, 13,* 3–8.

14. Freud, S. (1917). Mourning and melancholia. In J. Strachey (Ed.), *The standard edition of the complete psychological works of Sigmund Freud* (pp. 151–169). London: Hogarth.

15. Blatt, S.J. (1974). Level of object representation in anaclitic and introjective depression. *Psychoanalytic Study of the Child, 29,* 107–157.

16. Beck, A.T. (1967). *Depression: Causes and treatment.* Philadelphia: University of Pennsylvania Press.

17. Kessler, L.G., Burns, B.J., Shapiro, S., Tischler, G.L., George, L.K., Hough, R.L., et al. (1987). Psychiatric diagnoses of medical service users: Evidence from the Epidemiologic Catchment Area Program. *American Journal of Public Health, 77,* 18–24.

18. Goodnick, P.J., Henry, J.H., & Buki, V.M.V. (1995). Treatment of depression in patients with diabetes mellitus. *Journal of Clinical Psychiatry, 56,* 128–136.

19. Mancuso, C.A., Peterson, M.G., & Charlson, M.E. (2000). Effects of depressive symptoms on health-related quality of life in asthma patients. *Journal of General Internal Medicine, 15*, 301–310.
20. Burke, K.C., Burke, J.D., Reigler, D.A., & Rae, D.S. (1990). Age at onset of selected mental disorders in five community populations. *Archives of General Psy-chiatry, 47*, 511–518.
21. Weissman, M.M., Wolk, S., Goldstein, R.B., Moreau, D., Adams, P., Greenwald, S., et al. (1999). Depressed adolescents grown up. *Journal of the American Medical Association, 281*, 1707–1713.
22. Weissman, M.M., Wolk, S., Wickramaratne, P., Goldstein, R.B., Adams, P., Greenwald, S., et al. (1999). Children with prepubertal-onset major depressive disorder and anxiety grown up. *Archives of General Psychiatry, 56*, 794–801.
23. Kessler, R.C. (2002). Epidemiology of depression. In I.H. Gotlib & C.L. Hammen (Eds.), *Handbook of depression* (3rd ed., pp. 23–42). New York: Guilford.
24. Keller, M.B., Lavori, P.W., Mueller, T.I., Endicott, J., Coryell, W., Hirschfeld, R.M., et al. (1992). Time to recovery, chronicity, and levels of psychopathology in major depression: A 5-year prospective follow-up of 431 subjects. *Archives of General Psychiatry, 49*, 809–816.
25. Thase, M.E., & Sullivan, L.R. (1995). Relapse and recurrence of depression: A practical approach for prevention. *CNS Drugs, 4*, 261–277.
26. Solomon, D.A., Keller, M.B., Leon, A.C., Mueller, T.I., Lavori, P.W., Shea, T., et al. (2000). Multiple recurrences of major depressive disorder. *American Journal of Psychiatry, 157*, 229–233.
27. Kessler, R.C. (2000). Gender differences in major depression: Epidemiological findings. In E. Frank (Ed.), *Gender and its effects on psychopathology* (pp. 61–84). Washington, DC: American Psychiatric Publishing.
28. Kessler, R.C., McGonagle, K.A., Swartz, M., Blazer, D.G., & Nelson, C.B. (1993). Sex and depression in the National Comorbidity Survey: I. Lifetime prevalence, chronicity, and recurrence. *Journal of Affective Disorders, 29*, 85–96.
29. Nolen-Hoeksema, S. (1990). *Sex differences in depression*. Stanford, CA: Stanford University Press.
30. Nolen-Hoeksema, S. (2002). Gender differences in depression. In I.H. Gotlib & C.L. Hammen (Eds.), *Handbook of depression* (3rd ed., pp. 492–509). New York: Guilford.
31. Twenge, J., & Nolen-Hoeksema, S. (2002). Age, gender, race, SES, and birth cohort differences on the Children's Depressive Inventory: A meta-analysis. *Journal of Abnormal Psychology, 111*, 578–588.
32. Keller, M., & Shapiro, R. (1981). Major depressive disorder: Initial results from a one-year prospective naturalistic follow-up study. *Journal of Nervous Mental Disorders, 169*, 761–768.
33. Nolen-Hoeksema, S., Larson, J., & Grayson, C. (1999). Explaining the gender difference in depression. *Journal of Personality and Social Psychology, 77*, 1061–1072.

48. Wang, P.S., Simon, G., & Kessler, R.C. (2003). The economic burden of depression and the cost-effectiveness of treatment. *International Journal of Methods in Psychiatric Research, 12,* 22–33.
49. Kessler, R.C., Greenberg, P.E., Michelson, K.D., Meneades, L.M., & Wang, P.S. (2001). The effects of chronic medical conditions on work loss and work cutback. *Journal of Occupational and Environmental Medicine, 43,* 218–25.
50. Stolberg, R.A., Clark, D.C., & Bongar, B. (2002). Epidemiology, assessment, and management of suicide in depressed patients. In I.H. Gotlib & C.L. Hammen (Eds.), *Handbook of depression* (3rd ed., pp. 581–601). New York: Guilford.
51. Field, T. (1992). Infants of depressed mothers. *Developmental Psychopathology, 4,* 49–66.
52. Birmaher, B., Ryan, N.D., Williamson, D.E., Brent, D.A., Kaufman, J., Dahl, R.E., et al. (1996). Childhood ands adolescent depression: A review of the past 10 years. Part I. *Journal of the American Academy of Child and Adolescent Psychiatry, 35,* 1427–1439.
53. Kessler, R.C., Walters, E.E., & Forthofer, M.S. (1998). The social consequences of psychiatric disorders, III: Probability of marital stability. *American Journal of Psychiatry, 155,* 1092–1096.
54. Whisman, M.A. (1999). Marital dissatisfaction and psychiatric disorders: Results from the National Comorbidity Survey. *Journal of Abnormal Psychology, 108,* 701–706.
55. Greenberg, P.E., Kessler, R.C., Nells, T.L., Finkelstein, S.N., & Berndt, E.R. (1996). Depression in the workplace: An economic perspective. In J.P. Feighner & W.F. Boyer (Eds.), *Selective serotonin re-uptake inhibitors: Advances in basic research and clinical practice* (2nd ed., pp. 327–363). New York: John Wiley & Sons.
56. Johnson, J., Weissman, M.M., & Klerman, G.L. (1992). Service utilization and social morbidity associated with depressive symptoms in the community. *Journal of the American Medical Association, 267,* 1478–1483.
57. Hamet, P., & Tremblay, J. (2005). Genetics and genomics of depression. *Metabolism, 54*(5 Suppl. 1), 10–15.
58. Sullivan, P.F., Neale, M.C., & Kendler, K.S. (2000). Genetic epidemiology of major depression: Review and meta-analysis. *American Journal of Psychiatry, 157,* 1552–1562.
59. Kendler, K.S., Kuhn, J.W., Vittum, J., Prescott, C.A., & Riley, B. (2005). The interaction of stressful life events and a serotonin transporter polymorphism in the prediction of episodes of major depression: A replication. *Archives of General Psychiatry, 62,* 529–35.
60. Sadock, B.J., & Sadock, V.A. (2003). *Kaplan and Sadock's synopsis of psychiatry.* New York: Lippincott, Williams, & Wilkins.
61. Kendler, K.S., Thornton, L.M., & Gardner, C.O. (2001). Genetic risk, number of previous depressive episodes, and stressful life events in predicting onset of major depression. *American Journal of Psychiatry, 158,* 582–586.

62. Kamphuis, W., Lopes da Silva, F.H., & Wadman, W.J. (1988). Changes in local evoked potentials in the rat hippocampus (CA1) during kindling epileptogenesis. *Brain Research, 440,* 205–215.

63. Drevets, W.C. (2000). Functional anatomical abnormalities in limbic and prefrontal cortical structures in major depression. *Progress in Brain Research, 126,* 413–431.

64. Spreux-Varoquaux, O., Alvarez, J.C., Berlin, I., Batista, G., Despierre, P.G., Gilton, A., et al. (2001). Differential abnormalities in plasma 5-HIAA and platelet serotonin concentrations in violent suicide attempters: Relationships with impulsivity and depression. *Life Science, 69,* 647–657.

65. Rowe, W., Steverman, A., Walker, M., Sharma, S., Barden, N., Seckl, J.R., et al. (1997). Antidepressants restore hypothalamic-pituitary-adrenal feedback function in aged, cognitively-impaired rats. *Neurobiology of Aging, 18,* 527–533.

66. Holsboer, F. (2000). The corticosteroid receptor hypothesis of depression. *Neuropsychopharmacology, 23,* 477–501.

67. Smith M.A., Makino, S., Kvetnansky, R., & Post, R.M. (1995). Effects of stress on neurotrophic factor expression in the rat brain. *Annals of the New York Academy of Sciences, 771,* 234–239.

68. Nibuya, M., Morinobu, S., & Duman, R.S. (1995). Regulation of BDNF and trkB mRNA in rat brain by chronic electroconvulsive seizure and antidepressant drug treatments. *Journal of Neuroscience, 15,* 7539–7547.

69. Nestler, E.J., Barrot, M., DiLeone, R.J., Eisch, A.J., Gold, S.J., & Monteggia, L.M. (2002). Neurobiology of depression. *Neuron, 34,* 13–25.

70. Quitkin, F.M., McGrath, P.J., Stewart, J.W., Deliyannides, D., Taylor, B.P., Davies, C.A., et al. (2005). Remission rates with 3 consecutive antidepressant trials: Effectiveness for depressed outpatients. *Journal of Clinical Psychiatry, 66,* 670–676.

71. Berman, R.M., Narasimhan, M., & Charney, D.S. (1997). Treatment-refractory depression: Definitions and characteristics. *Depression and Anxiety, 5,* 154–164.

72. Sackeim, H.A., Hasket, R.F., Mulsant, B.H., Thase. M.E., Mann, J.J., Pettinati, H.M., et al. (2001). Continuation pharmacotherapy in the prevention of relapse following electroconvulsive therapy: A randomized controlled trial. *Journal of the American Medical Association, 285,* 1299–1307.

73. Rasmussen, K.G. (2003). Clinical applications of recent research on electroconvulsive therapy. *Bulletin of the Menninger Clinic, 67,* 18–31.

74. Belanoff, J.K., Rothschild, A.J., Cassidy, F., DeBattista, C., Baulien, E.E., Schold, C., et al. (2002). An open label trial of C-1073 (mifepristone) for psychotic major depression. *Biological Psychiatry, 52,* 386–392.

75. Macritchie, K.A., & Young, A.H. (2001). Emerging targets for the treatment of depressive disorder. *Expert Opinion on Therapy Targets, 5,* 601–612.

76. Monroe, S.M., & Hadjiyannakis, K. (2002). The social environment and depression: Focusing on severe stress. In I.H. Gotlib & C.L. Hammen (Eds.), *Handbook of depression* (3rd ed., pp. 314–340). New York: Guilford.

77. Mazure, C.M. (1998). Life stressors as risk factors in depression. *Clinical Psychology: Science and Practice, 5*, 291–313.

78. Constantino, M.J., Wilson, K.R., Horowitz, L.M., & Pinel, E.C. (in press). The direct and stress-buffering effects of self-organization on psychological adjustment. *Journal of Social and Clinical Psychology.*

79. Linville, P.W. (1987). Self-complexity as a cognitive buffer against stress-related illness and depression. *Journal of Personality and Social Psychology, 52,* 663–676.

80. Beck, A.T. (1964). Thinking and depression: Theory and therapy. *Archives of General Psychiatry, 10,* 561–571.

81. Beck, A.T. (1967). *Depression: Clinical, experimental, and theoretical aspects.* New York: Hoeber.

82. Young J.E., Klosko, J.S., & Weishaar, M.E. (2003). *Schema therapy: A practitioner's guide.* New York: Guilford.

83. Seligman, M.E.P. (1975). *Helplessness.* San Francisco: Freeman.

84. Abramson, L.Y., Alloy, L.B., Hankin, B.L., Haeffel, G.J., MacCoon, D.G., & Gibb,B.E. (2002). Cognitive vulnerability-stress models of depression in a self-regulatory and psychobiological context. In I.H. Gotlib & C.L. Hammen (Eds.), *Handbook of depression* (pp. 268–294). New York: Guilford.

85. Beck, A. T, Rush, A.J., Shaw, B., & Emery, G. (1979). *Cognitive therapy of depression.* New York: Guilford.

86. Hollon, S.D., Haman, K.L., & Brown, L.L. (2002). Cognitive-behavioral treatment of depression. In I.H. Gotlib & C.L. Hammen (Eds.), *Handbook of depression* (pp. 383–403). New York: Guilford.

87. Hollon, S.D., & Beck, A.T. (2004). Cognitive and cognitive behavioral therapies. In M.J. Lambert (Ed.), *Bergin and Garfield's handbook of psychotherapy and behavior change* (5th ed., pp. 447–492). New York: John Wiley & Sons.

88. Gloaguen, V., Cottraux, J., Cucherat, M., & Blackburn, I. M. (1998). A meta-analysis of the effects of cognitive therapy in depressed patients. *Journal of Affective Disorders, 49* 59–72.

89. Sullivan, H.S. (1953). *The interpersonal theory of psychiatry.* New York: Norton.

90. Meyer, A. (1957). *Psychobiology: A science of man.* Springfield, IL: Charles C. Thomas.

91. Weissman, M.M., & Markowitz, J.C. (2002). Interpersonal psychotherapy for depression. In I.H. Gotlib & C.L. Hammen (Eds.), *Handbook of depression* (pp. 404–421). New York: Guilford.

92. Klerman, G.L., Weissman, M.M., Rounsaville, B.J., & Chevron, E.S. (1984). *Interpersonal psychotherapy of depression.* New York: Basic Books.

93. Roth, A., & Fonagy, P. (2005). *What works for whom? A critical review of psycho-therapy research* (2nd ed.). New York: Guilford.

94. Abraham K. (1924). A short study of the development of the libido, viewed in the light of mental disorders. In *Selected papers on psychoanalysis* (pp. 418–501). London: Hogarth.

95. Bibring, E. (1953). The mechanism of depression. In P. Greenacre (Ed.), *Affective disorders* (pp. 13–48). New York: International.
96. Busch, F. N., Rudden, M., & Shapiro, T. (2004). *Psychodynamic treatment of depression.* Washington, DC: American Psychiatric Publishing.
97. Messer, S. B., & Warren, C. S. (1995). *Models of brief psychodynamic therapy: A comparative approach.* New York: Guilford.

Chapter 8

The Will to Die

Viola Mecke

Contentment is a stranger to the suicidal person. Striving for an elusive sense of inner peace brings only a weariness of life. Hope is murdered within the soul as problems loom larger with each day. Gratitude for life eludes the person. Meaningfulness in life is drowned under a dark sea of discouragement. Vital connections to others are buried beneath disappointments, and longed-for love seems unavailable. It is a bitter unquantifiable hunger.

Suicides arise from a "psychache"—a suffering in the mind that makes living appear desolate, dark, and dismal.[1] The suicidal person is driven by mental distress that is perceived as unbearable, deemed intolerable, and felt unacceptable. This mental distress is a bankruptcy of the soul, and solutions seem unavailable. Sometimes death has been an obsession from early childhood, a mental dream that is fantasized and then acted out for all to see. To others, the suicide seems a sudden and unreasoned act.

Sylvia Plath writes, "It is a love of death that sickens everything. . . . I lose life after life."[2] Death seems to gradually take over the thoughts and finally the actions of suicidal persons.

Edwin Shneidman explains that suicide is "a multifaceted event and those biological, cultural, sociological, interpersonal, logical, conscious and unconscious, and philosophic elements are present in each suicidal event."[3] These extenuating factors lay behind any suicidal act, and he concludes, "I believe suicide is a drama of the mind, where the suicidal drama is almost always driven by a psychic pain of the negative emotions—what I call psychache."[4] While each of these factors is considered important, they do not provide an understanding of the forces that drive the self-killing.

Suicide has stolen the lives of many people throughout the centuries and throughout the world. Suicide is a Latin word composed of three parts: *sui*, meaning the self, *cide*, to cut, and *caedere*, to kill; and then *suicidere* became the word for suicide.

The person who kills himself is often referred to as a victim. True, he is a victim of homicide, a victim of his own mind and actions. However, the word may not really fit, for the *Oxford English Dictionary* states that a victim is "a person who is put to death or subjected to torture by another. Victims are subject to "profound, ruthless and damaging forces from outside themselves."[5] The torture of the suicidal mind resides within itself. Even so, torture is often felt by suicide victims. That is, some external person is often the instigator of another's inner distress, either consciously or unconsciously. The wishes of these instigators become felt demands that the suicidal person destroy his life.

WHO ARE THE VICTIMS?

Death by illness or accident brings sorrow to the survivors. The loss of a life by suicide brings a grief that cuts through the soul of the survivors. In the year 2000, the National Institute of Mental Health reported that suicide was the 11th cause of death in the United States, the 8th cause of death for all U.S. men, and the 19th cause for U.S. females. White men accounted for 73 percent of all suicides and 80 percent of all suicides using firearms. Approximately 1.3 percent of all deaths in the United States in 2000 were from suicide.[6]

It is a sobering fact that suicide causes more deaths than homicide; there are five suicide deaths for every three homicides. Further, there are twice as many deaths due to suicide than deaths caused by HIV/AIDS.

Women attempt suicide three times as frequently as men, but men are four times more likely to die by suicide than women. This is related to the fact that men use firearms more frequently, although the use of guns is increasing among women.

Suicide rates are highest among whites and second highest among American Indians and Native Alaskan men. In all ethnic groups, the frequency of suicides rises sharply for men over 60 years of age. At all ages, more white men kill themselves than black men, and fewer black females commit suicide than white females.

In 2005 the international World Health Organization estimated that approximately 1 million people will die by suicide every year and it is the third leading cause of death for both sexes. The worldwide mortality rate of suicide is 16 per 100,000 persons, or one suicide every 40 seconds. The number of suicides appears to be increasing; there has been about a 60 percent increase in suicides worldwide in the last 45 years. Fifty-five percent of suicides occur before 44 years of age. Forty-five percent of suicides occur after the age of 45, with a disproportionate number occurring after 65 years of age. Traditionally, suicide rates have been highest among elderly males, but the rates for young people have increased so much that youth are now the group at highest risk in a third of all countries.[7]

In the United States, it is estimated that there may be 8 to 25 attempted suicides for every suicide death, suggesting that between 250,000 and 790,000 persons actually attempt to kill themselves every year. The National Center for Injury Prevention and Control in the United States reported that 132,353 individuals were hospitalized following a suicide attempt in 2002 and another 116,639 were treated in emergency departments of hospitals and released. The primary method suicide in the United States is with a gun, and about 69 percent of all suicides have involved the use of firearms. Suffocation with gas (carbon monoxide) or plastic bags, poisoning, and jumping from high places rank next in frequency.[8]

In the past, most suicides occurred by jumping or falling. In ancient Greece, Sappho, who was widely acknowledged for her love poems, was abandoned by her lover, Phaon.[9] She then leaped from the Leucadian Cliffs, dressed in wedding attire, praying to the gods to spare her life. High places continue to attract many suicidal people. A prime setting in the United States is the Golden Gate Bridge in San Francisco. Over a thousand persons have leaped to their death from that bridge. Beachy Head in England, which has a sheer drop of 550 feet to the sea, is the site of even more suicides per year than the Golden Gate Bridge.[10] Other places include the Maiden Rock of the Sioux Indians, craters of certain Japanese volcanoes, some waterfalls on the Island of Bali, and almost any bridge or cliff available to these disheartened souls.

To kill one's self can be done in many ways, psychically as well as physically. Murder of the soul happens sometimes just by giving up awareness of one's desires or pleasures. Other times murder of the self can be seen in accidents, gambling, alcohol and drug abuse, and other self-destructive actions.

SUICIDE THROUGHOUT THE LIFE SPAN

Suicide in Children Ages 1–10

Case 1: Tommy

It seems unbelievable that children under the age of 10 can think about killing themselves, let alone succeed to suicide. Yet they can and do. I had an experience with a little boy that sobered and saddened me. Tommy killed himself when he was five years old. I first saw Tommy when he was nine months old. He was brought to the clinic by his parents for an evaluation of his developmental status. The father stated that Tommy was retarded and should be placed in an institution for disabled children. He emphasized that Tommy certainly did not belong in their home, not with the older boy, age six, who was so bright and intelligent.

Tommy was an appealing, even beautiful baby with a non-expressive look in his eyes. Sitting on the floor in my office, he did not look at his parents, the toys, or me. His parents left the room while I carried out the evaluation. Tommy did not acknowledge their leave-taking, not by a look or a change of expression. Gradually Tommy warmed up to me, would touch the toys, and then responded to the playful challenges of the evaluation material. Surprisingly, he scored well within the levels of normal development in memory, in fine motor skills, and in following simple instructions.

Thinking the parents would be pleased, I shared the results of the evaluation with them. The mother, a drably dressed and seemingly depressed woman smiled wanly. Tommy's father became dour and grumbled that something must be wrong.

The parents returned when Tommy was 18 months of age and again when he was about 30 months old. Each time Tommy displayed appropriate physical and intellectual development for his age, albeit the fact that he had limited emotional reactions. At 30 months of age, he was entered into the nursery school of the clinic for more extensive observation. Tommy was at first quite shy but soon ran eagerly into the schoolroom and began to play with the other children as well as with the toys. Three months later, his parents withdrew him.

At four years of age Tommy swallowed his mother's psychotropic pills, which she kept at her bedside. He was rushed to the hospital where the emergency team was successful in keeping him alive. A year later, he again took his mother's pills, still kept at her bedside. This time Tommy was more successful, for he could not be resuscitated. He had killed himself.

The constant message that Tommy had heard from his father was that he was unwanted, that he should not have been born, and that, if he took the pills again, he would die. The hostile rejection by his father and the severe failure of the mother to protect him gave Tommy the loud message that he should be dead. He did what his father and mother wished. He made himself dead.

Certainly the question of whether or not Tommy knew what being dead meant can be asked. We do know that to be dead meant to be "gone" for Tommy. It was a certainty that he was unwanted and that his father would like it if he were not there. Tommy accommodated his father's wish. The quality of the attachment of his parents toward Tommy failed to foster his life; his father had a malevolent attachment, and his mother had, at best, an ambivalent attachment to him. These non-supportive attachments are at the base of many a suicide.

In this case, and in other cases of severe physical or emotional abuse, the child lives in fear and tension. Always in danger, the child becomes hypersensitive. When withdrawal becomes the safest posture, intellectual as well as the emotional development is impaired. The child accepts the hostility coming from others and learns to hate himself.

Tommy presents an unusual case, but there have been many other instances when a child set about to kill himself or herself.[11] While there are not many statistics on self-killing under the age of 10, the National Center for Injury Prevention and Control reported in 2002 that there were at least 20 deaths by suicide for these ages.[12] Most reports of childhood suicide come from clinical studies, so many may be unreported.

For children ages 10–14, the known suicide rate is about 248 deaths per year. Within this number, there are three times as many boys as girls, a ratio that is typical for older ages.

The inner turmoil of the child may be expressed with unexplained irritability, inability to concentrate, anger, or rebelliousness. In one study of children at risk for suicide, it was found that "suicidal children had high levels of psychomotor activity, an intense preoccupation with death, and parents who had suicidal ideation."[13] A different reaction was seen in Tommy, with his subdued withdrawal that left him only a depleted inner and outer world. His traumatic dis-attachments occurred at such a young age, there was little energy left for expression of any anxiety. The risk of suicide increases if the child is depressed or there is unalleviated stress for the child in the home.

Another sensitive indicator that suggests suicide may be on the mind of the child arises from an unexplained experience with death, such as a parent's death, whether by illness, suicide, or abandonment. A frequent reaction for a child is guilt over the loss of the parent, if the child assumes the death came about because of his or her own anger or badness.[14] The guilt arises from an ambivalent attachment to and an ungratified need for security. Sometimes the child may so yearn for the parent's love that he or she expresses wishes to join the parent by death—and thus gain the affection that is longed for. In this case, the child introjects death as a solution for loss and a means to quiet guilt. It is important to note that the introjection is not an identification with the person who died but with the action of dying itself.

Later in life, the person may kill himself or herself in an anniversary reaction to the death. Anniversary reactions occur when an adolescent or adult kills himself or herself during a time symbolic of the death, whether at a similar age, a similar time of the year, a similar incident, and so forth. To avoid such trauma lingering in the psyche, it is imperative that the child receive nurturance and security following the death and be provided sufficient emotional care to relieve the turmoil that may permeate the child's psyche. Without these assurances, the sense of being abandoned and the pull toward death may supersede other defenses of the child.

A further sensitive sign of a possible suicidal intention is the child's preoccupation with death. Normally, children of five to seven years of age are curious about death and have many questions about it. When the questions are answered satisfactorily for the child, the curiosity is abated. However, when the theme of death persists in the child's reality, in fantasies, or in play, some psychological intervention is advisable. The child needs and deserves the emotional support and intellectual understanding given for his or her appropriate age level to free him or her from the anxieties provoked by the loss.

An additional sensitive indication concerns the child who, through his or her own illness or accident, comes close to death. This child has suffered a primal experience of death, at least on the unconscious level, that keeps him or her anxiously fighting death and psychologically fighting to live. This psychological suffering is also seen in instances of severe physical or emotional abuse, in which the child's psyche is fraught with fears of being killed and of dying.

There are not that many children who kill themselves at this young age; when it happens, adults are astounded. For the youngster, it was a life without hope.

Suicide during Adolescence and Young Adulthood

Case 2: Sonny

Fifteen-year-old Sonny left a note for his parents: "To Mom and Dad, I know your life will be easier without me. Love, Sonny." The next morning his parents found the note when they opened his bedroom door to awaken him for school. There he was, swinging on the end of a rope, dead. Sonny's parents recalled that he had been unusually sweet the night before. He kissed them goodnight, told them that he loved them, and instructed his younger brother and sister to be good to their mother and father.

Sonny was a good boy. Intelligent and excelling at school, he seemed motivated for college and a profession. He was a quiet, studious child who never was into trouble—no smoking, drinking, or drugs. Sonny's parents were professional persons with a marriage that was contentious, competitive, and unsatisfying. Not only were the parents driven to achieve, they placed high expectations on the three children—Sonny (age 15), Kay (age 12), and Ron (age 8). To others, the family appeared as a cohesive, normally functioning family. But no one was happy.

Sonny was an unwanted child, conceived before the marriage of his parents. His mother was in graduate school at that time and was determined to continue her studies. After Sonny's birth, she left his care to babysitters and his father. Sonny grew up hungry for his mother's nurturance and love. She described him as a child who was always clinging to her. Sonny had been a lonely child, without friends. In high school, his loneliness increased, but his mother assured him that was to be expected. He killed himself during his sophomore year.

Sonny's suicide could have been prevented. From birth, Sonny suffered from the lack of a secure, nurturing bond with his parents. He could only react to his mother's rejection and his father's benign neglect. He suffered the cold, inner isolation that resulted from the lack of a warm, responsive mother who would provide a life-giving mirror of himself. There was no substance, no picture of himself in his inner being. That is, without the introjection of a constant, life-giving image of himself reflected back from another, his inner sense of self was empty, a nothingness. By adolescence, the inner emptiness was too much to bear, and death seemed more giving that life.

The attachment of his mother to Sonny was a negative attachment, if not actually a malevolent one. Andre Green described this type of mothering quite aptly. He wrote, "The non-presence of the mother becomes an object, if you will, one tenaciously occupying a central position in the child's psyche. Non-existence is paradoxically therefore the most intense psychological experience of the child."[15] The failure of attachment is often found in suicidal cases.

Sonny is one of a multitude of youth that kill themselves, youth who are unable to face the future with hope. Suicide is the third leading cause of death for adolescents, following unintentional injuries and homicide. In 2003 the suicide rate was 8.2 deaths per 100,000 teenagers age 15–19. There were five times as many males as females. The rate increases to 12.8 per 100,000 for 20–24 years of age with seven times as many males as females killing themselves.[16]

Adolescence is a challenging, often stressful period. It brings many changes for the young person—within the self, in the family, and in the sociocultural setting. Periods of emotional vacillation are frequent, and mood swings are normal. As self-awareness increases, it stimulates changes in the self-concept and heightens the perception of social relatedness. When the stress overwhelms the psychological strengths, it may damage the perception of the person and his or her relationships with others. The young person may pull away from stress through rebelling, running away, or drowning himself or herself in alcohol or drugs—all are a kind of self-demolition. When fear and anxiety are too oppressive and he or she pulls back into himself or herself, the withdrawal can be a foreboding of a depressive reaction; the ultimate withdrawal from inner turmoil is death, or suicide.

The special circumstances and emotional signs that can be used to identify those adolescents who may be prone to suicide include social isolation from family or friends, a dearth of personal attachments, and the lack of coping skills for everyday problems. The adolescent's most intense need is for a warm connection to others; and if the adolescent does not find it with parents, he or she seeks it with friends.

Suicide in Adulthood

Shneidman writes, "What is suicide but a damp and dismal November in the mind?"[17] Suicide marks a failure in the struggle for life and an inability to solve the problems that arise. The rate of suicide for the ages of 30 through 70 remains fairly stable, averaging about 6.97 deaths per 100,000 persons. It exists as a major health problem throughout the world. The reported rate of suicide varies from 6.4 per 100,000 in Mexico to 15.1 in the United Kingdom and 82.5 in the Russian Federation. The World Health Organization reports that there is about one suicide every 40 seconds and an attempted suicide every three seconds.[18] These statistics are startling and reveal that for many, inner distress makes death more inviting than life. The unsuccessful attempts may be tests that permit some chance of living. Among other tests-to-live are such suicidal behaviors as chronic alcoholism or substance abuse, pathological gambling, death-defying sports, reckless driving, playing roulette, and self-mutilation.[19]

Clinicians report that about 90 percent of suicidal persons merit the diagnosis of depression, bipolar disorder, or schizophrenia. Very often the diagnosis is given after death and may provide some comfort for the survivors but provide little insight into the act. The internal darkness of the suicidal person remains unexplained except that death was more inviting than life.

Situations that lead to self-killing represent personal conflicts and problem situations that appear common enough. Yet these persons feel problems are not resolvable and life cannot go on. The problems include (1) personal situations such as interpersonal losses or conflicts, a sense of isolation, a family history of suicide, a childhood history of physical or sexual abuse, or serious illnesses; (2) situational events with shame over an event, financial difficulties, or job problems; (3) personality factors such as hopelessness, violence, aggression, low self-esteem, depression, or preoccupations with dying; and (4) neurochemical factors such as a low cerebrospinal 5-hydroxyindolacetic acid level, low cholesterol levels, and physical illness.

The following excerpts from a few suicide notes illustrate some last thoughts of the suicidal person:

"All I do is suffer each and every day. Every moment is pain or numbness. How long can one go on without pleasure?"[20]

"It is a love of death that sickens everything."[21]

"Death, you lie in my arms like a cherub, as heavy as bread dough."[22]

"I have a feeling I shall go mad. I cannot go on longer in these terrible times. I shant recover this time. I hear voices and cannot concentrate on my work."[23]

"I must end it. There's no hope left. I'll be at peace. No one has anything to do with this."[24]

"When all usefulness is over, when one is assured of an unavoidable and imminent death, it is the simplest of human rights to choose a quick and easy death in place of a slow and horrible one." [25]

"Everyone seems so happy and I am so alone. . . . I'm so tired and lonely."[26]

It is apparent that each of these notes speaks of the agony of the soul, whether it is loss of love, hopelessness, illness, loneliness, or even revenge.

There are some indicators of a potential suicide that can alert others to the tragic action and apply particularly when more than one factor is present.[27] These include (1) a previous attempt or fantasized suicide; (2) anxiety, depression, exhaustion, or pervasive hopelessness; (3) availability of lethal methods; (4) expressed concern for the effect of suicide on family members; (5) preparation of a will and resignation after a prolonged, agitated depression; (6) a life crisis, such as illness or mourning for a loss; (7) a family history of suicide.

Suicide in Older Adults

How can we escape from you, life, except through death?

Our sorrows are endless. Endure? Escape?[28]

Death creeps closer with age. People think more often of dying as they become older and face the challenges that aging brings. Suicide is a way of hastening inevitable death. Although individuals over 65 make up 13 percent of the U.S. population, they account for 18 percent of all suicides. A demographic group with one of the highest rates of suicide is white men age 85 or older; there were 59 deaths per 100,000 in 2002 for this age group. This is more than five times the national rate of 10.6 per 100,000.[29]

Depression besets many an older adult.[30] It is estimated that about 2 million Americans age 65 and older have a depressive illness. Another 5 million have subsyndromal depression with some symptoms but not enough to meet the criteria for a full depressive disorder. Seven million of 35 million Americans over 65, or 20 percent, can be identified as depressed. Depression may occur concomitantly with a serious illness or may be a reaction to an illness. Since depression may be a forerunner of suicide, it is important that it be recognized and treated although the signs are often difficult to identify, even for physicians. While despair of life seems to increase in the aging population, depression is not a normal part of aging. The normal emotional expressions of sadness, grief, loss, and passing mood states are not indications of depression. Only when the sad, hopeless feelings become chronic and interfere with the individual's ability to function can a diagnosis of depression be considered.

The reasons for the increase of suicide in older aged persons are sad but understandable. Life becomes more difficult physically, psychologically, and socially as the older person is faced with more adjustments than before. Normal aging itself brings physical changes and a decrease in physical energy. Changes in social roles, retirement from employment, and economic worries loom larger, especially with burgeoning costs of medical care. Independence is lost, and a reliance on others becomes necessary. The lifelong accumulation of stress takes its toll and diminishes coping skills. Older people may find a weakening of the ability to handle anxiety as their ego becomes wearied and the ability to control their own lives lessens. Fears brought on by dependency and illnesses overshadow the pleasure of living. Despair may accompany the serious illnesses of age—such as heart diseases, stroke, diabetes, cancer, Parkinson's disease, and various forms of dementia.

Mostly, loneliness is an important factor. Loneliness as stark as winter cold and unbearable for many overwhelms the person as he or she is beset by loss of a spouse, family, and friends, and with them, the loss of affection and intimacy. The meaningfulness of living deliquesces.

A gradual fatigue of the ego occurs, and the social world becomes less appealing as capabilities decrease. The future holds the picture of aloneness, of illness, and of death. For many, death becomes a welcome friend. Sometimes sufficient aggressive energy remains to enable older people to take death into their own hands.

I remember the death of Bruno Bettelheim, a renowned psychotherapist for seriously disturbed children. Bedridden in a nursing home, beset by strokes, he nevertheless did not want to waste away to death. He saved some sleeping pills and then one night placed a plastic bag over his head and smothered himself to death. I compare this with my mother who also was in a nursing home for the last three months of her life. She was comatose for much of the day, but when I asked her about dying, she thought a minute and responded, "I want to die the natural way." Her sense of herself and her ego was strong enough even in the last couple days of her life to choose to experience a "natural" death. Her attachment to life was secure.

THE MORALITY OF SUICIDE

The dialogue among philosophers, social scientists, ethicists, mental health professionals, sociologists, and theologians has been continuous throughout the known history of mankind. The questions seem to focus on the following: (1) What is suicide? (2) Does a person have a right to take his or her own life? (3) Is it in accord with the rules of nature to kill one's self? (4) What is the damage incurred by others and by society with suicide?[31]

Suicide is generally defined as any self-caused death, whatever the reasons or means of self-killing. But, consider, if suicide has an ulterior motive, is it then suicide? If killing one's self has a different reason other than death itself, is it suicide? What if the suicide has the purpose of relieving physical pain, or release from psychological anguish, or revenge against or punishment of another, or martyrdom, or the service of apolitical or religious cause, or protection of someone else, and so forth? For our purpose, suicide is considered a voluntary death committed at one's own volition in a manner chosen by that person.

Philosophical discourses about suicide in our Western world often begin with the writings of Plato. Plato was convinced that suicide was wrong and suggested that individuals who commit suicide should be forbidden an honorable funeral and be buried without recognition in an isolated spot.[32]

Aristotle condemned suicide as an offense against not only the self but also against society. A suicide damages the welfare of the community because of the loss of a contributing member. To Aristotle, suicide is an act of cowardice that reneges on the responsibilities of life.[33]

The precepts governing suicide in ancient Greece were clear: "Whoever no longer wishes to live shall state his reasons to the Senate, and after having received permission shall abandon life. If your existence is hateful to you, die; if you are overwhelmed by fate, drink the hemlock. If you are bowed with grief, abandon life. Let the unhappy man recount his misfortune, let the magistrate supply him with the remedy, and his wretchedness will come to an end."[34]

The Cyrenaic and Epicurean philosophies (ca. 400 B.C.–270 B.C.) encouraged the person to make a decision about suicide without fears of the afterlife. One Cyrenaic, Hegasus, was expelled from Egypt because he successfully persuaded too many young people that suicidal death was preferable to life. Hegasus's attitude foretells the justification of suicide by martyrs who kill themselves for a cause—political or religious.

The Roman approach was more liberal and applauded suicide as an act of honor under certain circumstances. There were many Roman leaders who did choose to kill themselves; among them were Brutus, Crasus, Gracchus, Cato, Lucretia, Antony, Cleopatra, Nerva, Seneca, Nero, and Calpurnicus.

Attitudes about suicide changed with Christianity. Beginning with Augustine, suicide was a sin for which a person could not repent. Thomas of Aquinas supported Augustine's reasoning based on three principles: suicide is contrary to natural self-love; life is a gift given by God, therefore is sacred; and, as God is the giver of life, God alone can determine how long we should live.

Because suicide was seen as sin, the bodies of those who killed themselves were often desecrated, they were not permitted a burial in the community or church cemeteries, and survivors often lost any claim to the goods and possessions of the person. The traditional Christian view lasted well into the 17th century with few exceptions. Two notable exceptions were Thomas More and David Hume.[35]

In the late 16th–17th century, the rigidity of the Christian view that the devil and the suicidal person were in cahoots was questioned. John Donne, an Anglican bishop, wrote a book entitled *Biathanatos: A Declaration of that Paradoxe, or Thesis, that Self-homicide is not so naturally Sinne that it may never be otherwise,* in which he reasoned that suicide was not contrary to the laws of nature, of reason, or of God, because there is no clear condemnation of suicide in the Bible itself ; because other forms of self-killing were acceptable, such as martyrdom. or wartime killing. Shakespeare included about 52 suicides in his writing.

Present Views of Suicide

Many well-known and seemingly successful individuals from all walks of life have killed themselves, such as Virginia Woolf, Marilyn Monroe, Ernest Hemingway, Sylvia Plath, Anne Sexton, Admiral Boorda, Kurt Cobain, and Freddie Prinz. Morality no longer seems to be the question. In the late 19th and then in the 20th century, psychological sciences were beginning an intensive study of the effect of experiences on human life. The concern about suicide focused on the individual and the circumstances of the suicide. Among notable contributions were the works of Sigmund Freud, as he investigated the conscious and unconscious determinants of behavior. While Freud did not specifically attend to the problem of suicide, his contributions changed the direction of investigations. He wrote,

> There is no need to think such self-destruction rare, for the trend to self-destruction is present to a certain degree in very many more human beings than those in whom it is carried out. Self-injuries are, as a rule, a compromise between this instinct and the forces that are still working against it, and even when suicide actually results the

inclination to suicide will have been present for a long time before in less strength or in the form of an unconscious and suppressed trend.... Even a conscious intention of committing suicide chooses its times, means and opportunity.[36]

In the book *Man against Himself*, Karl Menninger dramatically pictured how an individual can be his own worst enemy. He asserted that unconscious motives, as well as conscious wishes, play a significant role in self-destructive behavior—from incidental accidents, to avoidable actions (as self-mutilation), to suicide. Menninger suggested that suicide included three basic elements: "There is the element of dying, the element of killing, and the element of being killed. Each is a condensation for which there exist complexes of motive, conscious and unconscious."[37]

It would be impossible to look at suicide without recognition of the contributions of Edwin Shneidman and his associates. After a lifetime of study, research, and therapy with suicidal persons, Shneidman's contributions have had worldwide reverberations. As a young psychologist, he was sent, serendipitously, to get some information about two patients who had committed suicide. Reading a suicide note left by one patient, he was challenged to understand the factors that led to suicide. He became intensely involved with the problems leading to killing one's self. In 1958, Shneidman, with his associates Norman Farberow, Robert Litman, and others, established the Los Angeles Suicide Prevention Center. It was a multidisciplinary crisis center that focused on providing immediate support and intervention to those persons considering suicide. These crisis centers now exist in most cities and throughout the world and are usually open 24 hours a day, 7 days a week.

His research identified the field of suicidology as an area of study in its own right. Suicide, to him, is the result of psychological pain; it is a matter of the mind. Shneidman was in agreement with Alfred Alvarez, who thinks that suicide is "a terrible but utterly natural reaction to the strained, narrow, unnatural necessities we sometimes create for ourselves."[38]

In a chapter entitled "This I Believe," Shneidman categorized four clusters of frustrated psychological needs that may underlie the tormented mind of the suicidal person:

1. Thwarted love, acceptance or belonging;
2. Fractured control, excessive helplessness and frustration;
3. Assaulted self-image and avoidance of shame, defeat humiliation and disgrace;
4. Ruptured key relationships and attendant grief and bereftness.[39]

The repeated theme of these needs points in the direction of damaged attachment bonds between the suicidal person and another.

The research into suicide has multiplied many times over these last fifty years. The areas of study have included the impact of gender, marriage, dysfunctional families, economic failures, and psychological illnesses on suicide.

DEPRESSION, MENTAL ILLNESS, AND SUICIDE

In the past few years, depression and other mental illnesses have been regarded as responsible for 95 percent of all suicides. Eighty percent of persons attempting suicide have the diagnosis of depression; another 10 percent have the diagnosis of schizophrenia. For persons with a diagnosis of depression, 15 percent are at risk for suicide; for those with an impulsive behavior, about 25 percent. In addition, about 25 percent of all depressives are alcohol-dependent, and this increases the possibility of suicidal attempts.[40]

Some researchers have suggested a genetic relationship with suicide, for often the risk of suicide is greater among those persons who have had a family member commit suicide. For example, there are quality studies suggesting a metabolic problem associated with suicides. A serotonin deficiency, which is a decrease in the metabolism of 5-hydroxyindoleacetic acid (5-HIAA), appeared in a group of patients who attempted suicide. The study reported that those who had used violent means to attempt suicide had a lower 5-HIAA level in the cerebrospinal fluid than did the depressed patients who were not suicidal.[41] Other studies have identified possible additional neurochemical contributors. However, there has been no conclusive evidence as of yet.

Another contemporary topic receiving much attention is the relationship between medications prescribed for depression and their potential role in compelling a person toward suicide. Again, while the U.S. Food and Drug Administration has responded with warnings about the need to take additional care in using the medications, especially for young persons, the evidence for these medications causing self-homicide has not been conclusive.

Some factors that put people at risk for attempted suicide include chronic depression, alcohol abuse or cocaine use, death of a partner, and separation or divorce.[42] The behaviors regarded as symptomatic of a person who is considering suicide include (1) a previous attempt at suicide; (2) severe anxiety or depression; (3) easy availability of firearms, medication, or other self-destructive means; (4) concern for the effect of suicide on family members; (5) verbalized suicidal threats or plans; (6) preparation of a will; (7) impending or recurrent life crises; (8) a family history of suicide; and, (9) pervasive pessimism or hopelessness.

Although these behaviors describe some observable characteristics of a suicidal person, most people endure life's pressures without suicide. The list does provide some awareness of the depth of distress of a person, but it needs to be used with caution, as a signal only. To rely on the results of present research, whether psychological or physiological, for the answer to the reasons behind suicide negates the individual and his or her unique situation. Diagnoses may alleviate the concern of a professional and some distress of the survivors, but neither is really satisfied. Shneidman stated, "Nowadays, the gambit used to make a field appear scientific is to redefine what is being discussed. The most flagrant current example is to convert the study of suicide, almost by sleight of hand, into a discussion of depression—two very different things. (One can lead a long unhappy life with depression, but acute suicidality is often quickly fatal.)"[43]

There is almost no worse experience for the psychotherapist than to have a patient who kills himself or herself. Even worse is the anguish of the survivors, for it is never really abated—and there are at least six significant survivors for each suicide. To live and to struggle with the loss through a suicide is to mourn and to grieve for life itself.

I leave this discussion with a question: Could there be a death drive that is activated by psychological and/or physiological circumstances?

THE INSTIGATION TO SUICIDE

It is reported that the psychoanalyst Otto Will warned, "In cases of suicide, ask who wanted the patient dead."[44] In reviewing the social relationships of the suicidal person, attention has been given to the suicides within dysfunctional families, perturbed marriages, and the loss of love. The problem of intimate attachments has, however, received little analysis. In the book *Fatal Attachments: The Instigation to Suicide*, I investigate the attachment patterns of those who do kill themselves, but more importantly of the person behind the suicide, that is, of the instigator.[45] It seems almost unreal that one would bring about the suicide or death of another, yet it is not uncommon. The common expression "Drop dead" is usually spoken in jest but is sometimes seriously intended. More frequent are the unspoken wishes that something should happen to take that person out of one's life. The instigator is a person who abets the suicidal act because of his own anxieties for life.

Instigation may be conscious or unconscious, overt or silent. Margaret Little identifies the dynamics of the instigators, although she is speaking of the suicidal person. She writes, "These patients are people who cannot in any circumstances take survival for granted. There exists in their unconscious memories and experiences of something which we must really regard as annihilation; in many cases there has been in early infancy some actual threat to life—illness of the infant or mother, hostility in the environment, . . ."[46] With instigators, their expectancy of annihilation or death is projected onto others, usually the person who is psychologically the nearest or dearest to them. The suicide of the other provides the instigator with a sense of power—over life—and temporarily allays the fears of his or her own demise. In turn, the suicidal person, seeking the love and the existential power of the instigator, introjects the death drive and acts out the suicide.

Little continues, "The fear of annihilation, however, is dynamic and all-pervading and therefore governs the patient's reactions and his behavior. . . . By reason of the life-and-death quality of the patient's experience, his concrete thinking and inability to make deductions, and the fact that events belonging to earliest infancy are being lived out in a grown-up body . . . contain a large element of actual danger (suicide, death or attack upon someone)."[47] This is the danger facing the instigator and makes for disturbed, pathological relationships with others.

Mecke identifies four types of instigators, individuals whose psyches have been so overpowered by an early experience with death that their own existence is strengthened through projection of death fears and wishes onto others.

Active external instigators deliberately incite suicide in another. For instance, the case of Tommy, whose father wanted him dead, can only be understood by an analysis of the background of Tommy's father. Tommy's father had been abandoned by his parents when an infant. He was left on a church doorstep when he became ill while his parents were escaping the Nazi scourge. The parents determined that the sick child's crying could put them in danger. Yet Tommy's father lived, with the anxiety of death pervading his unconscious, enlivened by his infantile illness and the abandonment by his parents. Tommy's father relived his death anxiety through Tommy's suicide and empowered his own will to live.

There are *passive external instigators*, who incite suicide consciously or unconsciously. They project the wish for another's death. Their mode of relating involves rejection, withdrawal, or abandonment from the person who is close to or intimate with them. The cold withdrawal is a defensive reaction against the intimacy that evokes their earlier anxieties about death. Seeking to regain the closeness, the suicidal person assimilates the death trauma and acts it out.

The *internal instigator* develops through identification with the death of a significant person during his or her childhood. For instance, if the death of a parent early in the life of the instigator is traumatic, it may result in an almost persecutory obsession with death. Usually the relationship was a problematic attachment. The suicidal act is a feeble attempt to correct the ungratified attachment and reconnect through death.

Provocateur instigators are external instigators whose angry push for another's death justifies their own existence. These instigators actively goad the social conscience and sabotage the life of others. This category includes cult death leaders, terrorist instigators, and others who use the person as a pawn.

The fatal attachment is defined by pathological relationship patterns that exist between the instigator and the suicide victim, and in reciprocal manner, from the victim to the instigator. The attachment patterns include malevolent attachments, negative attachments, nullified attachments, fantasized relationships, ambivalent attachments, self-attachments, usurped attachments, and exploitative attachment patterns.[48]

The suicidal person is really a victim—a victim of his or her own tortured mind when expected attachments have failed or been denied to him or her. True, the attachment that the person desires is not available, for it lingers from ungratified infantile longing for closeness. Suffering from the early loss of a positive, nurturing attachment and idealistically seeking it, the suicidal person tends to bond with someone whose own sense of survival is gained by the power of life over another.

PREVENTION OF SUICIDE

The first line of prevention of suicide would be to erase the personal, social, economic, and biological factors that play such a large part in making a person despondent. That herculean effort would include elimination of conditions such as poverty, divorce, and availability of instruments of violence followed by the development of a healthier lifestyle for the individual.

The next line of prevention would be to identify the person prone to suicide and to provide him or her the necessary therapeutic guidance to enhance his or her living and alleviate psychic pain. Alerting the suicidal person's social support system to the distress of the suicidal person would imply an intense commitment on the support system's part to deal with the failed attachment bonds. Psychotherapy is a sine qua non for recovering a pleasure in living; while it cannot replace a social support system, the therapist can alleviate the suicidal person's psychic pain and redirect him or her toward life.

THERAPEUTIC INTERVENTIONS

There is no doubt that there is help for the person who is in a crisis of suicide. First and foremost, it is important to recognize that the desperateness of the person is real and not an artifact of seeking attention. There are crisis hotlines in almost every city.

Psychotherapy with or without medication is effective and helps people through these critical and painful periods. There are different styles of psychotherapy, all of which provide benefits to the individual. In his book *An Autopsy of a Suicidal Mind*, Shneidman asked seven renowned psychotherapists to analyze a suicide letter written by a young medical doctor, age 33.[49] These therapists included psychiatrists—Robert Litman, John Maltsberger, Jerome Motto, Morton Silverman, and Avery Weisman; psychologists—Norman Farberow and David Rudd; and a sociologist—Ronald Maris. All are noted experts in the field of suicidology.[50] The eight therapists wrote from the unique perspective of suicidology, which included a *developmental* perspective that investigates the psychache as it developed throughout childhood and adolescence; a *crisis approach* in which the person gains a more positive outlook on current psychic or real-life distress; the *etiological* view that delineates how present and past problems led to feelings of suicide; a *family* perspective in which the dynamics of family interaction that led to such severe psychache are explored; a *psychoanalytic* view that analyzes the origins of feelings and reactions to life events; a *biological* view that speaks of the physiological causes underlying crises situations; and, a *cognitive psychology* approach that focuses on changing moods and thoughts in order to alter the person's approach to a crisis. Each therapist expressed a high degree of confidence that the approach could offer help for the psychache, could alleviate the troubled mind, and could provide hope and gratification for life itself. It behooves the person considering suicide to find a psychotherapist who can respond to his or her distress and own way of understanding life problems. As Shneidman emphasizes, the aim of therapy should be first of all to reduce the psychic pain, then to guarantee the inviolacy of the person so that he or she finds a "safe self" that includes the ability to protect the self, to remain separate and independent and not intruded upon by others. Finally, the goal is to help the person accept his or her pain as part of life and to aid him or her in the search for succor and acceptance.

NOTES

1. The term "psychache," used to describe the agony of the person, was introduced by Edwin Shneidman in "Suicide as Psychache," *Journal of Nervous and Mental Disease* 131 (1993): 147–49.

2. Sylvia Plath, *Sylvia Plath: The Collected Poems* (New York: HarperPerennial, 1981), 181.

3. Edwin Shneidman, *Comprehending Suicide. Landmarks in 20th Century Suicidology* (Washington, DC: American Psychology Association, 2001), 201.

4. Ibid., 202.

5. *The Shorter Oxford English Dictionary*, 3rd ed., ed. C. T. Onions (Oxford: Clarendon Press, 1977), s.v. "victim."

6. The following statistics are taken from a publication of The National Institute of Mental Health, "In Harm's Way: Suicide in America. A Brief Overview of Suicide Statistics and Prevention," National Institute of Mental Health, retrieved April 21, 2006 from http://www.nimh.nih.gov/publicat/harmsway.cfm.

7. World Health Organization, "Mental Health: Suicide Rates per 100,000 by Country, Year, and Sex," retrieved April 21, 2006 from http://www.who.int/mental_health/prevention/suicide_rates/en/.

8. The National Center for Injury Prevention and Control, "Suicide Prevention Strategies and Links," http://www.cdc.gov/ncipe/wisqars/fatal/help/helpfile.htm.

9. For the story of Sappho and Phaon, the reader is referred to J. A. Symonds, *The Greek Poets* (New York: Harper & Brothers, 1901), p. 308.

10. Simon Fanshawe, "Children on a Field Trip Understood the Suicidal Lure of Beachy Head," *San Francisco Chronicle*, January 24, 1999.

11. For further information on child suicides, the reader is referred to Cynthia R. Pfeffer, *The Suicidal Child* (New York: Guilford Press, 1986).

12. Office of Statistics and Programming, National Center for Health Statistics, Center for Disease Control and Prevention Data Source: Vital Statistics of the United States, www.cdc.gov/nchs/fastats/suicide.htm.

13. C. R. Pfeffer and others, "Suicidal Behavior in Latency-Age Children: An Outpatient Population," *Journal of the American Academy of Child Psychiatry* 19 (1980): 704.

14. C. R. Pfeffer and others, "Suicidal Behavior in Child Psychiatric Inpatients and Outpatients and in Nonpatients," in *Essential Papers on Suicide*, ed. John T. Maltsberger, MD, and Mark J. Goldblatt, MD (New York: New York University Press, 1996), 562–73.

15. Barbara Stimmel, review of *The Dead Mother: The Work of Andre Green*, ed. Gregorio Kohon, *Psychologist-Psychoanalyst* 24, no. 2 (Spring 2004): 48.

16. For these statistics, refer to National Institute of Mental Health, "In Harm's Way: Suicide in America" (see note 6).

17. Edwin Shneidman, *Autopsy of a Suicidal Mind* (Oxford: Oxford University Press, 2004), 160.

18. World Health Organization, "Mental Health Global Action Programme (MHGAP)," http://www.who.int/metal_health/actionprogramme/en/index.html.

19. R. W. Maris, "Suicide," *Lancet* 360 (2002): 319–26.

20. This quote is taken from a suicide letter written by a young medical doctor and reported in Shneidman, *Autopsy of a Suicidal Mind*, 165.

21. Plath, *Sylvia Plath: The Collected Poems*, 181.

22. Anne Sexton, *The Complete Poems*. Boston: Houghton Mifflin, 1981), 357.

23. Virginia Woolf, "Virginia Woolf, 1882–1941," retrieved April 21, 2006 from www.classic-shorts.com/bios/biowoolf.html.

24. Freddie Prinz, "Brain Candy Celebrity Quotes: Dying Words," retrieved April 21, 2006 from www.corsinet.com/braincandy/dying3.html.

25. Charlotte Gilman, Gilman was a writer who chose to die by chloroform rather than to die by cancer. Available from "Brain Candy Celebrity Quotes: Dying Words," retrieved April 21, 2006 from www.corsinet.com/braincandy/dying3.html.

26. This note and the following were selected from suicide notes collected by Art Kleiner at a coroner's office. "Suicide Notes," http://www.well.com/user/art/ suicidenotes.html.

27. H.I. Kaplan and B.J. Saddock, "Psychiatric Emergencies," in *Synopsis of Psychiatry, Behavioral Sciences/Clinical Psychiatry* (Philadelphia: Lippincott, Williams & Wilkins, 1998), 871.

28. Aisopos (a 4th century A.D. poet), "Aesop's Fables," in *Greek Lyric Poetry*, trans. Willis Barnstone (New York: Schocken Books, 1967), 231.

29. National Institute of Mental Health, "In Harm's Way: Suicide in America" (see note 6).

30. The reader is referred to the information that follows: "Older Adults: Depression and Suicide Facts" as reported in Medical Moments, http://www.medicalmoment .org/_content/risks/dec03/187856.asp.

31. I do not attempt to cover the rich history of the philosophy of, attitudes about, and resulting actions from suicide. There are excellent books that provide thoughtful overviews and analyses of the cultural responses to suicide, including *The Savage God: A Study of Suicide* (see note 33) and George Minois, *History of Suicide: Voluntary Death in Western Culture* (Baltimore: Johns Hopkins University Press, 1995).

32. Plato, *The Laws*, trans. Loeb Classical Library (Cambridge, MA: Harvard University Press, 1989), ch. 9.873C.203.

33. Aristotle, "The Nicomachean Ethics," trans. W. D. Ross, *The Internet Classics Archive*,, http://www.classics.mit.edu/Aristotle/nichomachaen.html.

34. Libanius, quoted in Alfred Alvarez, *The Savage God: A Study of Suicide* (New York: W. W. Norton and Company, 1990), 79.

35. As found in Gary B. Ferngren, "The Ethics of Suicide in the Renaissance and Reformation," in *Suicide and Euthanasia: Historical and Contemporary Themes*, ed. B. Brody (Dordrecht, The Netherlands: Kluwer, 1989), 160–61.

36. Sigmund Freud, *Standard Edition of the Complete Psychological Works*, vol. 6 (London: Hogarth Press, 1953–1965), 178–85 (quotation from 1901).

37. Karl Menninger, *Man against Himself* (New York: Harcourt, Brace and World, 1938), 5.

38. Alvarez, *The Savage God: A Study of Suicide*, p. 11.

39. Shneidman, *Comprehending Suicide*, 202–3.

40. Kaplan and Saddock, *The Synopsis of Psychiatry*, 870.

41. This is an area of research that is under intense investigation now. The source for this information came from M. Asberg, L. Traskman, and P. Thoren, "5-HIAA in the Cerebrospinal Fluid: A Biochemical Suicide Predictor?" in John T. Maltsberger and Mark L. Goldblatt, *Essential Papers on Suicide*, 342–55.

42. Office of Statistics and Programming, NCIPC, CDC. Web-Based Injury Statistics Query and Reporting System (WISQARS). Center for Disease Prevention, "Healthy Youth! Health

Topics: Injury and Violence (Including Suicide)," *Center for Disease Prevention*, http://www.cdc.gov/healthyouth/injury/index.htm. ; Kaplan and Saddock, Table 33.1–1 Factors Associated with Suicide Risk, 870; Suicide and Mental Health Association International, "Worldwide Suicide Information," *Suicide and Mental Health Association International*, http://suicideandmentalhealthassociationinternational.org/about.html.

43. Shneidman, *Comprehending Suicide*, 200.
44. This quote by Otto Will is taken from Shneidman's foreword to Maltsberger and Goldblatt, *Essential Papers on Suicide*, 6.
45. Please refer to Viola Mecke, *Fatal Attachments: The Instigation to Suicide* (New York: Praeger, 2004) for case histories and intensive analyses of the role of instigators in suicide.
46. Margaret Little, "On Basic Unity (Primary Total Undifferentiatedness)," in *The British School of Psychoanalysis: The Independent Tradition*, ed. Gregorio Kohon. (New Haven, CT: Yale University Press, 1986), 136.
47. Ibid., 139.
48. Each of these attachment patterns are discussed and exemplified in *Fatal Attachments: The Instigation to Suicide*, chapter 4.
49. Shneidman, *Autopsy of a Suicidal Mind*, p. 200.
50. Ibid., 202.

BIBLIOGRAPHY

Aisopos. "Aesop's Fables." In *Greek Lyric Poetry*. Translated by Willis Barnstone. New York: Schocken Books, 1967.

Alvarez, Alfred. *The Savage God: A Study of Suicide*. New York: W.W. Norton and Company, 1990).

Baechler, J. (1979). Suicides. Oxford: Blackwell Publications) Canadian Association for Suicide Prevention (October 2004) Blue Print for a Canadian National Suicide Prevention Strategy. Canadian Association for Suicide Prevention. <Prevention@suicideprevention.ca>

Fanshawe, Simon. "Children on a Field Trip Understood the Suicidal Lure of Beachy Head." *San Francisco Chronicle*, January 24, 1999.

Ferngren, Gary B. "The Ethics of Suicide in the Renaissance and Reformation." In *Suicide and Euthanasia: Historical and Contemporary Themes*, edited by B. Brody, 160–61. Dordrecht, The Netherlands: Kluwer, 1989. Freud, Sigmund. *Standard Edition of theComplete Psychological Works*. Vol. 6. London: Hogarth Press, 1953–1965.

Kaplan, H.I., and B.J. Saddock. "Psychiatric Emergencies." In *Synopsis of Psychiatry, Behavioral Sciences/Clinical Psychiatry*, 8th ed. Philadelphia: Lippincott, Williams & Wilkins, 1998.

Little, Margaret. "On Basic Unity (Primary Total Undifferentiatedness)." In *The British School of Psychoanalysis: The Independent Tradition*, edited by Gregorio Kohon. New Haven, CT: Yale University Press, 1986.

Maris, Ronald W. "Suicide." *Lancet* 360 (2002): 319–26.

Mecke, Viola. *Fatal Attachments: The Instigation to Suicide.* New York: Praeger, 2004.

Menninger, Karl. *Man Against Himself.* New York: Harcourt, Brace & World, 1938.

Minois, George. *History of Suicide: Voluntary Death in Western Culture.* Baltimore: Johns Hopkins University Press, 1995.

Pfeffer, C. R. *The Suicidal Child.* New York: Guilford Press, 1986.

Pfeffer, C. R., Herbert R. Conte, and Robert Plutchik. "Suicidal Behavior in Latency-Age Children: An Outpatient Population." *Journal of the American Academy of Child Psychiatry* 19 (1980): 703–10.

Pfeffer, Cynthia R., Robert Plutchik, Mark Mizruchi, and Robert Lipkins. "Suicidal Behavior in Child Psychiatric Inpatients and Outpatients and in Nonpatients." In *Essential Papers on Suicide,* edited by John T. Maltsberger, MD, and Mark J. Goldblatt, MD, 562–73. New York: New York University Press, 1996.

Plath, Sylvia. *Sylvia Plath: The Collected Poems.* New York: HarperPerennial, 1981.

Plato. *The Laws.* Translated by Loeb Classical Library. Cambridge, MA: Harvard University Press, 1989.

Sexton, Anne. *The Complete Poems.* Boston: Houghton Mifflin, 1981).

Shneidman, Edwin. *Autopsy of a Suicidal Mind.* Oxford: Oxford University Press, 2004).

———. *Comprehending Suicide. Landmarks in 20th Century Suicidology.* Washington, DC: American Psychology Association, 2001.

———. "Suicide as Psychache." *Journal of Nervous and Mental Disease* 131 (1993): 147–49.

Symonds, J. A. *The Greek Poets.* New York: Harper & Brothers, 1901.

Chapter 9

Helping Adolescents with Self-Injurious Behavior: Cutting in Developmental Context

Lori Goldfarb Plante

Self-injurious behavior such as the cutting and burning of one's skin is an increasingly prevalent phenomenon among adolescents with a range of difficulties and diagnoses.[1,2] Self-injurious behavior involves the deliberate infliction of injury without the intent to kill oneself. Most commonly, adolescents will inflict non-life-threatening cuts or burns on their arms or legs thereby providing a visible marker of their distress. While teenagers are vulnerable to a range of high-risk behaviors, the intentional infliction of wounds through cutting is becoming an increasingly prevalent syndrome among adolescents.[2] Understandably, the discovery of a teenager with self-inflicted wounds raises horrified alarm in parents, friends, and teachers and often requires immediate psychotherapeutic intervention.

While self-mutilation has been practiced by individuals and cultures throughout history, modern psychiatric attention to self-injurious patterns of cutting and burning emerged in the 1960s[3,4] and burgeoned in the 1980s.[5,6] Viewed by some as a discrete impulse control disorder[7,8] and by others as just one of many impulsive behaviors exhibited by individuals with a range of disturbances such as anorexia nervosa, bulimia, eating disorders, depression, and borderline personality disorders,[9] the sine qua non of this form of self-injury is a repeated pattern of direct, intentional bodily harm without suicidal intent. The most commonly cited purpose of self-injury is affect regulation, in that adolescents report reductions in anxiety, tension, depression, guilt, and loneliness.[8,10] The syndrome most often begins in early adolescence and often persists for many years, even well into adulthood.

Who are the teenagers most prone to these self-injurious behaviors? First, females are more likely to engage in self-injurious behavior of this kind than their male counterparts,[1,9] consistent with patterns indicating that males tend to utilize more lethal methods than females in a range of self-injurious acts.[2] Teenagers with depression, eating disorders, adjustment disorders, social difficulties, sexual conflicts, and often simply normative problems related to adolescent development can all seek catharsis, control, and communication through self-destructive physical acts. Few simple acts garner the type of attention and response from others that the appearance of bloody, self-inflicted wounds in one's loved one evokes. Surprisingly, cutting is becoming an increasingly prevalent phenomenon, and it is plaguing teens, parents, and schools. The prevalence of cutting in adolescents has been estimated at 1,000 per 100,000, compared to estimates of between 14 and 750 per 100,000 in the general population.[9] In a recent national study, cutting rates among patients presenting to community hospitals increased from 4.3% to 13.2% between 1990 and 2000.[2] The incidence among adolescent inpatients has been cited as a startling 40%.[10]

Indeed, cutting is frequently the most visible sign of other severe associated problems. For example, females who repetitively cut themselves also suffer from an eating disorder such as anorexia or bulimia in 40% of cases. Similarly, 62% of self-cutters have a history of sexual or physical abuse.[8,11] Thus, cutting serves to focus, contain, cleanse, broadcast, and ultimately relieve a wide range of underlying emotional disturbances. Not only does cutting raise the specter of overt suicide risk, it also can result in infection, permanent scarring, and an intractable pattern of self-mutilation. Superficial cutting, usually on the arms and legs, is probably the most common and widespread form of self-injury and will comprise the focus of this chapter.

WHY ADOLESCENTS INFLICT SELF-INJURY

Why would a completely normal appearing and acting teenager choose to inflict cuts or burns on himself or herself? What purpose could it possibly serve? Surprisingly, there are usually healthy strivings underlying these seemingly pointless acts, and untangling them becomes imperative in both understanding and intervening in the developmental struggle behind the self-destructive behavior. The need to understand cutting as not merely self-destructive but ultimately in the service of the adolescent's emerging sense of self is critical to effective intervention. In other words, these destructive acts fall under the common adolescent theme of "Doing all the wrong things for the right reasons." It is these underlying, often unconscious conflicts that not only drive such behavior but hold the keys to stopping it.

In addition, social contagion appears to account for some of the increased prevalence of cutting.[12,13] Observation of peers engaging in self-injury can result in contagion through modeling of these behaviors as an appropriate coping device. Much like the social contagion aspects of overt suicide attempts and eating disorders and the renowned suggestibility of teenagers, the increased awareness of self-injury among one's peers may provoke engagement in such acts.

UNDERSTANDING THE ADOLESCENT IN DEVELOPMENTAL CONTEXT

The almost universal challenges of adolescence can be summed up as centering around three central themes: (1) identity formation, (2) autonomy and independence, and (3) intimacy and sexuality. Identity formation is the ultimate development of an acceptable and realistic sense of who one is, how one relates to others, and what activities and interests form the structure of one's life. Identity is rarely solidified by the end of the teen years, often evolving over the course of one's lifetime, but a consistent sense of self that emerges intact through the dramatic transition from childhood to adulthood poses a particularly daunting task. Identity confusion can result in both the normative and more problematic appearance of troubling symptoms such as depression, anxiety, moodiness, anger, school failure, and self-doubt.

Autonomy and independence are gradually achieved in the tightrope walk between maintaining critical parental attachments and yet a sense of competent independent functioning. The young adolescent is called upon to become less dependent on parents for both intimacy and decision-making assistance as he or she simultaneously ventures more earnestly into friendships, sexual relationships, and autonomous pursuits outside the home. It is a seesaw of emotional peril and exhilaration for both the adolescent and his or her parents. As adolescents transition through their teen years, they are expected to become increasingly capable of responsible and independent functioning. Accordingly, their parents are required to relinquish control and tolerate the diminished closeness they can enjoy with their children.

Intimacy and sexuality are of course lifelong themes for all of us, but adolescents are especially challenged as a result of pubertal changes and the onset of overtly romantic and sexual involvements. An imperative developmental goal is the ability to relate intimately and rewardingly to others, and where appropriate, to integrate a responsible and healthy sexuality into one's intimate relationship. Adolescents are caught in the throes of intense sexual desires, needs for acceptance and affiliation, and the often confusing task of defining one's sexual orientation and identity. These challenges during a time of decreasing parental connection and increasing freedom make for an often tumultuous and stressful period of development.

Thus, as adolescents grapple with challenges related to the formation of identity, autonomy, and intimacy, distress and confusion are understandable by-products. However, for some adolescents, these challenges prove so painful or overwhelming as to compel them to behave in self-damaging ways. Drug abuse, school failure, promiscuity, and the like are quintessential pitfalls of adolescence. Increasingly, self-injury is becoming a mode of coping with overwhelming distress that the adolescent is otherwise unable to contain.

WHAT MOTIVATES SELF-INJURY? DOING ALL THE WRONG THINGS FOR THE RIGHT REASONS

The quelling of intensely negative emotions is often cited as the most immediate goal of self-injury. In fact, its usefulness in quelling distress renders many teens reluctant to discontinue it.[14] The adolescent who is overwhelmed by longing, sadness, hurt, self-loathing, anxiety, or a host of other emotions commonly resorts to cutting as a means of refocusing emotional pain onto a physical act over which he or she has control. Thus, many adolescents report that cutting helps them feel: numb, calm, in control, relieved, or otherwise less distressed.

Case Example: Denise is a 17-year-old high school senior who often has failing grades and is not sure what she will do after graduation. Recently, she experienced a miscarriage after becoming pregnant by a "friend with benefits" whom she now hates. She feels alone and inadequate and cannot tolerate the depth of her anxiety and despair. Cutting has become a ritual that helps to drain these feelings, as it reliably leaves a calmer, trancelike numbness in its wake. She was once briefly hospitalized for threatening to commit suicide and often feels intense remorse over the litany of scars that cover her arms, legs, and neck. Yet, she is not able to control the impulse to cut herself when feeling emotionally overwhelmed; it is the only thing that provides any relief.

A second goal of self-injury can be the conscious or unconscious wish to alert others to one's distress. The sight of bloody scars is literally a red flag to parents, friends, and teachers, who are inevitably alarmed by these obvious and disturbing signs of a troubled adolescent. Importantly, because the teen is often in conflict over the desire to be independent yet still reliant on outside support, the scars are often displayed for "accidental" discovery as opposed to a direct plea for help. Indeed, while the scar screams out the teen's desire for help, often the self-injurer is decidedly resistant or even defiant to intervention. The cutting then becomes the battleground upon which the dependence-independence conflict is fought within the adolescent as well as between himself or herself and others. It is this conflict that can make self-injury such a complicated and intractable problem in teens.

Case Example: Marta, 13, has always seemed to be the "perfect" child, with everything going for her. She is bright, attractive, athletic, sociable, and an excellent student. Her parents, teachers, and friends have come to expect great things from her. What they don't know, however, is that Marta doesn't really feel very smart and she worries that in high school her inadequacies will be revealed. No one seems to realize the anxiety and pressure she feels before tests or track meets. Also, many of her friends already have boyfriends and some sexual experience, and she feels unready and frightened by the complexities of entering into such relationships. Furthermore, she hates the good girl reputation she has at school. She begins cutting partly to illustrate her invisible suffering and to broadcast to others her hidden complexities in a way that words just don't seem to convey.

A third goal of self-injury can be to punish or reject hated aspects of oneself. Commonly, poor body image and low self-esteem create such internal rage and misery as to lead the teen to harm himself or herself in this manner. The cutting serves to provide a sense of cleansing and relief that helps the teen regain equilibrium and a temporary sense of redemption. By symbolically excising the hated traits, the teen is in a sense saying, "I will not accept this and therefore it is no longer a part of me." Self-injury can take on the type of magical thinking qualities that drive the anorexic to starve or the bulimic to purge: by ridding oneself of the hated feeling, the cutting ritual serves to restore a sense of greater peace and acceptance.

Case Example: Allana is 15 and has been struggling with bulimia for two years. She has been at trouble both at home and at school for smoking marijuana and for drinking so much she has twice passed out. Allana is preoccupied with her weight and often feels out of control with her pattern of binging and purging. She is furious at her self for giving in to these urges and hates the body that torments her so. She has a host of cigarette burns that she has inflicted primarily as a form of self-punishment for what she views as her hideous behavior. It is a form of penance she has developed, which rewards her with less distress in the forms of guilt and shame.

Often, a fourth goal of cutting is the declaration of autonomy and power. As parents campaign to make the adolescent stop the loathsome behavior, a dynamic develops wherein the teen discovers a newfound source of tremendous power. Parents and others will plead, demand, panic, threaten, and otherwise try to help the teen stop injuring himself or herself, but alas, the teen alone maintains the power to cut or not to cut. This sense of control over others can be a misdirected and passive means of expressing independence and a dramatic statement to the effect, "I am not your little girl anymore; I have my own mind and will make my own choices." Thus, the cutting can serve as a vivid assertion that the teen is demanding more freedom and autonomy and as a demonstration of inner strength and resolve. Helping the adolescent reassert these healthy strivings through positive choices and active negotiation with parents can greatly assist the teen's ability to relinquish the cutting.

Case example: Jamie is 16 and frantic to break loose from her parents' suffocating restrictions on her social life. They don't understand her urgent need to be with her friends and outside the stifling house virtually all the time. She cannot stand to be separated from her friends and left out of all the drama, and once when grounded for the weekend, she carved a gash in her wrist out of rage and frustration. Once her parents found out, they were suddenly terrified and no longer so confident in their parenting. They seemed afraid that if she wasn't happy, she would harm herself, and they became more tentative with their authority and more apt to let her have her way. Cutting was certainly one way they could see that she would not let them control her: she was calling the shots now. But at the same time, why was she so unable to be alone without feeling anxious and depressed, and so afraid that her friends might abandon her?

Fifth, and perhaps most difficult to grasp, is the adolescent's attempt to express his or her changing identity in the act of self-injury, replete with complex emotions, thoughts, and conflicts that revolve around more adult themes than ever previously experienced. The adolescent is often displaying to friends and others both the pain and the intriguing nature of his or her nascent maturity. The scars garner a curiosity and a mystique that often appeal to the teen in the quest to declare himself or herself no longer a child but a highly unique, hip, and complex person. Thus, as the teen struggles with the enormous distress of conflicts regarding autonomy, sexuality, and a changing sense of identity, the cutting and scarring represent the relinquishing of childhood's innocence and dependency and the advent of full-blown adolescence.

Case example: Kay, 15, is in love with her best friend Diane. She has never had such strong feelings before for a boy or a girl and longs to begin a romantic relationship with Diane. She isn't sure if she's gay or bisexual, but something unexpected and powerful has taken hold of her. Unfortunately, Diane has made it clear to Kay that she loves her as a friend but does not share her romantic feelings, insisting that she prefers boys. Kay feels isolated and rejected and yet emboldened by the force of her newfound romantic and sexual desires. She is not like everyone else, and it is painful and wonderful all at the same time. Overwhelmed with frustrated longing, Kay cuts her arms and wears tank tops to school. Some people comment, but mainly her schoolmates simply take notice and look at her with new intrigue in their eyes. Kay is declaring her newly unfolding identity and the competing feelings of pride and distress it entails.

Self-injurious behavior is therefore often much more than simply the expression of pain or a cry for help. While it is easy to dismiss this disturbing behavior as the hostile, manipulative actions of an exasperating teen, it is absolutely imperative that parents and clinicians understand the primary motives as being rooted in otherwise healthy developmental conflicts related to identity, autonomy, and intimacy. For cutting not to remain the entrenched battleground upon which these titanic adolescent struggles are fought, the deeper meanings and ultimately healthy strivings need to be uncovered and drawn out. Thus, self-injury is a negative behavior perversely employed toward the ultimate goal of successful adolescent development.

INTERVENTION AND TREATMENT STRATEGIES

Cutting is understandably feared to indicate that a teen is suicidal. However, cutting is rarely an exit strategy and is most commonly a misguided effort to both cope with and communicate despair. The appearance of bloody scars on an adolescent's body understandably elicits alarm and immediate attention from others—often the desired response motivating the cutting in the first place. Parents and others may assume that the adolescent is suicidal and may implement various forms of crisis management or hospitalization. Indeed, true suicidal intent and risk needs to be fully assessed once cutting becomes apparent, but it is thankfully not meant to be a lethal act in itself. Successful treatment most commonly hinges on the calm articulation and recognition of the adolescent's conflicts, an avoidance of a power struggle with the cutter, and the development of alternative strategies to both cope with painful emotions and attain truly desired outcomes. All treatments need to assess suicidality on an ongoing basis, employ "no-suicide" contracts, and involve medical professionals to assess the risk of infection, general health, coexisting eating or substance abuse disorders, and the potential usefulness of psychotropic medication in the patient's overall care.

CRYING OUT IN PAIN: AN EFFORT TO CALM AND CONTAIN PAINFUL EMOTIONS

The first intervention with an adolescent who is discovered cutting is to express concern over their obvious pain. Often, helping parents to not panic and overreact is critical to the teen's ability to communicate his or her distress directly and relinquish cutting as a coping mechanism. Only when the teen feels confident that others are trying to assist and not control him or her will he or she engage in a nonbelligerent dialogue. It is critical that parents, friends, and clinicians all acknowledge the stark reality of the cutting behavior: only the teen has control over the behavior. In other words, no one can make the teen stop cutting; he or she is in charge.

When cutting is used to quell intense emotional distress, it is important to glean information about what circumstances bring on the urge to cut. When, where, and why is it most likely to occur? Once the teen can make the association between a painful event or thought, the need to cut, and the emotional relief gained by cutting, intervention can proceed. Often, teens are quite open to discussing alternative strategies for coping with overwhelming distress. These can include journaling, calling a friend, taking a walk, listening to an inspiring song, or other individual strategies useful to the teen. The notion that the teen has a choice over whether or not to cut is extremely important. Only then can he or she begin to take responsibility for his or her actions and their outcomes and build a bigger arsenal of coping strategies.

CRYING OUT TO OTHERS

Cutting is usually a means of communicating with others. It elicits intense reactions, particularly from parents who become alarmed at the realization that their beloved child is mutilating himself or herself, often permanently. The implicit threat of suicide mobilizes parents, teachers, friends, and ultimately clinicians. The self-injurer suddenly wields terrible power in their defiance of admonishments to cease and desist the bloody behavior. At once the cutter seems to be saying, "Help me, I'm suffering" yet at the same time declaring, "You have no control over me and can't help me." Therein lies what is frequently the central struggle for the adolescent self-injurer as he or she seeks to overcome a classic developmental impasse: the need to stay dependent at an unsteady time of life, yet the simultaneous need to seize autonomy and independence from parental figures.

The inherent irony of this mixed message makes intervention a delicate and difficult task. Parents and clinicians must strike a balance between offering support and setting limits yet demonstrating clear recognition of their lack of choice in the teen's actual injurious behavior. Teenagers need to know that their parents are available to support them, yet they are compelled to assert that everything is their choice and their own doing. The teen needs to hear the difficult message that adults are concerned and dedicated to helping, but for better and for worse, the teen holds all of the choices and control. With the clear caveat that suicidal risk will be swiftly addressed through hospitalization to assure safety, minor self-injury cannot be stopped by command or force. The teen needs to perceive that others are reaching out to assist him or her in achieving his or her goals and are not simply demanding that he or she behave.

Clinicians and parents need to contain their own anxiety regarding the self-injurious behavior to calmly and nonjudgmentally convey their ability to tolerate the teen's intense emotions and offer competent assistance. As parents avoid panic and overt distress, the power and the intensity of the cutting often abates. Without effecting dramatic reactions in others, the teen's need to advertise his or her message through self-injury is no longer reinforced, leaving the teen freer to choose other modes of expression and communication.

CRYING OUT A NEW IDENTITY: VALIDATING GROWING DEPTH AND COMPLEXITY

When a teen is shown an interest in his or her private emotional and social life, he or she can begin to give voice to newly discovered parts of himself or herself. Passions around romantic and sexual feelings are newly experienced; the longing to win the acceptance and approval of peers, newly imperative; and the ability to think complexly, suddenly strengthened by brain development advancing abstract thinking abilities. Reflecting and validating these areas of rapid growth assists the teen's self-understanding and self-esteem. The therapist in particular can then assist the adolescent in redirecting his or her changing identity toward productive as opposed to destructive forms of self-expression. What are the teen's thoughts about his or her sexual orientation? How might he or she approach conflicts with friends in a more successful way? How might he or she negotiate maturely with parents around a desired freedom or privilege? What might be other ways of managing the unbearable stress of academic expectations? These are but a small sprinkling of the larger issues that adolescents need to confront and where clinicians need to focus their work. The self-injurious behavior is, after all, secondary to conflicts in these areas and needs to fade into the background as more active coping with developmental challenges takes hold.

Case illustration: Sharon, age 14, is furious that her parents won't let her go the upcoming concert with all of her friends. They don't understand how important this is to her, and they insist she can't go unless adults will be there to supervise. She storms off to her room, slams the door, and cries. This is her best chance to get together with Josh, the guy she's had a crush on, and if she's not there, Tanya will definitely go after him. She's not even sure that Josh likes her; she's not as thin as some of the other girls and not as "fast" as boys like him might prefer. Sharon has never felt this kind of longing for a boy, much less so many inexplicable feelings of desire, fear, love, and anger. She can't stand it!

Sharon hates herself right now. She hates her parents and the horrible way she feels. There isn't even anyone who understands her distress, least of all her parents. She thinks about those girls at school known as "cutters" who are either rumored or known to cut themselves. They seem mysterious, different, and obviously in some sort of distress. Sharon walks into the kitchen and takes a paring knife from the drawer. She takes it back to her room, thinking how utterly clueless her parents are. On the back of her forearm she prepares to inscribe her signature of distress. Will it hurt? Who cares, nothing is as bad as how she feels. This pain will be her doing; she can control it. She steels herself, intent on numbing herself to any pain or awareness of her own perverse behavior, and coolly observes the striking red beads of blood as they erupt beneath her barely penetrating knife blade. She's mesmerized, transfixed, and squeezes the cut to make the blood drip onto her desk. Slowly she realizes that she feels calmer now, stronger, and more in command of her pain. This cut tells the story of her internal quagmire of frustrations, and it can only be read by those to whom she reveals it. It seems an appropriately perverse way of expressing this confluence of confusing emotions, and cutting quickly becomes a preoccupation for Sharon, resulting in a litany of scars on her arms and stomach.

DEFINING THE CONFLICTS AND INTERVENING EFFECTIVELY

This episode of Sharon's reveals a great deal about the 14-year-old issues that overwhelm her. First, she desires more freedom and independence, but her parents constantly obstruct her in their efforts to assure her safety. Second, she does not know how to communicate her burgeoning emotional investment in peer relations and culture. She is not a little girl anymore, yet her parents don't seem to recognize the changes in her. Third, Sharon is not yet equipped to calm or cope with the intensity of these new emotions. Thus, with her identity, independence, and intimacy needs all feeling hopelessly thwarted, she turns to self-harm as an expression of her torment.

When her parents discover that their daughter has dozens of self-inflicted scars, they are shocked and appalled. In fact they are terrified, worried, and yet angry that she has chosen to do this seemingly ridiculous, destructive thing. They confront her with their concerns, and the intensity of their reaction stuns even Sharon. She feels immediately attacked and defensive and withdraws into a posture of defiance and then distance. Her parents are frightened that she might be cutting herself again in her room, behind the locked door, and they feel help-less to intervene short of threatening or beseeching her to stop. Might she even try to kill herself, they wonder? What should they do?

Parents reflexively react to threats to their children with intense emotional and protective instincts. It is extremely difficult for parents to remain calm and cogent when faced with the revelation that their daughter is engaging in truly disturbing behavior. Not only do they want the behavior to cease imme-diately, they are alarmed by the implications of emotional instability inherent to self-injurious behavior. Suddenly, concerns literally related to life and limb are brought into focus. Naturally, then, parents need professional guidance and support in treating a self-injurious teen.

After several consultations with a psychologist, Dr. Galvan, Sharon and her parents began actively confronting the developmental issues underlying the red flags of her cutting behavior. An initial evaluation was undertaken by Dr. Galvan to not only assess Sharon's psychological and behavioral status, but importantly, her suicide risk and immediate danger from any related self-destructive activi-ties (e.g., drug or alcohol use, sexual risk-taking, anorexia or bulimia). Sharon strongly denied any intentions, thoughts, or plans to seriously injure or harm herself, and a "no-suicide" contract was developed in which Sharon promised to contact Dr. Galvan if she ever did feel the urge to more seriously harm herself. A medical exam was recommended to assess the severity of her wounds and rule out any current risk of infection.

Sharon and Dr. Galvan discussed her current life context including her social, emotional, familial, and academic environments. Sharon was able to describe her intense frustration with her parents along with deep-seated feelings of self-doubt regarding her appearance and competence. Her feelings for Josh and pressing needs for acceptance by both female and male peers were notable for their urgency and the anxiety they generated. In short, Dr. Galvan and Sharon began to understand the key conflicts underlying her misery and the correspond-ing need to injure herself. These conflicts are multiple. First on her developing self-image as a maturing and social adolescent, with all its inherent anxieties.

Second, the classic developmental struggle, fraught with ambivalence galore, for the teen to separate and become more independent while the parents ease up controls had begun in earnest. Third, the confluence of intense, confusing emotions at a time of rapid hormonal change rendered Sharon unable to effectively cope. She needed alternative strategies for contending with emotional distress that did not involve self-harm and that more successfully achieved her goals.

Critical to any effective intervention with teenagers is concurrent consultation with parents. The adolescent's journey is inextricably linked to his or her parents, and they each must adapt to the rapid developmental changes facing them both. While teens struggle with their own challenges, parents suddenly face a loss of control, a loss of intimacy, and a new set of behaviors and emotions emanating from their previously predictable child. It is a process of enormous give and take; mutual gains and losses; huge successes and dismal setbacks. Thus, the parents need consultation and support in order to assist their teenager's successful transition through adolescence.

Sharon's parents met with Dr. Galvan and conveyed their worries and many questions. They had never seen her so moody before; never dealt with her current level of defiance; and felt unsure where and how to set limits. Dr. Galvan helped them understand the normal developmental transition that they, too, were undergoing, as their parental roles were shifting with Sharon's evolving needs. They became better able to understand the conflicts underlying her seemingly senseless fits of emotion, for example, the age-appropriate insistence on spending more time with friends and the growing ambivalence around parental control and dependency. Sharon's parents needed to first ground their understanding of Sharon's self-injurious behavior in the context of age-appropriate developmental challenges. This understanding better equipped them to support Sharon's appropriate expressions of autonomy and independence while maintaining a loving, supportive but less hovering presence. This started with the very difficult task of accepting that Sharon was the only person in control of her own cutting and that for the time being, they needed to convey their concern yet contain their own intense emotional responses.

Sharon felt truly validated and supported by this intervention with her parents. As the notion of a two-way street of negotiation and communication took hold, Sharon finally felt that she had some avenues through which to assert her needs with her parents. She also understood a bit better that her parents were only doing what loving parents tend to do: reacting protectively and only reluctantly relinquishing intimacy and control with their daughter.

This explicit articulation of the developmental tasks facing both Sharon and her parents provided a framework within which they could better understand the individual and collective challenges facing them. This helped to externalize and diffuse conflicts in the sense that they could now grasp the real issues at the heart of their struggles. That is, the inexorable process of development was the ultimate culprit in their midst rather than merely the angry behavior of a disturbed adolescent or the controlling actions of insensitive parents. Sharon and her parents were thus better able to humanize themselves and each other in this difficult process, and to see each other more as allies than adversaries.

Sharon insisted to Dr. Galvan that her self-injurious behavior gave her an important sense of identity and control. The central work of treatment involves assisting the teenager in finding more productive means of self-expression and control while acknowledging the even more daunting nature of the real-life challenges that cutting merely assists her in actively avoiding. For Sharon, she felt particularly anxious about her ability to attract a boyfriend and earn a secure social niche among her friends. She witnessed major changes in many of her friends, who were suddenly dressing more provocatively, becoming more aggressive in pursuing friends and boyfriends, and seemed to Sharon to be light-years ahead of her in tackling the sexuality and independence aspects of adolescence. At the same time her body was developing, but to her the result was primarily a feeling of being fat and therefore unattractive and inferior. Her self-esteem and sense of control were diminished by the changes she observed both within and outside herself.

On one hand, Sharon wanted her parents to let her go to concerts and stay out late and generally stop treating her like a child. But on the other hand, she was also nervous about going to the concert and contending with the scores of teenagers, drugs, and rowdy elements characteristic of heavy metal concerts. Similarly, she wanted a later curfew but was aware that after ten o'clock many of her friends started hooking up with boys and she wasn't sure how she felt about that. While she wanted her parents to stop nagging her about homework, she herself was deeply troubled by her poor grades. Thus, it was critical that Sharon learn to recognize and assume more responsibility for her own very natural personal fears and conflicts. Only then could she implement more effective, more honest solutions and choices. As Sharon's parents learned to listen to the quiet conflict underlying her loud protestations, they were better able to understand Sharon as simultaneously a vulnerable child and a maturing young woman struggling with increasing pressures and demands.

While both Sharon and her parents' psychological understanding and communication improved, the need remained to assist Sharon immediately with a means of confronting so many stressful challenges without resorting to self-injury. Cognitive-behavioral interventions that actively target specific thoughts and behaviors can be essential in the treatment of self-injurious behavior. These interventions tend to connect the precipitating cause, emotional response, and subsequent destructive behavior in the adolescent's consciousness as a related sequence that he or she can learn to interrupt.

The first step in this process often involves the teen recording aspects of the self-injury sequence in a log. When did you experience the urge to cut? What were you feeling at the time? How did your body feel? What events, feelings, or thoughts preceded the urge? What was the intended goal of the self-injury? What would be the intended and unintended messages communicated to others through the self-injury? What action did you finally take? What was the result? These questions can be addressed on a log sheet or journal and then carefully reviewed during therapy sessions. There the adolescent can begin to develop the self-knowledge that can empower him or her to make changes and alternative choices.

Alternatives to self-injury are a cornerstone of treatment. There are many actions the teen can take in response to emotional distress; for example, the teen can confront the person inspiring his or her anger, or call a sympathetic friend, or take a walk, or cry, or simply do nothing and weather the emotional storm knowing that it will indeed pass. Teenagers need to build a new arsenal of coping skills now that the childhood options of running to one's parents or throwing a tantrum no longer seem age-appropriate. Working with the teen to define his or her own set of alternatives to self-injury focuses the responsibility and the means for coping squarely on the teen and can empower him or her to actively choose not to cut.

Common alternatives to self-injury include journaling, exercising, listening to music, leaving the room, taking a bath, drinking tea, watching television, calling a friend, contacting the therapist, looking at photos with positive memories, cuddling with the family dog or cat, or writing a letter to the friend, teacher, or family member toward whom the teen may feel frustrated or enraged. Individualizing the list as much as possible helps the adolescent identify with his or her own options and take ownership over the process.

Sharon began a log of every occasion on which she felt a compelling urge to harm herself. She recorded the time, location, bodily sensations, emotions, and thoughts accompanying the urge. She also forced herself to think about what precipitated these feelings, how she expected the cutting to bring relief, and what she might ultimately be seeking to communicate through the cutting and visible scarring. She would then record at least five alternatives to actually engaging in the cutting. Finally, she would record what action she ultimately did take and the outcome.

For Sharon, strong feelings of anger, self-doubt, and longing tended to precede the episodes of self-injury. When she felt furious, her body felt hot and full of energy; when she felt lonely her body felt inert, tired, and miserable. She learned to differentiate between these various feelings and sensations and put words to them. This exercise alone helped her feel less overwhelmed and helpless in the face of an emotional storm as she could break down the weighty burden into more identifiable pieces. She also learned to associate the events, thoughts, and interactions that preceded these intensely distressing emotions. Was she stressed out about the midterm exam? Was she feeling rejected? Was she making negative judgments about her physical appearance? Was she feeling thwarted by her parents in achieving a desired freedom? Once the picture became clearer, Sharon was able to imagine alternatives to cutting that would achieve her goals without injury and possibly with even greater success. Her alternatives included (1) journaling about her thoughts and feelings; (2) writing a letter to her parents expressing her feelings and needs; (3) calling a friend and asking for support and reassurance; (4) playing a mindless computer game; (5) physically removing herself from her room to another location; and (6) listening to music.

Dr. Galvan made it clear that these alternatives would take some time and experimentation to work as well as her habit of self-injuring. Each week they reviewed her log and discussed the recorded sequences. Importantly, Dr. Galvan worked with Sharon toward better understanding the healthy, positive meta-issue driving the urge to cut, such as a desire to feel loved, a desire to make independent decisions, or self-doubt regarding perceived limitations. Once Sharon could see, for example, that her fears of rejection were better overcome through active communication and engagement with her friends than by the quick fix of cutting, she could make more positive choices.

Sharon particularly found journaling to be a satisfying means of both soothing herself and expressing her thoughts and feelings. In so doing, Sharon was able to see in black and white the evidence of her own internal and interpersonal struggles and the maturing parts of her that were heroically grappling with the challenges inherent to adolescence. She could keep these insights wholly private or share selections with her therapist, a friend, or even a parent with whom she had trouble communicating. She also found that by simply leaving her room she could "change the channel" as it were and allow the emotional storm to subside while she watched television, prepared a snack, or sat on the front step. She also learned to rely on a friendship with Joanna that was fast becoming more intimate as she contacted her more frequently in times of distress.

Sharon was gradually accepting that only she could and must surmount not only the cutting but the larger struggles compelling it. As the focus shifted to her goals for intimacy, competence, and realistically defining herself as a complex individual with strengths and limitations, Sharon engaged less and less often in self-injury. Once her parents and friends no longer responded with alarm and urgency to fresh scars, the cutting became a less powerful tool for communicating and increasingly became viewed by Sharon as the unpleasant and useless coping strategy it was. The focus became her struggles, her goals, and her choices, and she herself, the only beneficiary or victim of them. Simultaneously, Sharon's parents had begun accepting their lack of control and were stepping back from inserting themselves into Sharon's struggles. It became clearer to Sharon that she wanted and needed her parents' support but that she had to assume responsibility for either making good independent decisions or seeking out their assistance. This, ultimately, signifies true healthy development as the teen becomes more competently independent while remaining securely invested in supportive relationships with parents and peers.

LARGER SOCIAL AND CULTURAL FACTORS

Since time immemorial people have engaged in body art, adornment, scarring, and other symbolic rituals involving trauma or visible marking of the skin. In many American cultures, tattoos and piercings are employed much like clothes or hair styles to signify affiliations with subgroups of peer culture and disassociation with mainstream mores. Self-injury can be a truly private act, but more often the evident scarring conveys significant meaning in each person's cultural context.

While it is beyond the scope of this chapter to address the in-depth social forces acting upon youth in diverse socioeconomic and racial groups, clearly our broader society's ever-increasing focus on appearance makes the skin an ideal billboard for advertising identity. For youths who self-injure, the message is that of a sense of damage, daring, and exquisite pain. Fresh wounds scream more urgently and immediately than the gradually developing evidence of anorexia, bulimia, depression, or sexual abuse, therefore affording the teen immediate and urgent attention.

Media also increasingly highlight sensationalized, aberrant behavior. The explosion of reality television attests to the public's fascination with dysfunction, exhibitionism, and the exposure of private lives. Few behaviors are as shocking as a young person intentionally carving himself or herself bloody, immediately declaring himself or herself a spectacle of pain and fascination. In an ever-competitive society it may be more difficult to distinguish oneself through one's accomplishments than through the demonstration of victimization or dysfunction. "Body art" consisting of tattoos or multiple piercings, has increasingly become commonplace among adolescents and is generally a more socially acceptable means of self-expression than cutting.

Social contagion has been recognized as a significant influence in the spreading epidemic of cutting. Studies have concluded that even a majority of self-harm incidents on an adolescent psychiatric ward may have been induced by contagion.[12,13] This spread of self-injurious behavior was even observed in adolescents who had previously been unaware of this behavior existing. Self-injury may even be more socially contagious than suicidal behavior among adolescent inpatients.[13] The compelling need for adolescents to identify with peers and try out all sorts of ill-fated activities readily explains the spreading use of cutting as a means of coping with and expressing pain.

In short, the meaning and message behind self-injury can only be deciphered in the context of each adolescent's peer, family, and cultural milieus. This is precisely why intervention often requires more than a laser focus on the teen's seeming pathology and on aspects of his or her environment that can be drawn on as resources or addressed as detriments. A biopsychosocial approach emphasizes the need to integrate biological, psychological, and social factors into a meaningfully individualized treatment strategy. As a result, group psychotherapy, family therapy, and medication can be essential components of a comprehensive intervention.

In Sharon's case, a number of relevant social and environmental factors contributed to her distress. First of all, as an average student in a high achieving, highly educated and successful family, Sharon viewed herself as a de facto failure in her parents' eyes. Second, her parents had been contending with a severe strain in their marriage, and the tense, unhappy home environment created a discomforting feeling of anxiety for Sharon. Third, Sharon's peers were suddenly embracing pop culture with a vengeance, and she was feeling pressure to grow up, behave sexually and dress in more provocative ways than she felt comfortable. Finally, Sharon felt new pressure to be competitively thin and attractive and saw herself as a contender in this social realm but as hopelessly unexceptional in school or sports.

Dr. Galvan recommended couple's therapy for Sharon's parents and conducted several family sessions in which her parents could validate her perceptions yet reassure her that they were working on things. Sharon was also referred to group treatment with a psychologist who conducted an appropriate group of 14- and 15-year-old adolescents with similar difficulties. Sharon was also encouraged to establish a relationship with her academic counselor toward the goal of better defining her own goals and aspirations and assisting her in finding meaningful volunteer work or paid employment.

CONCLUSIONS

The increasing prevalence of self-injurious behavior among adolescents demands particularly sensitive and even sophisticated intervention by clinicians and families. The cutting needs to be viewed as the complex manifestation that it is and not just the weird, provocative behavior of an unruly adolescent.

Frequently, interventions focus immediately on demands that the adolescent cease the behavior without providing needed alternatives or insights. This leaves the adolescent feeling stranded and misunderstood, often only escalating his or her despair and infliction of injury. Critical to any effective treatment is an understanding of the teen in the context of his or her developmental stage. In addition to in-depth understanding, competent limits, comprehensive treatment options and medical oversight need to be implemented.

Perhaps most surprising to both parents and teenagers is the revelation that cutting represents positive, healthy strivings screaming to be surmounted. Reframing the cutting in the context of the teen's age-appropriate conflicts with an emphasis on his or her innate positive strivings helps to shine a light on what is right about the teen as opposed to what is wrong. Avoiding the head-on collision of criticizing and condemning the teen's behavior provides an avenue for far greater success in enlisting the teen's openness and cooperation.

REFERENCES

1. Olfson, M., Gameroff, M., Marcus, S., Greenberg, T., & Shaffer, D. (2005). National trends in hospitalization of youth with intentional self-inflicted injuries. *American Journal of Psychiatry, 162*(7), 1328–1334.
2. Conterio, K., & Lader, W. (1998). *Bodily harm.* New York: Hyperion.
3. Graff, H., & Mallin, R. (1967). The syndrome of the wrist cutter. *American Journal of Psychiatry, 124,* 36–42.
4. Gruenbaum, H., & Klerman, G. (1967). Wrist slashing. *American Journal of Psychiatry, 124,* 527–534.
5. Pattison, E., & Kahan, J. (1983). The deliberate self-harm syndrome. *American Journal of Psychiatry, 140,* 867–872.
6. Favazza, A. (1987). *Bodies under siege: Self-mutilation in culture and psychiatry.* Baltimore: Johns Hopkins University Press.
7. Morgan, H. (1979). *Death wishes? The understanding and management of self-harm.* New York: Wiley.
8. Favazza, A., and Conterio, K. (1989). Female habitual self-mutilators. *Acta Psychiatry Scandinavia, 79,* 282–289.
9. Favazza, A. (1998). The coming of age of self-mutilation. *Journal of Nervous and Mental Disease, 186*(5), 259–268.
10. Darche, M. (1990). Psychological factors differentiating self-mutilating and non-self-mutilating adolescent inpatient females. *Psychiatric Hospital, 21,* 31–35.
11. Briere, J. (1996). *Therapy for those molested as children.* New York: Springer.
12. Rosen, P., & Walsh, B. (1989). Patterns of contagion in self-mutilation epidemics. *American Journal of Psychiatry, 146,* 656–658.

13. Taiminen, T., Kallio-Soukainen, K., Nokso-Koivisto, H., Kaljonen, A., & Helenius, H. (1998). Contagion of deliberate self-harm among adolescent inpatients. *American Academy of Child and Adolescent Psychiatry*, 37(2), 211–217.

14. Briere, J., & Gil, E. (1998). Self-mutilation in clinical and general population samples: Prevalence, correlates, and functions. *American Journal of Orthopsychiatry*, 68(4), 609–620.

Chapter 10

Reading, Writing, and Therapy: Mental Health Issues Among College Students

Julie B. Jampel

Jan* matriculated at a large eastern university after growing up in the Midwest with her two older sisters and younger brother. She did well academically in high school and spent her time at home hanging out with a small group of friends. There was nothing in her personal history to suggest that she would have a difficult time adjusting to college and campus life. However, two months after she arrived on campus, she still had not met any fellow students with whom she felt comfortable, she struggled to keep up with her French class, and she was gaining weight from eating too much in her residence hall at dinner. She began to feel overwhelmed and believed she made a poor choice in selecting a college so far from her family and high school friends. When she sat down in a therapist's office at her university counseling center in November of her freshman year, the first thing she said was, "I don't know why I'm so unhappy here. I've never had this trouble before."

Why was Jan's experience at college so different from her experience in high school? How do her goals and circumstances as a college student differ from those of a younger adolescent? Many things have changed for Jan. She left the home her parents made for her and now needs to make her own decisions and set her own guidelines—including, for example, how much she will eat when presented with the wide variety and abundance of foods in her residence hall.

---

* All names in this chapter have been altered for privacy.

She also left a group of friends who grew up with her in the same neighborhood; now she meets people from many different backgrounds and parts of the country. Previously a good student among kids representing a wide range of abilities, she currently finds herself among many other good and even better students. When Jan used to think of her future after high school, she thought of college and saw herself as a student for another four years. Now when she thinks of her future, she sees . . . question marks. What will she do professionally? What role will she serve in society?

Some of the issues Jan faces as she begins her college years have been well documented by developmental and clinical psychologists. Erik Erikson's psychosocial stages of development in adolescents and young adults highlight two of Jan's struggles—identity versus role confusion and intimacy versus isolation.[1] Jan skimmed through the college course catalogue shortly after she arrived on campus, as she had begun to think about which field of study she wanted to claim for her major. She was pretty sure she favored the humanities, but she enjoys art history as much as English literature, and she also likes cultural anthropology, one of the social sciences. She felt overwhelmed by her multiple interests, and she felt confused when she thought about her career possibilities. Did she want to be a writer, a curator in an art museum, a teacher or professor, or perhaps a researcher or relief worker in another country? She felt a bit hopeless about choosing a path amid so many options. Jan also felt pessimistic about establishing—with a new group of peers and eventually within a family of her own—the comfort and familiarity she enjoyed with her family and friends from home.

Alan, an 18-year-old freshman from New England, grappled with different, but no less distressing, identity concerns when he enrolled at a small college in his home state:

Alan was shy and did not date much in high school. Shortly before Thanksgiving, he asked a young woman from his economics class out for dinner. Despite feeling self-conscious, he had a good time. He felt confused and worried, though, because he was attracted to a guy in his calculus class. Did this mean he was gay or bisexual? Alan didn't know how to understand his sexual desires, and he began to feel anxious much of the time. He also stopped going to church, even though he had previously attended church regularly with his parents and younger brother, and he felt guilty about not going.

Although students seek out university counseling centers for all kinds of reasons, students like Jan and Alan are typical in that they struggle to manage developmental conflicts—that is, they grapple with issues related to growing up and becoming their own person. Over the course of the academic year, there are two surges in presentations that reflect developmental issues. Through case examples, these will be discussed below.

HOMESICK FRESHMEN, SENIORS ADRIFT

From September through November, many freshmen seek services because they miss their families and hometowns and feel miserable at college. Sometimes this expresses itself as acute separation anxiety, in which a student cannot function on campus because he or she is intensely longing to return home to be with family and friends, and to the student it feels as though being home is the only way to quell the anxiety. Other times it expresses as a milder anxiety and dysphoria; a student wishes to be home because college life does not seem to be working out as planned or does not meet expectations. A student may not have made any friends on campus, for example. A student in this situation can function at college, but he or she feels unhappy and wants to return home. By late November, these presentations have largely stopped. A few students may have left school and gone home; most students, however, have adjusted by the end of their first semester.

What factors influence homesickness in freshmen? Two factors stand out—a history of separation anxiety and high expectations for instant adjustment to college. Sue, for example, told her counselor that she had always left sleepover parties early when she was in elementary school, and she had cried so long and hard when her parents took her to overnight camp at age nine that they returned just a few days later to bring her home. She spent the first week of college in her room crying and calling her mother multiple times each day. She did not attend classes and did not eat much, as she had no appetite. After encouraging Sue to stick with it for 10 days, her mother came to see her, and together they sought help from the counseling center. Sue's separation anxiety had gone untreated before; with treatment, she adjusted to being at college and to being away from her mother, although reaching this point took most of her freshman year.

In contrast to Sue, Jill had no history of separation anxiety. In fact, change and transition had always gone well for Jill. She entered college thinking she would love all of her classes and would become close friends with a group of girls by the end of the first week. When this didn't happen, she grew worried and discouraged. As she told her counselor, she had expected that she would be sitting around eating pizza with a bunch of friends by now, like the picture in her college brochure. With the support and perspective of her counselor, Jill was able to relax and give herself more time to meet her goals. She developed some friendships, and she really enjoyed a couple of her classes; she no longer expected to love all of them.

Whereas freshmen need to transition from home to college, seniors need to transition from college back out into the world. For some seniors, decisions come easily. They know they want to attend graduate school or get a particular type of job. They apply for various jobs or graduate programs, and they start looking for housing when they know where they'll be living. Things fall into place. For other students, though, the college years have not resulted in a sense of direction. These students still don't know what they want to do after graduation, and they haven't found a field that really interests them. They don't know where they want to live, either. Each spring, with graduation looming, these seniors appear at university counseling centers hoping to find answers. They might feel anxious about the future, sad that college is ending, or confused about their next steps. Amy, a senior who sought services in early April, reported feeling all three. She noted that she felt as though she no longer had a purpose or place in life. She would have to smile during graduation for the sake of her parents and two siblings, but that would be an act. In the waiting room she had seen a magazine cover in which a young actress was smiling broadly. She believed that the actress truly had something to smile about—she had appeared in a couple of movies and seemed to have a promising career ahead of her—whereas Amy had no clue about what she wanted to do for the rest of her life. She was often tearful and seemed alone as well as lost. One of her roommates was going to medical school in the fall and would work as a research assistant at a local hospital over the summer. Amy did not even have a summer job lined up, despite pressure from her parents to find one. She didn't see how she was going to break out of this rut, and she felt pretty hopeless. She wasn't sleeping well at night and had recently fallen behind in one of her classes. Her difficulties were multiplying.

Amy went through four years of college without discovering a field of study or work that she really loved. Matt, on the other hand, assumed he was going to law school after graduation—until he returned from a semester abroad at the end of his junior year. Being in South America changed him, he said, and he wasn't sure who he was anymore. He wanted to go back to South America to teach children living in poor areas. Part of him still wanted to earn money and have a comfortable life, like his parents, yet that didn't seem as satisfying as it once had. He tried to talk with his parents about these changes over the summer and again during winter break, raising the idea of at least waiting a year or two before applying to law school, until he was more certain of what he wanted. His parents were against waiting; they refused to support him if he went back to South America for a year to teach. Matt felt stuck and demoralized. He began seeing a therapist halfway through his senior year. He smoked marijuana a couple of times to relieve the tension he felt about his situation, as well as the guilt he felt about not filling out law school applications. With his therapist's help, he was able to communicate his distress to his parents, and he decided to spend a year in New York City teaching English to Latino children.

Although Matt did not see his marijuana use as a problem, substance abuse is a serious problem for some students. Alcohol and drug use are embedded in adolescent and young adult culture, as individuals "experiment" with alcohol, drugs, and other risky behaviors. What factors make drug and alcohol use a serious problem on college campuses nationwide? This question will be explored in the next section.

DRUGS ON CAMPUS

In 1997, a freshman at the Massachusetts Institute of Technology died of alcohol poisoning a little more than a month after he arrived on campus.[2] He drank about 15 shots in an hour while pledging a fraternity. In 2004, a 21-year-old student at Minnesota State University consumed 16 shots in an hour the night of his 21st birthday. He was participating in a drinking binge known as "power hour"[3]—consuming 21 shots in an hour to celebrate reaching the legal drinking age. These students were among the 1,400 college students aged 18–24 who die an alcohol-related death each year.[4] This figure includes accidental deaths stemming from alcohol use, such as those from drunk driving, as well as deaths due directly to acute alcohol poisoning. In addition, many more college students suffer injury and illness due to alcohol use. Date rape often involves alcohol, as the perpetrator, victim, or both may be drunk at the time of the attack.

Drinking does not occur only at parties. Some students drink to relieve stress and overwhelming emotion. Lisa, a sophomore, suffered from severe generalized anxiety. Her legs would frequently twitch while she sat in her therapist's office, and her whole body reflected her immense anxiety. She reported drinking several beers per night in an effort to manage and quell the intensity of the anxiety. This helped her feel better at night, although she ended up feeling worse each morning. It also reduced her academic productivity, which concerned her. She used alcohol as a "medicine," and her drinking subsided when she began taking an antianxiety medication prescribed by a psychiatrist on campus.

Less obvious examples of students who drink for some form of relief include shy students who have a drink or two to increase their spontaneity and comfort in social interactions and harried students who drink to unwind from their whirlwind days. Students may use drugs other than alcohol for similar reasons. Illegal drugs such as marijuana, stimulants, and hallucinogens can be found on most college campuses. Furthermore, in a practice called "pharming," students may take Ritalin or Adderall—prescription drugs used to treat attention deficit hyperactivity disorder—to increase their academic performance.[5] These drugs may help students stay focused and alert for longer periods of time, leading to more productive study sessions and perhaps to better grades. However, the drugs also have side effects; some, like dry mouth, are merely bothersome, whereas others, such as high blood pressure, are potentially more serious.[6]

The developmental, academic, and social stresses of college life yield an environment ripe for substance use. Other factors, too, may increase the likelihood that a college student will develop a substance abuse problem. A family history of substance abuse can increase risk. Also, just as younger adolescents do, college students may take drugs to rebel against parental and other forms of authority, to explore new or risky behaviors, and to fit in with peers. Consider the case of Sam:

> A junior in college, Sam had been smoking marijuana on and off since his senior year in high school. He first tried it out of curiosity, then continued because he enjoyed the way it made him feel—less self-conscious around other people and more euphoric and "tuned in" with his friends. He also liked the fact that his parents would disapprove if they knew about it. In college, he continued to smoke but did not see it as a problem. He stayed up late on nights when he smoked, and sometimes he chose to smoke and hang out with friends rather than keep up with his schoolwork. Since his freshman year, Sam's grades had slipped from mostly Bs to mostly Cs. He sought out a counselor when he had an adverse reaction to marijuana one day. His heart raced, his mind felt foggy, he believed his roommate was staring at him, and he felt a sense of impending doom. He met with the counselor only once, yet he told the counselor that he was quitting marijuana immediately because he couldn't stand this reaction. It scared him; Sam didn't know a person could feel this way "just from smoking pot."

Like many college students, Sam was uninformed about the effects of drug use, especially chronic use. While he recognized his adverse reaction right away, and it scared him, he didn't notice some of the subtler signs of use, such as changes in his sleep and study habits and ultimately his poorer academic record. Binge drinkers, too, often seem either unaware or unconvinced of the dangers of drinking large amounts of alcohol in a relatively short period of time. Even if they recognize the dangers, they may decide to ignore them for several reasons. They may enjoy the feeling of taking risks, or perhaps they feel a greater sense of invulnerability than is warranted. They may also believe that not conforming to social norms and peer pressure is worse than risking bodily harm. It's possible that they think their peers know how to look after them, as the 21-year-old student from Minnesota State University apparently did.[3] Clearly, substance use fills many social and emotional needs among college students and can represent a major problem for campus safety. Food, too, can serve a variety of social and emotional needs. Combined with developmental factors, issues with food and eating can lead to eating disorders, a common diagnosis among college students.

EATING DISORDERS ON CAMPUS

There are three main patterns of disordered eating: eating too little (anorexia), eating too much (binge eating), and eating too much, followed by trying to rid the body of the food or calories (bulimia). Of these, anorexia can be the most frightening. The onset of anorexia "is often associated with a stressful life event, such as leaving home for college."[7] This may help explain why the average age of onset is 17 years, with peaks at ages 14 and 18 (p. 543).[8] Consider Joan's story:

> Joan began thinking she was overweight at age 16, when she compared herself to popular teenage actresses. She began a low-fat diet, lost a little weight, and felt great physically. She got a lot of compliments from her friends and classmates. She dieted on and off to maintain her new weight through the rest of high school. When she got to college, even though her weight was normal for her height, she worried that she was still too heavy to get a boyfriend. She began another low-fat diet and then gradually started reducing the amount she ate even further. She eliminated all forms of dairy, including low-fat dairy and anything containing cheese. She started having a small bowl of cereal without milk for breakfast, a "big" salad without dressing for lunch, and nothing or a piece of fruit for dinner. Eventually she was significantly underweight. When she examined herself in the mirror, she felt that her thighs and stomach were still too big and unattractive. She obsessed about tiny flaws. She lost more weight. Her friends had long stopped complimenting her, and her roommate was worried because she looked much too thin but still barely ate. Joan had stopped getting her period months ago and felt weak.

Joan didn't seek therapy because she was too thin; in April of her freshman year, she sought it because she was so unhappy, particularly with herself and her body. She hoped the therapist would be able to tell her how to lose weight even more effectively. Instead, the therapist thought she was dangerously thin and sent her to a hospital for a thorough medical evaluation. The hospital ended up admitting her for dehydration. Joan was placed on leave from college; she spent the rest of that academic year and the following one on leave, struggling to return to normal weight. Joan was fortunate in that she received good treatment and recovered. The long-term mortality from anorexia nervosa among individuals admitted to university-affiliated hospitals is over 10 percent, with starvation, suicide, and electrolyte imbalance being the most common causes of death (p. 539).[8] This mortality data is for true anorexia nervosa, which requires a 15 percent loss of body weight for diagnosis. Most college students exhibit milder but still serious forms of anorexia, and the disorder is more common in females than it is in males.

Individuals with bulimia—again mostly females—have repeated episodes of binge eating, and these binges are followed by an effort to rid the body of the excess food or calories. The binges feel out of control and scary. Vomiting, intense exercise, use of laxatives, or periods of severe calorie restriction between binges represent methods for eliminating or negating the excess food. Bulimia, like anorexia, involves a significant preoccupation with food, body size, and weight, although the degree of cognitive distortion of one's body size may be less with bulimia. Also like anorexia, bulimia can lead to a host of medical problems, including dental problems from vomiting.

College students with anorexia are easier to identify because they look emaciated. However, bulimia is more likely to become a community problem in a college residence hall. Roommates may notice that some of the food they keep in their rooms gets taken, even though they may not be able to say with certainty who took it. Vomit may be noticeable to others in a communal bathroom. This can be quite distressing for the residents of the hall, but again, they may not know who to approach about cleaning it up. Students with bulimia often feel a good deal of shame about their symptoms and try to hide their disorder. They delay seeking help, thinking they can handle it on their own. In other cases, students with bulimia may not be ready to commit to treatment because they fear gaining weight if they do. Resident hall advisors sometimes consult with university counselors because they have an unidentified bulimic student on their hall; the student's behavior, while hidden, is upsetting to others, and everyone feels frustrated about how to deal with the problem when the student in question refuses to seek treatment or is unknown.

Overeating, given all the food available to students in residence halls and nearby stores and restaurants, is common among college students. Food serves many purposes; it not only nourishes and fuels the body, but it may also provide comfort, feel good, and be associated with love, as when a student's mother bakes his or her favorite cookies right before the student goes home for winter break. Food is often part of social gatherings, and groups of students studying together may order in pizzas or bagels. Binge eating—a type of overeating that is characterized by (1) consuming a large amount of food in a relatively short period of time and (2) feeling out of control while it's happening—can leave one feeling disgusted, ashamed, or physically uncomfortable from the fullness. Because individuals with binge-eating disorder do not purge afterwards, they are prone to being overweight and thus may suffer from the health consequences of obesity.[5]

All three forms of disordered eating are associated with depression. Deb, a sophomore with bulimia, describes her feelings this way:

I feel so disgusted with myself. I'm fat, my thighs are horrible, I've got pimples, my hair is a mess. When I binge—usually by eating whatever is around, like chips, microwave popcorn, crackers, other snacks—I try to make up for it by eating very little the next day. I'll feel better for a little while, but then I get hungry, or I'll feel frustrated about something, and I'll binge again. I feel so incompetent and stupid. I can't do anything right. I don't have a boyfriend, but who would want to be with me? Nobody likes ugly, incompetent people.

Deb says all of this in a quiet, pained, resigned voice. She sought help from a therapist at the urging of her parents, particularly her mother, who was worried about her poor self-esteem. Feelings like Deb's are not limited to students with eating disorders, of course. Depression is common among the college-age population, and suicide is a serious concern on campuses nationwide.

DEPRESSION AND SUICIDALITY AMONG COLLEGE STUDENTS

Estimates of the rates of major depressive disorder in America vary, with the lifetime risk ranging from 10 to 25 percent for women and from 5 to 12 percent for men (p. 339).[8] The incidence in adolescent and adult females is two times that in adolescent and adult males, although the rates are equal in boys and girls before puberty. The highest rates of depression are reported in women and men aged 25–44 years, with the mid-twenties representing the average age of onset. A family history of depression increases risk, as major depressive disorder occurs 1.5 to 3 times more frequently among the first-degree biological relatives of a person suffering from the disorder than it does among the general population (p. 339).[8]

There is some evidence that the age of onset is currently decreasing (p. 340).[8] This has implications for college mental health services, as many undergraduate and graduate students are in their early and mid-twenties. Depression in college students can express itself in many ways. Consider just a few, described below:

Beth, a junior, came to the university counseling center because she had been feeling sad and depressed, with occasional thoughts of suicide. She was also worried about a 4-year-old half-sister who lives with her father and stepmother. Her father is an alcoholic; he emotionally and verbally abuses her when he is drunk. Beth wants to protect her little sister as well as herself but feels helpless.

Carl, a sophomore, came to the university counseling center because of his ongoing depressed mood. He is not interested in his classes or friends, and he has trouble falling and staying asleep. His father had died suddenly of a heart attack a few years ago, and subsequent to his father's death, there were three more deaths in Carl's extended family.

Pat, a senior, came to the university counseling center due to worsening and daily suicidal thoughts. Her plan was to disguise her suicide as an accidental drowning. Only the thought of her mother crying kept her from doing it. She feels responsible for her parents' chronic marital discord, has never been involved in an intimate relationship, and has few friends on campus.

Mary, a graduate student, reported a long history of depressed feelings; she needed help getting out of the "hole" she sometimes fell into and was worried about falling into repeatedly. By the time she sought services, her depression had already resulted in poor performance in several of her classes.

All four of these students arrived at college with a history of depressed feelings, although the feelings may have increased in intensity since their arrival. Pat and Mary take medication for their depression. Teenagers who take antidepressant medication in high school find that they can perform and function well enough to apply to and attend college once they graduate. Without the medication, their resultant poor functioning in high school may prevent them from participating in college life. Thus, university counseling centers are now seeing more students who come to college with preexisting conditions of depression and other mental disorders. The number of students who need treatment or follow-up services for mental health conditions has increased dramatically in recent years. In 2001, an increase in severe psychological difficulties was reported by 85 percent of the counseling center directors participating in a national survey.[7] In the decade between 1989 and 2001, furthermore, the following increases among college students were reported: the number of cases of documented depression doubled, the number of suicidal students tripled, and the use of psychiatric medications increased 15 percent, from 10 to 25 percent of college students.[9]

Having a preexisting condition is not the only reason for the increase in depression among college students. Other factors that increase the stresses and pressures college students feel, such as world events and economic trends, in turn may increase symptoms of depression and other mental disorders. A poor economy, for example, may affect students in several ways. It may increase marital discord in the student's family, or the student may feel guilty about the expense of college. A poor economy may also reduce the number of job openings available when the student graduates, thereby increasing anxiety about finding suitable employment. The examples of depressed students outlined above illustrate a variety of other environmental stressors that contribute to depression. These include alcoholic and abusive parents, chaotic family environments, and the death of a parent or other important person in the student's life.

The reasons that college students think about and sometimes attempt suicide are likewise varied and influenced by the times in which the students live.

A student with chronic depression may despair of ever feeling better or of ever overcoming the hardships he or she experiences on a daily basis. Another student may feel trapped by the pressures he or she faces and may see no other way out. A student may feel guilty or ashamed about something, even to the point of considering suicide. It's also possible that a student may feel overwhelmed by so much rage that he or she seeks to punish another person by attempting suicide. Regardless of the particular motivation, suicide is a serious problem on college campuses. During the fall of 2003, three New York University students independently killed themselves by jumping from tall buildings on their university campus.[10] The stories that receive wide publicity—such as the three N.Y.U. suicides—are alarming, yet they represent only a fraction of the suicides committed by college students. One survey noted that about 10 percent of college students report thinking seriously about killing themselves; for college students, suicide is the second leading cause of death and is responsible for the loss of about 1,100 lives a year.[11]

Although it is impossible to identify all at-risk students, reaching as many of these students as possible through outreach and prevention efforts is crucial. The roommates or friends of a suicidal person, rather than mental health professionals, may be the first to learn of a dangerous situation. Indeed, sometimes roommates or friends seek university counseling services to consult about a third person, who may be severely depressed or talking about suicide. Unfortunately, these individuals are not always comfortable providing the name of the student in question. They may worry about betraying their friend's confidence, or they might be worried about making too big a deal of the situation, especially if the suicidal student downplays his or her concern. In this way, outreach designed to (1) educate the university community about depression and suicide and (2) increase familiarity with mental health services and personnel on campus can be lifesaving. Other efforts to identify and intervene with students at risk for suicide have been enacted by various universities. These efforts include the use of anonymous mental health questionnaires, encouraging faculty and staff to contact deans or university counselors if they notice signs of depression or troubling changes in a student's behavior, putting counselors in residence halls, and mandating counseling sessions for at-risk students.[12] It is important to note that the increased attention to the mental health issues of college students over the past few years has focused on undergraduates. Graduate students, in contrast, have received relatively little attention, even though they are often more isolated than undergraduates and are subject to enormous stress (e.g., intense competition, relative isolation in research laboratories, financial worries, and anxiety about employment).[13]

UNIVERSITY MENTAL HEALTH SERVICES: IMPEDIMENTS TO TREATMENT

Mental health services on a college campus are often conceptualized as a particular type of specialty within the field of clinical practice. This specialty encompasses three main factors. The first emphasizes the developmental and environmental aspects of colleges and college students. The second emphasizes the boundaries and context inherent in university settings, which are concerned primarily with education rather than with mental health. The third factor emphasizes the range of flexibility and scope of services needed to respond in different ways to different student or organizational needs.[14] Colleges and universities vary in the mental health services they offer to students and to faculty and staff as well. Some colleges provide assessment, consultation, crisis, and referral services only. Others provide treatment, either short-term or long-term, in addition to the services listed above. Unfortunately, it is true that university counseling centers cannot reach all of the students who potentially need mental health services. Some of the reasons for this are outlined below.

Stigma

For some people, therapy is synonymous with exploration and getting to know oneself better. For many people, though, therapy is associated with severe mental illness. Some students do not want to be associated with a service they think is for crazy people. These students might feel embarrassed or ashamed if someone they knew saw them walking in the door of the counseling center. They might not think their problems are serious enough to take up a counselor's time, or—for those students who are really struggling to function—they might not want to admit the extent of their difficulties to themselves. They might believe their symptoms indicate a personal flaw—laziness or ineptitude, for example—rather than an illness. These attitudes are present not only in the troubled student but are reflected by parents and peers as well. A parent might tell a depressed student who complains of not being motivated to complete schoolwork that the student should get a grip and try harder. Friends might worry about confronting a depressed student because they don't want the student to think they believe he or she is crazy or weird. In other words, a lack of understanding of mental disorders is prevalent in American society; the stigma associated with depression and other mental disorders is also embedded in society.

Societal change comes slowly. There is both greater understanding of mental disorders and greater acceptance of the need for treatment of these disorders than there was a generation ago, and the children of today's college students may feel more comfortable about therapy than their parents did. However, educating the university population through pamphlets or Web sites about depression and anxiety, eating disorders, and substance abuse may make it easier for some students to see past the stigma and seek treatment. It also may make it easier for roommates, friends, and professors to approach students and encourage them to seek help. Advertising the university counseling center as a casual place where students can ask questions, discuss a problem, or receive help for depression likewise may help students feel more comfortable walking in the doors, even if they are still concerned that someone might see them.

Fear

Another factor that keeps students from utilizing university counseling services is fear. Some might have had unpleasant or unhelpful experiences with therapy in the past, and they may be skeptical or leery of being in therapy now. They may be afraid of taking medications or of finding out that they are truly suffering from a serious condition. Students who have never sought mental health services before may be unaware of the confidential nature of most services. They may be scared to come for treatment because they think their parents or professors will find out. Students sometimes decline referrals for private therapy for this reason; they don't want the insurance statements or therapist's bills to end up in their parents' mailbox. Other students worry about having a mental health record; they fear it will somehow hurt their employment prospects.

Educating the university population about confidentiality policies and the circumstances under which confidentiality is broken may help some students realize their fears are far-fetched, thereby increasing the likelihood that they will obtain help. When it is necessary to involve parents or others in a student's treatment—when a student is seriously suicidal or requires hospitalization, for example—offering to help the student communicate with his or her parents may alleviate some of the fear.

The Nature of Mental Illness

Sometimes it is the student's symptoms themselves that prevent him or her from getting needed help. A student in the midst of a manic episode, for instance, may report feeling energized and euphoric rather than troubled. A student with paranoid thinking may not trust mental health personnel, among others, and therefore will not pursue counseling. Ann, a sophomore, saw a therapist only after being persuaded to do so by her academic advisor. Consider the reasons she gave for not seeking help sooner:

After being in treatment for three months and taking antidepressant medication, Ann's depressive symptoms improved significantly. She told her therapist
that she didn't seek help on her own, even though she had thoughts about suicide
at the time, because she didn't think anyone could help her or understand her.
She felt hopeless, and that applied to treatment as well as to her schoolwork and
other areas of her life. She also didn't have the energy. It would take a lot of effort
to call for an appointment and then show up for it, she explained, and she just
didn't have that energy, especially since she didn't think it would help anyway.

In this case, Ann's depressive disorder itself—specifically the depressive
symptoms of hopelessness and exhaustion or lack of energy—prevented her
from getting the treatment she needed to combat the disorder. Ann's situation
highlights the important role played by others in the university community.
A student may feel that it's useless to seek treatment, but roommates, friends,
and particularly persons in a position of authority (such as professors and
deans) may be able to convince the student to try it anyway.

Cultural Prohibitions among International Students

It is especially difficult for university counseling services to attract international students, and many international students do not receive help until a
crisis forces someone else in the university community to compel the student
to get treatment. As Dr. Richard Kadison, chief of the Mental Health Service
at Harvard University Health Services, points out, "When the worries become
overwhelming, international students are the last to seek help. It seems that
talking about stress and its effects on health is an American phenomenon that
many international students do not understand" (p. 64).[15] Students from some
cultures may feel that having emotional problems represents a personal failure,
and they may worry about shaming themselves and their families. Students
from certain cultures may feel prohibited from talking about their families,
their feelings, or other "private" matters, especially with people outside of their
families.

Furthermore, language barriers may prevent some international students
from obtaining counseling. Cultures that do not emphasize emotional expression may not have a lot of words for emotion concepts, and thus a student
from such a culture may not know how to talk about what is happening to him
or her. Other students may find it exhausting or difficult to talk for extended
periods in English if it is not their first language. Finally, some cultures have
"culture-bound syndromes" associated with them (p. 843).[8] For example, the
Diagnostic and Statistical Manual of Mental Disorders (DSM–IV) defines a
syndrome called "brain fag" as a "term initially used in West Africa to refer to

a condition experienced by high school or university students in response to the challenges of schooling. Symptoms include difficulties in concentrating, remembering, and thinking. Students often state that their brains are 'fatigued.' Additional somatic symptoms are usually centered around the head and neck and include pain, pressure or tightness, blurring of vision, heat, or burning (p. 846)."[8] Some of the symptoms of brain fag sound like those of depression or anxiety. The *DSM–IV* identifies 25 culture-bound syndromes. In addition to language barriers, the absence of any of these syndromes from counseling center pamphlets and advertising may lead international students to believe that the service providers will not understand or be sensitive to their concerns.

There are several ways that university counseling centers can try to increase access for international students. Students from other cultures may be more likely to seek services if they know there are counselors on staff who are fluent in languages other than English. Also, as suggested above, culturally inclusive pamphlets, Web sites, and other advertising may increase use by international students. Finally, universities often have special student centers that are geared toward international students, Latino students, or African American or Asian American students. Strong liaison relationships between counseling center staff and the staff of these student centers can facilitate needed referrals to the counseling center.

The impediments to treatment previously discussed—stigma, fear, the nature of mental illness, cultural prohibitions, inadequate funding, and lack of visibility—all pertain to the students in need of services. The following factors pertain to the counseling facilities themselves.

Inadequate Funding

Often, colleges and universities do not prioritize student mental health services, especially in difficult economic times. Inadequately funded counseling centers cannot hire the staff needed to serve the university population effectively. While increasing numbers of students currently need mental health services on campus, even those counseling centers with relatively large staffs may feel the strain of not being able to respond as fully as they would like to this demand. In one informal survey, university counseling center directors cited the lack of funds for adequate staffing as their chief complaint.[5] If a college student has to wait a long time for an appointment with a counselor, it is not only potentially dangerous for that student, but it is a turnoff as well. The student may be less likely to follow through than if he or she is offered an appointment within a couple of days. This is especially true for a student who was reluctant to contact the counseling center in the first place.

Several outside sources of funding have stepped in to ease the financial burden colleges and universities face in providing adequate mental health services. The Jed Foundation, for example, is a nonprofit organization whose mission is to reduce the frequency of suicides committed on college campuses. The organization is named for Jed Satow, a college student who at age 20 killed himself in the late 1990s.[11] The Campus Care and Counseling Act, furthermore, passed by the Senate in the fall of 2004, allocates $10 million in grants to college mental health services to "help with prevention of and early intervention with behavioral and mental health problems such as depression, eating disorders and substance abuse."[16]

Lack of Visibility

University counseling center staff serve dual roles. They are clinical practitioners for students and other members of the university community who need their services. They are also members of that community. On the one hand, they need to preserve the confidentiality and protect the boundaries of their treatments. On the other hand, they need to be engaged in the life of the campus. If counseling center staff are too isolated, the services they offer will be less visible to the students who need them. Faculty and other staff may also be less likely to refer students for evaluation or treatment if they perceive the counseling center as distant and uninterested in campus life. Printed and electronic media, such as brochures and Web sites, are of limited utility if the counselors themselves are nowhere to be seen. To maximize usage of mental health services, counselors need to attend to both roles.

CONCLUSIONS

College students seek counseling services for all sorts of reasons. A freshman might feel homesick or anxious about separating from her family and high school friends. A senior might feel lost and directionless, unsure of who he is and what he wants to do after graduation. One student might abuse drugs or drink to excess; another might binge on large amounts of food and end up feeling bloated and ashamed. Still others might feel depressed—unable to study or socialize—and some might feel dangerously suicidal. College students, whether struggling with developmental concerns or new or preexisting mental disorders, represent a particular clinical population, and college campuses represent a specialized treatment setting. Can university counseling services reach these students? Can they minimize the stigma and quell the fear that a struggling student might feel? Are they accessible to roommates, friends, professors, and deans—those who might recognize that a student needs help even when the student cannot see it? Do they offer and advertise culturally sensitive and knowledgeable services? Are they adequately funded and visible on campus? By addressing the needs of college students and by intervening quickly and effectively, college mental health centers foster the intellectual, social, and emotional growth needed for a productive, fulfilling adulthood.

REFERENCES

1. Erikson, E. H. (1968). *Identity: Youth and crisis.* New York: W. W. Norton.
2. Sontag, D. (2002, April 28). A suicide at M.I.T. *New York Times Magazine, 94,* 57–61.
3. Gegax, T. T. (2005, June 6). An end to 'power hour.' *Newsweek, 145,* 28.
4. National Advisory Council on Alcohol Abuse and Alcoholism. (2002, April 3). Summary of meeting. Retrieved June 6, 2005, from http://www.niaaa.nih.gov/about/min4–02.htm
5. Kadison, R., & DiGeronimo, T. F. (2004). *College of the overwhelmed: The campus mental health crisis and what to do about it.* San Francisco: Jossey-Bass.
6. Khan, M. (2003, July 13). Researching two new campus drugs. *Boston Globe,* p. A5.
7. Gallagher, R. (2002). *National survey of counseling center directors 2002.* Pittsburgh, PA: International Association of Counseling Services.
8. American Psychiatric Association. (1994). *Diagnostic and statistical manual of mental disorders* (4th ed.). Washington, DC: Author.
9. Hoover, E. (2003, December 5). More help for troubled students. *The Chronicle of Higher Education,* p. A25.
10. Arenson, K. (2003, October 21). At N.Y.U., not all want to talk about deaths, but reminders are never far away. *New York Times,* p. B6.
11. Gately, G. (2005, April 17). Colleges target mental health. *Boston Globe,* p. D18.
12. Arenson, K. W. (2004, December 3). Worried colleges step up efforts over suicide. *New York Times,* p. A1.
13. Butler, C. K. (2005, April 11). The pressure mounts. *U.S. News & World Report, 138,* 54–56.
14. May, R. (Ed.). (1988). *Psychoanalytic psychotherapy in a college context.* New York: Praeger.
15. Kadison, R., & DiGeronimo, T. F. (2004). *College of the overwhelmed: The campus mental health crisis and what to do about it.* San Francisco: Jossey-Bass.
16. Dittmann, M. (2004, September). Campus Care and Counseling Act passes U.S. Senate. *Monitor on Psychology, 35,* 17.

Chapter 11

Pedophile Priests: What Do We Know about Catholic Clergy Who Sexually Victimize Minors?

Thomas G. Plante

Since the mid-1990s, more than 130 people have come forward with horrific childhood tales about how former priest John J. Geoghan allegedly fondled or raped them during a three-decade spree through a half-dozen Greater Boston parishes. Almost always, his victims were grammar school boys. One was just 4 years old. Then came last July's disclosure that Cardinal Bernard F. Law knew about Geoghan's problems in 1984, Law's first year in Boston, yet approved his transfer to St. Julia's parish in Weston. . . . The St. Julia's assignment proved disastrous. First, Geoghan was put in charge of three youth groups, including altar boys. In 1989, he was forced to go on sick leave after more complaints of sexual abuse. . . . Even so, the archdiocese returned him to St. Julia's, where Geoghan continued to abuse children for another three years.

The affable Geoghan usually befriended Catholic mothers struggling to raise large families, often alone. His offers to help, often by taking the children for ice cream or praying with them at bedtime, were accepted without suspicion. That is how 12-year-old Patrick McSorley, who lived in a Hyde Park housing project, allegedly became a Geoghan victim in 1986. . . . According to McSorley, Geoghan . . . learned of his father's suicide and dropped by to offer condolences to his mother, who is schizophrenic. The priest offered to buy Patrick ice cream. 'Felt a little funny about it,' McSorley recalled in an interview. 'I was 12 years old and he was an old man.' Riding home after getting ice cream, McSorley says, Geoghan consoled him. But then he patted his upper leg and slid his

hand up toward his crotch . . . then he put his hand on my genitals and started
masturbating me. I was petrified. McSorely added that Geoghan then began
*masturbating himself.**
                    —Michael Rezendes and the Boston Globe Spotlight Team, *Boston*
                                                        Globe, January 6, 2002

THE PEDOPHILE PRIEST CRISIS IN THE ROMAN CATHOLIC CHURCH

An incredible amount of media attention over the past several years has highlighted the "pedophile priest" crisis in the American Roman Catholic Church.† Beginning with the January 6, 2002, *Boston Globe* Spotlight Team investigative report,[1] this story was *New York Times* front-page news for 41 days in a row. Just about every newspaper, magazine, and television news show across the United States (and in much of the world) reported and commented on the many unfolding cases of Catholic priests who were accused of sexually abusing children and teens during the past few decades. Very few stories have received the kind of intense and sustained focus by the mass media and popular press for so long.

Many outraged citizens called for the immediate resignation or defrocking of not only the priests accused of such egregious sexual misconduct but also the various bishops, cardinals, and other religious officials who were responsible for supervising and managing these men and assigning them to their priestly duties.[2] A flood of lawsuits was filed on behalf of the victims and victim advocacy groups totaling well over a billion dollars in claims. Several Church dioceses across the United States, such as the one in Boston, threatened to go bankrupt by filing for Chapter 11 protection. Laws were quickly altered in many states to extend the

---

* John Geoghan, 68, was murdered in prison during August 2003. Patrick McSorley, 29, committed suicide during February 2004. Cardinal Law, 72, resigned during December 2002 and is now archpriest of the Roman basilica of St. Mary Major.

† Parts of this chapter were published in the following outlets: T. G. Plante, "Introduction," in *Sin against the Innocents: Sexual Abuse by Priests and the Role of the Catholic Church*, ed. T. G. Plante (Westport, CT: Greenwood, 2004), xix–xxix; T. G. Plante, "Conclusion: What Do We Know and Where Do We Need to Go?" in *Sin against the Innocents: Sexual Abuse by Priests and the Role of the Catholic Church*, ed. T. G. Plante (Westport, CT: Greenwood, 2004), 183–92; T. G. Plante, "After the Earthquake: Five Reasons for Hope after the Sexual Abuse Scandal," *America*, January 15, 2004, 11–14; T. G. Plante, "Another Aftershock: What Have We Learned from the John Jay College Report?" *America*, March 22, 2004, 10–12; T. G. Plante and C. Daniels, "The Sexual Abuse Crisis in the Roman Catholic Church: What Psychologists and Counselors Should Know," *Pastoral Psychology* 52 (2004): 381–93.

statutes of limitations so that additional victims could come forward with their accusations even decades later.

The clergy sexual abuse crisis also impacted the Roman Catholic Church in other countries as well, with similar accusations made against a number of priests and Church officials in Ireland, Australia, the United Kingdom, and elsewhere. Many Catholic Church leaders in these countries also had to contend with relentless and unflattering media attention, numerous accusations of victimization, and many lawsuits.

Catholics and non-Catholics alike have been furious with Church officials for not better protecting unsuspecting children and families from sex-offending priests. This is especially true since many Church officials knew of earlier incidents of priests abusing children yet chose to transfer these men to other unsuspecting parishes in different locations. Many have felt that the Church considered itself above the law and arrogant in the manner in which they handled these concerns over the years.[2] Many have suggested that the Church has lost its moral compass and authority. How could the public listen to Catholic bishops pontificate on topics such as unjust wars, the gap between rich and poor, sexuality, abortion, gay marriage, and other hot topics when the sexual abuse scandals were in the headlines? Calls for reform have also been voiced about other complex, challenging, and controversial issues with the Roman Catholic Church such as the prohibitions against women priests, married priests, and homosexual priests.[3] Energized new lay advocacy groups (e.g., Voice of the Faithful) emerged and grew very quickly. It is unlikely that the American Catholic Church has ever experienced a more difficult crisis.[1]

Given the recent media attention and crisis, it may be a surprise to hear that the problem of clergy sexual abuse among Catholic priests is not a new problem at all. In fact, the American media reported on this issue in fits and starts several times before the 2002 crisis in Boston. For example, throughout the 1990s it was well known that a sizable percentage of priests had sexually abused minors.[3,4] Books and articles had been published in both professional and popular press outlets about priest sex offenders. Several notable and sensational cases have dominated press attention in the past. These include the exploits of Fr. James Porter in New England as well as Fr. Gilbert Gauthe in Louisiana. Furthermore, comments about clergy sexual abuse were recorded hundreds and even well over a thousand years ago by the Church itself. For example, St. Basil (330–379) stated, "A cleric or monk who seduces youths or young boys ... is to be publicly flogged. ... For six months he will languish in prison-like confinement ... and he shall never again associate with youths in private conversation nor in counseling them" (p. 183 n.49).[5] Therefore, sexual abuse committed by Catholic priests is not a new story that only became public in the media storm of 2002.

The recent crisis, however, has drawn attention to the notion of or phrase "pedophile priest." Many have wondered about these men of the cloth who sexually violate children. What do we know about these "pedophile priests?"[6]

WHAT DO WE KNOW ABOUT "PEDOPHILE PRIESTS"?

The most comprehensive study of pedophile priests ever conducted was completed by the John Jay College of Criminal Justice in 2004 and was funded by the Unites States Council of Catholic Bishops.[7] The John Jay Report, as it has become known, was the most comprehensive and independent investigation of the problem of clergy sexual abuse ever conducted. In fact, it is reasonable to suggest that it was the most comprehensive independent investigation on the sexual abuse of children of its kind conducted for any major organization religious or otherwise.

The report concluded that 4 percent of Roman Catholic priests or other male Catholic clergy such as religious brothers and deacons have had a sexual experience with a minor (e.g., anyone under the age of 18) during the past 52 years with a total of almost 10,700 victims. The 4 percent figure translates into 4,392 clergy against whom credible accusations of child sexual abuse were made. It was also noted that 4.3 percent of these men were diocesan priests primarily working in pastoral settings in church parishes while 2.7 percent were religious order priests (e.g., Franciscans, Jesuits, Dominicans) who generally were not working in local parishes but rather in parochial schools, colleges, and universities, health facilities, and elsewhere.

The majority of the abusive behavior included touching minors inappropriately under their clothes (57%) with a sizable number of incidents involving oral sex (27%) and penile penetration or attempted penetration (25%). About half (51%) of the victims were between the ages of 11 and 14 with only 15 percent aged 16 or above. The vast majority of victims (81%) were male.

Unlike the most egregious cases frequently reported in the press, the majority of these clergy sex offenders had only one credible allegation of abuse against them (56%). However, 149 priests had more than 10 allegations against them, resulting in the reported abuse of 2,960 victims, or 27 percent of the total. Remarkably, only about 150 men accounted for almost 30 percent of all know sexual abuse cases in the past half century. These 150 serial offenders clearly accounted for much of the damage to so many children.

A large majority (almost 70 percent) of these abusive priests were ordained before 1970. The report concluded that most of the abusive behavior occurred in the 1970s and dropped significantly during the 1980s and 1990s.

WHY THE PHRASE "PEDOPHILE PRIEST" IS A MISNOMER

Although the term "pedophile priest" has received a great deal of media attention and acceptance in the general public, it does not truly inform people about the nature of the sexual misconduct. The *Diagnostic and Statistical Manual of Mental Disorders*, 4th edition, or *DSM–IV*, published by the American Psychiatric Association, defines pedophilia as "sexual activity with a prepubescent child (generally age 13 or younger)" (p. 527). Unfortunately, the John Jay Report did not investigate the victims of clergy sexual abuse based on pre versus post pubescence [4,8]. Rather, they reported that 81 percent of victims were boys between the ages of 11 and 14. This age range would likely include many children from both pre- and postpubescent developmental stages. However, research conducted elsewhere and published in scholarly books and journal articles suggests that the majority of clergy sexual offenders do not victimize prepubescent children and are therefore not technically considered pedophiles.[3–8] Rather, they would be considered "ephebophiles," or adults who target teenage postpubescent youngsters. Ephebophilia may be considered illegal in most states, as well as a sin or morally wrong, but it is not considered a psychiatric diagnosis according to the *DSM–IV* noted above. Therefore, a substantial number of "pedophile priests" are not pedophiles at all. Perhaps a case example may well illustrate this point.

Case 1

Fr. A is a 50-year-old priest teaching at an all-boys Catholic high school. Fr. A serves as the school swim coach. Prior to and following swim meets, Fr. A massages his student swimmers. He has physical therapy and physical education training as well. Furthermore, he was trained in "spiritual massage" at a theological training institute. On one occasion, one of his student teenage swimmers gets an erection. Fr. A. decides to massage the student until climax. After an investigation, it appears that Fr. A had similar experiences with two other students during his 23-year career at the school. His three reported victims were all about 15 years old.

Fr. A is an ephebophile and not a pedophile. One might argue that these diagnostic differences are "splitting hairs" and do not ultimately matter. However, both research and clinical practice suggests that the difference between pedophilia and ephebophilia is very important in terms of diagnosis, treatment, and attending to possible risk factors for abuse.[9] First, the difference between these two groups of sexual offenders helps better inform which youth population is most at risk. For example, the young altar boy may be less at risk than the teenage high school student for priests experiencing ephebophilia. Parents might worry about the safety of their 8-year-old altar boy son but be not at all worried about their 15-year-old son who attends a Catholic high school. These parents may not realize that their teenager might be at much higher risk for sexual victimization by priests than their young 8-year-old son is. Second, pedophilia has been found to be more resistant to treatment than ephebophilia. Therefore, all things being equal, the odds are that successful rehabilitation is more likely with ephebophiles than with pedophiles.[9]

The word "priest" is also somewhat of a misnomer as well. Catholic clergy who have been accused of sexual misconduct with minor children are not always priests. Many are religious brothers who may also take vows of obedience, poverty, and chastity but who are not ordained as priests. Therefore, they do not perform the Mass ritual and many other priestly duties. They might teach parochial school, coach sports, assist with Mass and other religious activities, and wear priestly attire. Some of the accusations have been made against deacons. Deacons are not priests and are often married men.

Thus, although the phrase "pedophile priest" has been used to describe the clergy abuse problem in the Catholic Church, a better phrase might be "sex-offending Catholic clergy." This new phrase is more accurate but perhaps not as catchy.

WHY WOULD A PRIEST SEXUALLY VIOLATE A CHILD?

The above statistics in the previous sections may shed some light on the frequency of sexual abuse by priests as well as provide some information about likely victims. However, these statistics tell nothing about what might be going on in the hearts and minds of sex-offending clergy. How could a man of the cloth, a religious, moral, and ethical leader, engage in such awful anwd harmful behavior with a vulnerable child? What do we know about the inner workings of these men? Years of both research and clinical practice provide some insights into the internal workings of the sex-offending clergy.

Sex-offending clergy come in various styles of offending.[10] Some are considered "situational" offenders. These men might describe themselves as primarily interested in adults as potential sexual objects of their desire (either heterosexual or homosexual attractions). They may be appropriately sexually attracted to adults whether they act on these attractions or not. They may not seek out children or teens to offend yet find themselves offending these youngsters during particular circumstances. These circumstances may include unsupervised access and closeness to potential victims, consuming alcohol or drugs, periods of high stress and low self esteem, "falling in love" with a minor to whom they feel particularly close or connected, anonymous sex with strangers who they think are adults but are actually under age, and so forth. Another case example may prove useful.

Case 2

Fr. B is a newly ordained young parish priest from another country. He lives in a rural area with an elderly pastor in a church rectory setting. Most of the parishioners in his church are conservative elderly Catholics. He often feels lonely and isolated. During periods of stress, he finds himself driving to a major city several hours away where he engages in anonymous homosexual sex with other consenting adults. He reports feeling terribly guilty and distraught about this behavior. However, he feels somewhat compelled to do this every few months. On one occasion, his anonymous partner was a 17-year-old boy and thus not a legal adult. Police caught them in the act.

Fr. B is a homosexual who is attracted to other adults. However, during periodic anonymous homosexual sex, a minor was involved.

Other offenders are more "preferential." They prefer children as sexual objects and seek them out. They are generally not sexually attracted to adults at all. They may engage in "grooming behavior" by working to secure the trust of a child (and perhaps his or her family) over time before sexual victimization ultimately unfolds. These men may development friendships with the child and family, do favors for them, and shower them with attention, gifts, treats, and the like. After trust is well established, sexual abuse begins. Another case example illustrates a preferential offender.

Case 3

Fr. C find himself sexually attracted to young boys and girls around the age of nine. He enjoys cuddling and wrestling with them, attending church-sponsored camping trips and other outings, and helping out with the church youth group. Fr. C was accused of fondling several children during a camping trip. Fr. C has a long history of depression and alcohol problems as well. The children reported smelling alcohol on his breath during the victimization. Fr. C reports feeling uncomfortable with adults and finds himself sexually aroused by younger children. He often finds himself watching children on playgrounds and at fast food restaurants. He reports that this sexually arouses him.

Sex-offending clergy usually experience psychiatric comorbidity as well.[4,9,11] This means that they suffer from at least one psychiatric disturbance such as clinical depression, a personality disorder, substance abuse problems, addictions of various sorts, or even brain injury. They often struggle with a range of behavioral, emotional, and psychiatric concerns. These additional disorders may make them more vulnerable to acting inappropriately with youth.

Information assembled from insurance claims as well as psychological reports and research suggests that sex-offending clergy tend to experience poor social skills, immaturity, social isolation, and low self-esteem. A sizable number come from troubled family backgrounds that included abuse and neglect when they were young.[8,9]

The overall profile suggests that priests and other Catholic clergy who sexually abuse children may do so for a variety of reasons, and they generally experience a number of personal demons that might contribute to their behavior. Although their psychiatric problems do not excuse their victimization of vulnerable children, it does help to better understand these men who abuse. In doing so, we are better able to evaluate, diagnosis, treat, and prevent abuse of children and teens.

Case 4

Fr. D worked as a parish priest in a very low-income setting in Mexico. He taught in a church school as well. Fr. D has a long history of personality and alcohol problems. He was sexually and physically abused himself as a child while living in an orphanage. Furthermore, when he was 10 years old doing some school-related volunteer work, he was sexually abuse by a priest who was working as a hospital chaplain. During a drinking episode with teens from the school, he sexually molested a boy. After an investigation, several other boys reported similar experiences with Fr. D. In total, about eight boys were abused by Fr. D during alcohol-related overnight trips. Fr. D reports that he is heterosexual in orientation but chooses boys because they are available and he has easy access to them. Furthermore, he is somewhat phobic about females, stating that they might get pregnant. Fr. D well illustrates that many sex-offending priests experience psychiatric problems that contribute to their abusive behavior.

HOW DO PEDOPHILE PRIESTS COMPARE TO NON-PRIESTS WHO SEXUALLY ABUSE CHILDREN?

Tragically, we know that sexual abuse of minors is also not limited to the behavior of Roman Catholic priests.[12,13] Although solid and reliable statistics are not easy to obtain, it is very clear that sexual abuse committed by male clergy is certainly found among Protestant, Jewish, Muslim, and other religious leaders. For example, the Anglican Church in Canada (and most notably, British Columbia) has experienced a large number of credible accusations of sexual misconduct with minors against their non-Catholic priests. These accusations have led to press reports and lawsuits similar to those in the United States. Unfortunately, no equivalent comprehensive John Jay Report has been conducted or published focusing on other clergy groups. Therefore, reasonable estimates secured from lawsuits, police reports, available research reports, and treatment facilities are the best we can do at this point in time. While the Roman Catholic Church has easily received the most media attention, sexual abuse of minors exists at alarming rates among others who have access to and power over minors and who are usually trusted with the welfare of children (e.g., physicians, psychologists, social workers, school teachers, Boy Scout leaders, coaches, school bus drivers). For example, it has been well established that in mental health professions, between 1 and 7 percent of female professionals and between 2 and 17 percent of male professionals sexually exploit their patients.[14] These figures, however, predominantly reflect adult victims, and the prevalence of child and teen victims among these professions is too poorly researched to draw clear conclusions. Sexual abuse committed by people in the helping professions is all too common. Quality research, for example, has demonstrated that about 5 percent of school teachers have experienced credible accusations of child sexual abuse.[15] Sadly, sexual abuse of children and adolescents can be found in every area of the world and in every profession. Those who have trusting relationships with children and ready access to them can do the most harm. Those with a great deal of power and authority and with little accountability can do enormous harm to many, regardless of their religious tradition and role.

Furthermore, it has been well established from a wide variety of solid research studies that approximately 17 percent of all American women and 12 percent of American men report that they have had an unwanted and abusive sexual experience with an adult while they were still minors.[16] Amazingly, about one in six adult Americans reports that as a child or adolescent, he or she was sexually abused by an adult. Sadly, there is a great deal of sexual exploitation of minors by adults regardless of religious persuasion, profession, and role. Of course, we'd expect much better behavior from clergy than from the general population. Tragically, we must admit that the sexual exploitation of children is and perhaps always has been fairly common.

WHAT DO PEDOPHILE PRIESTS HAVE TO DO WITH HOMOSEXUALITY?

Since 81 percent of clergy abuse victims in the Roman Catholic Church are male, many have wondered about the role of homosexuality in the clergy abuse crisis. In fact, some (including several bishops) have called for the elimination of all homosexuals from the priesthood in an effort to stop the sexual victimization of boys by priests. Some of these bishops, such as former United States Catholic Conference of Bishops president Fr. William Gregory, have made public statements that homosexual priests are at least partially to blame for the sexual abuse crisis in the American Catholic Church.[1] Official Catholic Church policy does not allow homosexual men to become priests. Vatican spokesman Joaquin Navarro-Valls recently reiterated this policy by stating that homosexuals cannot be ordained into the Catholic priesthood.[17] However, best estimates suggest that about 30–50 percent of Catholic priests and seminarians in America would describe themselves as being homosexual in orientation.[18]

Many seminaries, novitiates, and dioceses maintain a "don't ask don't tell" policy or do not enforce Church teachings in this matter.[19] This "don't ask don't tell" policy has led to the creation of a quiet gay subculture in the priesthood. A recent survey of 1,200 priests found that 55 percent recognized a gay subculture within the Catholic Church.[17]

Tragically, homosexual priests have become scapegoats in this area. Although the majority of clergy abuse victims are males, homosexuality cannot be blamed. First, many of the pedophile priests report that they are not homosexual. This is also true of many non-clergy sex offenders who victimize boys. Many report that they may target boys for a variety of reasons that include easier access to boys (e.g., working as a coach in an all-boys Catholic school), pregnancy fears with females victims, and more easily established trust and access with boys (and perhaps with their parents). Second, homosexuals in general have not been found to be more likely to commit sexual crimes against minors compared to heterosexuals. Sexual orientation is not predictive of sex crimes. Thus, eliminating all homosexual men from the Catholic priesthood would not stop a subset of men from sexually abusing minors.

WHAT DO PEDOPHILE PRIESTS HAVE TO DO WITH CELIBACY?

Thus far, no reliable research exists to conclude that Catholic priests are much more likely than male clergy from other faith traditions (or men in the general population) to sexually abuse children. Therefore, males who marry or engage in sexual relationships with consenting adults are not significantly less likely to sexually victimize children compared with Catholic priests. Furthermore, if someone could not have a sexual relationship with another person for any reason, such as religious vows, the inability to find an acceptable partner, or marital and relationship discord, children and teens would not necessarily become the object of his desire. Rather, consenting adults would. Thus, allowing priests to marry would not eliminate the inclination of some of these men to sexually victimize minors.

In 1970, the two primary reasons for priests leaving the priesthood were because of disagreements with authoritative Church structures and their desire to marry. In 2000, the most prominent reason for leaving was a desire to marry, while institutional criticism was not a significant factor any longer. In a recent survey, 56 percent of priests thought that celibacy should be optional while 12 percent stated that they would likely marry if celibacy were no longer manda-tory.[17] Overall, the current main reason for priest resignations and disagreements with Church policies is the issue of celibacy.[17] A recent poll in Boston reflects the beliefs of many Catholics. The survey found that 74 percent of Catholics in the Boston area disagree with the Church that priests should remain celibate.[20]

If Catholic priests could marry there would clearly be a significant increase in the potential pool of applicants to the priesthood. This would also be true if females could become priests in the Catholic Church. However, the increased number of priests would not necessarily eliminate the few men who have a predilection to sexually abuse minors. This is most evident in the fact that most sex offenders in the community are not priests at all and are often married men.

WHY HAS THERE BEEN SO MUCH ATTENTION ON SEXUAL ABUSE BY PRIESTS?

If priests are not more likely to sexually abuse minors than men from the general population or clergy from other faith traditions, then why has there been so much relentless attention on sexual abuse committed by Catholic priests and little if any attention to abuse perpetrated by other male clergy members or other respected groups in society? There are a variety of important factors that likely contribute to the laser beam attention the American Catholic Church has received regarding this awful problem. First, about 25 percent of the American population identify themselves as being Roman Catholic.[21] Additionally, many people (both Catholics and many non-Catholics alike) have received elementary, secondary, or university education through Catholic schools, colleges, seminaries, and universities. Furthermore, over 7 million Americans per year receive social and medical services from Catholic Charities, while Catholic hospitals are the largest nonprofit health care provider in the United States, with over 800 facilities treating over 70 million patients each year.[22] This figure alone represents almost one-third of the entire American population! Therefore, an enormous subset of Americans have had or continue to have direct contact with priests, other Catholic clergy such as religious sisters and brothers, and the Catholic Church in general in at least some capacity regarding education, health care, social service, or spiritual matters. Because of the large number of people affiliated with the Catholic Church and its social, educational, medical, and religious services and programs, many people either personally or professionally interact with the Catholic Church and Catholic clergy including priests. Therefore, they are more likely to be interested in and focused on these concerns among a group that they have had personal experiences with in the past or present.

Second, the clergy abuse crisis in the American Catholic Church is a crisis of priests (including religious superiors such as bishops making decisions about wayward priests under their charge) behaving very badly.[23] This includes the behavior of priests and other male Catholic clergy (e.g., brothers, deacons) who have sexually abused minors the behavior of Church leaders such as bishops for inadequate supervision and terrible decisions regarding how to best manage priests who behave in awful ways. Furthermore, the problem seems, on the surface, so easily preventable since it is a behavioral problem that is so obviously wrong, immoral, illegal, and against priestly vows. Additionally, no one would expect this kind of horrible behavior to occur on the part of a moral and religious clergy member and leader in the community. Before the media attention regarding sex-offending clergy, a priest was perhaps the last person on earth one would expect would be a sex offender. In general, we also would expect much better behavior from Catholic clergy than from clergy of other religious traditions who could be seen as being more "like us" because they are usually married. Priests appear to be much more removed from everyday life due to their commitment to chastity, poverty, and obedience, and they seem to maintain a special calling or relationship with God that one would expect might prevent them from engaging in sexually abusive behaviors with children or anyone. One has a very long way to fall if one is up high on a pedestal.

Third, the Catholic Church has had a long history of acting in a defensive and often arrogant manner regarding this and many other issues.[3] The defensive and arrogant posture has likely contributed to both Catholics and non-Catholics alike becoming furious with the Church and its leaders. In many cases, Church officials have not treated abuse victims and their families with concern and compassion.[2] This inability to be pastoral has led victims and victim advocacy groups to become enraged with the Catholic Church and its leadership. Many religious superiors such as bishops have not managed so many of these cases very well. For example, Cardinal Bernard Law of Boston was accused of allowing priests who had allegations brought against them to continue to serve in the Church in a variety of parishes for years without informing these churches of the allegations.[1]

Fourth, unlike most other religious traditions and most secular organizations in the United States and elsewhere, the Catholic Church does not use lay boards of directors to hire, fire, and evaluate priests or other Church leaders. Local bishops (as well as other religious superiors) do not have to answer to local boards, community members, or even to each other. They must answer individually to the Vatican, thousands of miles away, which is often preoccupied with the many needs and challenges of the world's 1 billion Catholics in just about every location on the globe (with 80 percent now below the equator). Furthermore, bishops and other religious superiors are not elected to their jobs with any kind of democratic process but are assigned. These assignments do not come with term limits and are not subject to renewal by the local lay community. Therefore, if a particular religious superior such as a bishop makes terrible decisions about how to manage problematic priests or others, the Church does not have the checks and balances associated with most organizations that might help to nip in the bud potential problems. Bishops do not get fired or recalled for poor performance. Other than legal limits imposed by local, state, and federal laws, Church leaders do not have to please a variety of groups in order to remain in their position of power and influence. Each bishop must please (or at least not upset) his boss, who is located in Rome and will likely not be in touch with the day-to-day operations and decisions of so many bishops across the globe. Therefore, without useful checks and balances, problems can easily spread like a virus out of control.

The Catholic Church is by far the largest continuously operating organization in the world, representing 20 percent of the 6 billion people on the planet. It is not a small, insular, and obscure cult or church. It impacts billions of people. The Catholic Church has also assumed an ethical voice of moral authority for 2,000 years. The Church's often unpopular positions and standards on sexual behavior such as contraception use, sexual activity among the unmarried, homosexuality, and divorce make sex crimes committed by their priests even more egregious.[6,18] When priests err, sin, and fall from grace, it is perceived as a much bigger drop than for ministers from other religious traditions who are perceived as much more like the general population. The intriguing secrecy and inner workings of the Catholic Church also make the story of sexual abuse committed by priests fascinating and of great interest to the media and the general population.[1] Finally, many of the 25 percent of Americans who identify themselves as being Catholic often have mixed feelings about their Church. Many of the millions of Americans who have experienced Catholic education or were raised in the Church have stories of priests and nuns who were overly strict and difficult to deal with. Many have felt that they couldn't measure up to the impossibly high standards of the Church. Perhaps the Gospel verse attributed to Jesus—"He who is without sin may cast the first stone"—is a poignant perspective of the media and public's view on clergy sexual abuse. Those who present themselves as being morally superior to others find the fall from grace much more notable than the fall by average persons.

WHY CAN WE BE HOPEFUL?

One of the striking findings from the John Jay Report was the fact that the bulk of clergy sex offenders were ordained around 1970.[7] The vast majority of the priests accused of sexually abusing children during the past 50 years tend to be in their late fifties and sixties and the reported abuse occurred over 20 years ago. Although sexual abuse committed by priests and others has occurred for centuries and, sadly, will not stop immediately or in the future, the best available data suggests that there may be a cohort effect about priests who were ordained around 1970 that puts these men at higher risk for offending minors.

Why would this be so? There are several factors that likely make these priests more vulnerable for sexual transgressions. First, many of these men, like generations before them, entered into religious life as teenagers. Thus, the majority entered seminary when there were still youngsters. They were unable to work through the numerous complex psychological and behavioral issues regarding sexual development, maturity, and expression that others are more likely to work through. Issues about sexual development and expression as well as impulse control matters were usually not really evaluated or discussed before entering seminary or even introduced once they entered religious life. If a seminarian had concerns about anything sexual, he was often told by his superiors to take a cold shower, work hard, and pray.

These young men also entered seminary during a highly remarkable Church and cultural upheaval centered around both Vatican II and the sexual revolution in the United States. It seemed that up was down and down was up during these tumultuous times. Furthermore, there was a great exodus from seminary during the late 1960s and early 1970s with 1973 being the peak year of priests and seminarians leaving their vocation. It was a major turning point in the history of the American Catholic Church as well as in America itself. Traditional boundaries, rules, and expectations were broken overnight. For example, research suggests that about 23 percent of male psychotherapists were sexually involved with at least one of their patients during these years.[24] This figure is closer to 2 percent today.[25] Overall, it is not a surprise that the majority of those accused of sexual misconduct are priests who are elderly men who committed their offenses around 1970. If this cohort theory is correct, then we can expect a much lower proportion of new abuse cases both now and in the future.

NEW CHURCH POLICIES AND PRACTICES

Long before the clergy sexual abuse crisis in Boston and elsewhere hit the press in 2002, many significant changes had already occurred in the selection and training of priests to help minimize clergy sexual abuse from occurring. First, entering seminary students have gotten much older in recent decades, with the current average age of entry being about 30.[26,27] Many of these men have had successful and satisfying intimate relationships and have grown and matured in many areas of their lives before entering religious life. Seminaries, dioceses, and religious orders now routinely hire well-qualified psychologists to conduct complete psychological testing evaluations for those seeking admission to seminary. Criminal and other appropriate background checks are now standard operating procedures for applicants as well. Seminaries now offer training in sexuality, strategies for maintaining appropriate professional and sexual boundaries, and ways to best manage impulse control–related problems and issues. Troubled seminarians and priests are usually quickly referred for evaluation and treatment by their religious superiors when symptoms first emerge. None of these changes were in place for earlier generations of priests.

The current crisis has forced all dioceses to follow new national guidelines from the United States Conference of Catholic Bishops about managing clergy sexual abuse allegations as well as procedures for the evaluation and treatment of both abuse victims and perpetrators.[28,29] Religious orders have followed suit as well. All dioceses and religious orders now have committees comprised mostly or entirely of laypeople that evaluate and consult on allegations of clergy misconduct. Many of these committees now include women, parents, victims of clergy abuse, and people who have a great deal of professional expertise in child sexual abuse such as psychologists, psychiatric nurses, police officers, criminal or family lawyers, and so forth. Many of these committees also include non-Catholics. Although these committees are advisory to the local bishop or religious superior, Church leaders would be foolish if not crazy to ignore the collective wisdom of these multidisciplinary group members. Finally, recent comprehensive research such as the John Jay Report provides the much-needed information to help better inform prevention and future policy decisions to protect children.[7] While these needed changes cannot entirely eliminate the possibility of child sexual abuse committed by priests, they are enormous movements in the right direction that will at least minimize the possibility of future abuse.

THE AWAKENED LAITY

The recent clergy abuse crisis has awakened the sleeping American Catholic laity. Groups such as Voice of the Faithful (VOTF) are a case in point. VOTF began as a grassroots organization of Catholics in the Boston area following the 2002 clergy abuse crisis in that diocese. It very quickly grew to member branches across the United States and around the world. It now includes over 40,000 members across the globe. The rapid growth, influence, and engagement of VOTF have been remarkable. Historically, the American Catholic Church has often experienced a fairly passive and uninvolved laity. Church policies that maximize decision making among the clergy and only offer minor advisory roles for the laity have not encouraged very active involvement and interest among average Catholics. The recent abuse crisis resulted in the laity getting assertively involved with the Church. This is very good news since it provides at least some degree of checks and balances to Church authorities and a lively, active, and involved laity can only be ultimately productive for the Church.

WHAT IS NOW IN THE LIGHT MUST STAY IN THE LIGHT

Now that the problem of clergy sexual abuse and words such as "pedophile" and "ephebophile" have become household words, it is almost impossible for priests to find themselves in situations where sexual abuse can easily occur. Parents, church employees, and the public are much less trusting of priests being alone with a child or teen. Policies have been developed that no longer allow priests to have unlimited and unsupervised access to children. A priest or bishop would be unreasonable in this day and age not to ensure that all children are safe in the company of priests. Furthermore, the media, VOTF, and others are watching much more closely now. In a nutshell, priests simply don't have the kind of unlimited trust and access to children that they once had. This is unlikely to change in the foreseeable future. We clearly live in different times and with different sensitivities. Now that the spotlight has been pointed on clergy sexual abuse, these issues cannot be hidden any longer. We have come to realize that some priests and bishops behave badly, and we won't forget that the priesthood, like all human groups, is not immune from troubled men who can inflict harm on others.

CONCLUSION

Church leaders could have done more over the years to prevent sexual abuse committed by priests from occurring. This is true in the now-famous Boston case that sparked the frenzy of attention on this problem in 2002. Victims and their families could have been treated with more care, respect, and compassion as well. Offending clergy could have been treated quickly and relieved from any duties that placed them in unsupervised contact with potential victims. However, the American bishops, with Vatican approval, now have policies in place to better respond to allegations of clergy sexual misconduct and to prevent at-risk clergy from having access to vulnerable children and others.[28,29] The media focus on sex-offending clergy has acted as a catalyst to examine this terrible problem more closely and to develop interventions at both individual and institutional levels. The problem of sex-offending clergy is certainly complex and lacks simple answers. Yet, at stake is the moral and spiritual authority of the Roman Catholic Church as well as the health and well-being of countless priests and laypersons. Hopefully, the Church will get it right this time and perhaps be a model for other organizations to create a climate and environment where sexual abuse of children won't happen.

REFERENCES

1. Boston Globe Investigative Staff. (2002). *Betrayal: The crisis in the Catholic Church.* New York: Little Brown.
2. Clohessy, D., & Wegs, M. (2004). Survivors network of those abused by priests (SNAP): An action plan. In T.G. Plante (Ed.). *Sin against the innocents: Sexual abuse by priests and the role of the Catholic Church* (pp. 97–100). Westport, CT: Greenwood.
3. Sipe, A.W.R. (1995). *Sex, priests, and power: Anatomy of a crisis.* New York: Brunner Mazel.
4. Plante, T.G. (Ed.). (1999). *Bless me Father for I have sinned: Perspectives on sexual abuse committed by Roman Catholic priests.* Westport, CT: Praeger/Greenwood.
5. Boswell, J. (1980). *Christianity, Social Tolerance, and Homosexuality: Gay People in Western Europe from the Beginning of the Christian Era to the Fourteenth Century.* Chicago: University of Chicago Press.
6. Jenkins, P. (2001). *Pedophiles and priests: Anatomy of a contemporary crisis.* New York: Oxford University Press.
7. John Jay College of Criminal Justice. (2004). *The nature and scope of the problem of sexual abuse of minors by Catholic priests and deacons in the United States.* New York: Author.
8. Plante, T.G. (Ed.). (2004). *Sin against the innocents: Sexual abuse by priests and the role of the Catholic Church.* Westport, CT: Greenwood.
9. Byrant, C. (1999). Psychological treatment of priest sex offenders. In T.G. Plante (Ed.), *Bless me Father for I have sinned: Perspectives on sexual abuse committed by Roman Catholic priests* (pp. 87–110). Westport, CT: Praeger/Greenwood.
10. Praesidium. (2001). *Creating safe environments: Training for members.* Arlington, TX: Author.
11. Rossetti, S.J. (Ed.). (1995). *Slayer of the soul: Child sexual abuse and the Catholic Church.* Mystic, CT: Twenty-Third Publications.
12. Francis, P.C., & Turner, N.R. (1995). Sexual misconduct within the Christian church: Who are the perpetrators and those they victimize? *Counseling & Values, 39,* 218–227.

13. Ruzicjka, M.F. (1997). Predictor variables on clergy pedophiles. *Psychological Reports, 81,* 589–590.
14. Schoener, G., Milgrom, J., Gonsiorek, J.C., Luepker, E., & Conroe, R. (Eds.). (1989). *Psychotherapists' sexual involvement with clients: Intervention and prevention.* Minneapolis, MN: Walk-In Counseling Center.
15. Shakeshaft, C. (2004). *Sexual abuse of students in schools: What schools must do to provide a safer environment for our children.* San Francisco: Jossey-Bass.
16. Laumann, E.O., Gagnon, J.H., Michael, R.T., Michaels, S. (1994). *The social organization of sexuality.* Chicago: University of Chicago Press.
17. Hoge, D. (2002). *The first five years of the priesthood: A study of newly ordained Catholic priests.* Collegeville, MN: Liturgical Press.
18. Cozzens, D. (2002). *Sacred silence: Denial and the crisis in the Church.* Collegeville, MN: Liturgical Press.
19. Sipe, A.W.R. (1990). *A secret world: Sexuality and the search for celibacy.* New York: Brunner Mazel.
20. Paulson, M. (2002, February 10). Catholics favoring priesthood changes. *Boston Globe,* A1.
21. Association of Statisticians of American Religious Bodies. (2000, September 18). *Religious congregations and membership in the United States.* New York: Author.
22. Catholic Charities USA. (2000). *Annual report.* Alexandria, VA: Author.
23. Plante, T.G. (2004). Bishops behaving badly: Ethical considerations regarding the clergy abuse crisis in the Roman Catholic Church. *Ethics and Behavior, 14,* 67–73.
24. Pope, K.S. (1994). *Sexual involvement with therapists: Patient assessment, subsequent therapy, forensics.* Washington, DC: American Psychological Association.
25. Pope, K.S. (1998). Sexual feelings, actions, and dilemmas in psychotherapy. In G.P. Koocher, J.C. Norcross, & S.S. Hill III (Eds.), *Psychologists' desk reference* (pp. 450–456). New York: Oxford University Press.
26. Plante, T.G., & Daniels, C. (2004). The sexual abuse crisis in the Roman Catholic Church: What psychologists and counselors should know. *Pastoral Psychology, 52,* 381–393.
27. Plante, T.G., & Boccaccini, M. (1998). A proposed psychological assessment protocol for applicants to religious life in the Roman Catholic Church. *Pastoral Psychology, 46,* 363–372.
28. United States Conference of Catholic Bishops (2002). *Charter for the protection of children and young people.* Washington, DC: Author.
29. United States Conference of Catholic Bishops (2002). *Essential norms for diocesan/eparchial policies dealing with allegations of sexual abuse of minors by priests or deacons.* Washington, DC: Author.

Chapter 12

Specific Phobia: A Common Problem, Rarely Treated

Christine D. Scher, Dana Steidtmann, David Luxton,
and Rick E. Ingram

Webster's New Universal Unabridged Dictionary defines a phobia as "a fear
or anxiety that exceeds normal proportions or that has no basis in reality;
an obsessive or irrational dread" (p. 1082).[1] Although useful, this definition
does not fully capture the nature of phobias as understood by most mental
health professionals. Indeed, when defining categories of emotional distress,
mental health professionals tend to rely upon widely used classification systems that are based on careful study of various phenomena. One such widely
used classification system is the fourth edition of the *Diagnostic and Statistical
Manual of Mental Disorders (DSM–IV).*[2] This official classification system of
the American Psychiatric Association provides criteria that are used to diagnose a wide range of mental health problems, including phobias. Although the
DSM–IV defines many different types of phobias, including agoraphobia and social phobia, the focus of this chapter will be specific phobias, one of
the most common forms of psychological distress.

According to the *DSM–IV*, specific phobias are characterized by "marked
and persistent fear of clearly discernible, circumscribed objects or situations"
(p. 405). There are several different categories that the *DSM–IV* identifies as
evoking phobic responses: animals, natural environments, blood-injection-injury,
situational, and other. When exposed to the feared object or situation, a phobic
person will almost always experience anxiety. Thus, in many cases, phobic persons simply avoid the target of their fear. In addition, in order to be diagnosed

with specific phobia, a phobic person must experience some disruption of his or her normal functioning or must be upset about having the phobia.

The various categories of specific phobias deserve further discussion, as they convey the breadth of the problem as well as suggest the personal toll that phobias can take. The first category, animals, includes all manner of living creatures. People with fears of spiders, cockroaches, and bees fall into this category, as do people fearing snakes and lizards. People fearing rats and mice are also included, as well as those who fear dogs and cats. The category of natural environments includes fears of all aspects of nature, including water, lightning and thunder, tornadoes, earthquakes, and heights. The blood-injection-injury category includes situations such as having blood drawn, receiving an injection (or watching someone else receive one), and viewing an open wound. Excessive fears of medical procedures would also be included in this category, as would hearing or participating in discussions of medical procedures. This latter group of phobias is rather unique in that it often elicits a physiological response in which heart rate increases, followed by a drop in heart rate and blood pressure and subsequent fainting.

The situational category includes experiences that are not necessarily part of a natural environment. This category includes various forms of transportation such as buses, airplanes, and subways, as well as tunnels, bridges, elevators, and enclosed places. People who are commonly called claustrophobic would fit here. In Southern California, a not uncommon phobia involves fear of driving on freeways, and thus, also fits this category of phobic experiences.

The final category is what is leftover and includes objects or situations that do not fit neatly into any of the previously discussed categories. Examples include fear of clowns or other costumed people, fears of choking, vomiting, or being unable to breath, and fears of loud noises. As should be apparent from this discussion, there are myriad objects and situations that may be the focus of specific phobias. Moreover, extreme fear upon encountering such phobic objects, or avoidance of these objects, has the potential to be quite impairing—a topic we discuss next.

ARE PEOPLE REALLY IMPAIRED BY PHOBIAS?

An Internet search using the word "phobia" quickly reveals that specific phobias have the capacity to negatively affect the lives of those who suffer from them. Web sites have been developed to help address the needs of people with fears of flying, needles, and dental procedures, among others. The impact of phobias is also reflected in the scientific literature. Several recent case studies (i.e., studies of individuals) have emerged that report on the impairment specific phobias can cause. For example, one report focused on the blood-injection-injury phobia of an airline pilot. Although the pilot had had previous symptoms indicative of such a problem, she sought treatment only after fainting while on duty, as coworkers discussed a medical procedure. She was not permitted to return to work until her phobia was successfully treated with behavior therapy.[3] This type of therapy will be discussed when we talk about treatments for phobia.

Another report focused on an elderly man who developed a phobia surrounding his implanted heart defibrillator. After receiving his third defibrillator, the man reported symptoms of anxiety and depression as well as concerns about his defibrillator discharging. He also began avoiding situations that he believed might lead to a defibrillator discharge, such as driving and walking. He was treated for his phobia with a combination of cognitive therapy and stress-management techniques.[4] These types of treatment will also be discussed.

A third report focused on a middle-aged man with a fear of heights. Because of this fear, the man avoided many situations, including elevators, stairs, and routes to work that involved bridges or other heights. Although the man had feared heights for 30 years, he sought treatment only after his fear decreased his enjoyment of a recent vacation to a hilly location and began to more severely impact trips to work. Like the previously described airline pilot, this man was treated with behavior therapy.[5]

We also personally know of cases where people are impaired by phobias. Several years ago, one of the authors worked with a talented graduate student. A paper they wrote was accepted for presentation at a scientific meeting in Hawaii. Only later did the author find out that the graduate student had a phobia, a fact that was revealed at the airport when she could not bring herself to board the plane. One might think that her phobia was a fear of flying, but it was not. She was claustrophobic and could not tolerate the idea that the airplane door would be closed and there could be no escape once they were flying over the Pacific Ocean. On a day-to-day basis, she found ways to deal with her phobia, but it also cost her a trip to Hawaii that the university had graciously agreed to pay for. To our knowledge, she never sought treatment for this problem.

Such case studies are supplemented by additional scientific work that examines, in large groups of people, impairment resulting from specific phobias. For example, one recent study examined the impact of having a phobia on life satisfaction. The study found that adults with specific phobia have less life satisfaction compared to those who did not have the problem. Phobias clearly do impair people's lives, but two additional points are notable. First, specific phobias were associated with a smaller decrease in life satisfaction when compared to several other disorders, including dysthymia (a form of depression), post-traumatic stress disorder (PTSD; an anxiety disorder that develops in response to traumatic events), and social phobia (an anxiety disorder that centers around fears of social and performance situations such as attending parties, talking on the telephone, and writing in public). Second, only people who had a disorder in addition to specific phobia reported substantially decreased life satisfaction.[6] It is probably the case that people are able to successfully enough avoid feared objects that they can minimize disruption in their lives.

Another study examined the economic impact of simple phobia, a predecessor of the specific phobia diagnosis. Costs of disorder due to a variety of factors were examined, including the use of physician and nonphysician mental health professional services (e.g., the services of a family physician, psychiatrist, or social worker) and workplace difficulties. Simple phobia was related to an increase in use of psychologists' services. However, it did not affect service usage of other mental health professionals or physicians, nor did it affect productivity at work or rates of absenteeism. Other disorders examined, including PTSD, panic disorder (an anxiety disorder characterized in part by sudden bursts of fear), and agoraphobia (an anxiety disorder that often is seen along with panic disorder), resulted in greater economic costs.[7] Thus, although clearly problematic for many people, phobias are not associated with the extent of impairment that is seen in some of the other anxiety disorders.

The information just summarized suggests that specific phobias can indeed be impairing. However, in terms of decreases in life satisfaction and economic costs, there are several other disorders that have greater impact. Perhaps this is why two of the people presented in case studies did not seek treatment until many years after initially noticing symptoms. Indeed, many people with specific phobias do not seek treatment, despite the potential of these phobias to cause distress and impact functioning.

HOW COMMON ARE SPECIFIC PHOBIAS?

Two large-scale studies conducted in the United States suggest that specific phobias are not uncommon in the general population. The first of these, the Epidemiologic Catchment Area (ECA) study, examined the prevalence of simple phobia at five sites: New Haven, Baltimore, St. Louis, Durham, and Los Angeles. Based on data from the latter four sites, 11.3 percent of people met diagnostic criteria for simple phobia at some point during their lives. Persons identified as black had approximately double the rates of simple phobia compared to persons identified as white or Hispanic. Women had approximately double the rates of simple phobia compared to men. When considering sex and ethnic or racial identity together, black women had the highest rates of simple phobia at 24.4 percent.[8,9]

The second study, the National Comorbidity Survey, also examined the prevalence of simple phobia. The percent of people who met diagnostic criteria for simple phobia at some point during their lives was identical to that of the ECA: 11.3 percent. Also similar to the ECA study, women had over double the rates of simple phobia compared to men. Moreover, this sex difference was apparent when examining rates of simple phobia over the past month. The study revealed that 5.5 percent of people met diagnostic criteria, with women having nearly four times the rate of simple phobia compared to men. With regard to ethnic or racial identity, being black or Hispanic was related to an increase in the number of phobias. When examining all groups, heights and animals were the most common types of fears.[9,10]

The consistent sex difference in rates of specific phobias is of particular interest to mental health professionals. Several possible explanations for this difference have been advanced. For example, men may tend to underreport their fears, perhaps in an attempt to conform to a stereotypically masculine gender role. Another possible explanation is that women are more likely than men to seek treatment for their fears. This explanation would also account for greater sex differences in samples of people seeking treatment compared to samples of people recruited from the larger community. Women may also develop specific phobias at increased rates due to greater opportunities to learn fear. For example, women may be more likely to see examples of other women acting fearfully (e.g., through television and film) than men are likely to see examples of other men acting fearfully. This type of learning, often termed "modeling" or "observational learning," can be quite powerful, as will be discussed later in this chapter. In sum, there are quite varied possible explanations for the sex difference in specific phobia, and additional research attention will likely be focused on this issue.[9]

WHAT CAUSES PHOBIAS?

An edition of a popular science magazine contained a full-page color photograph of an infant lying inside the loosely wrapped coil of a python. The baby looks comfortable and calm and shows no signs of the terrifying reaction that many people would feel in the same situation. It looks as though the baby doesn't even notice the snake. The image is striking, if not a little disturbing. Why isn't the infant afraid? Is it a digitally altered photograph? But in fact the photograph was *not* altered. Although it was a specially trained python, the baby actually sat inside the snake's coil without any sign of fear. This is a dramatic example of how learning can affect the development of fears and phobias. Many of our fears are learned, and the young infant in the photograph had not yet learned the fear of snakes. In fact, learning appears to play a central role in the acquisition and maintenance of phobias. In addition, there are a variety of other components believed to play a role. Although many of the individual theories have been around for years, contemporary researchers are now attempting to integrate the various lines of thinking and research into a more comprehensive theory of phobia etiology. Before turning to this comprehensive approach, it is useful to describe the individual theories in more depth.

Learning Theories

For a good part of the last 50 years, learning has been a predominant theory of phobia etiology. Even before that, psychologists found out that they could create strong fear in children. One of the most famous examples is the experiment in the early 20th century involving "Little Albert," a young boy who was taught to fear a white rat. Initially, Albert showed no fear when exposed to rats. Then, he was repeatedly shown a white rat just before he would hear a very startling loud noise that made him cry. After multiple trials, he began to scream and cry as soon as the rat was presented, even if no sound was made—he now feared the rat itself, rather than the unpleasant sound.[11] Such an experiment could not be conducted today because it is recognized as unethical to create a phobia that was not present to begin with. Nevertheless, this experiment demonstrates that intense fears can be learned.

Since the Little Albert experiment, more specific details about how learning leads to phobias have been discovered, and several specific learning pathways have been proposed. For example, it has been suggested that, just as with Little Albert, fears can be learned through traumatic experiences with feared objects.[12] In some instances it may only take one or two negative experiences with an object for an intense fear to begin developing.[12,13,14] This has been referred to as a conditioning model because the fear is conditioned, or learned, through a negative experience.

Although the conditioning pathway is one way in which phobias begin to develop, it does not account for all instances of phobia acquisition. Many people with phobias have not had traumatic experiences with the feared stimuli. Thus, it has also been proposed that some phobias are learned vicariously.[12] That is, children may grow up learning from a parent, teacher, friend, or even television that certain things are to be feared. Thus, it has been proposed that another pathway to phobia acquisition is learning fear through *copying* a fear someone else is displaying. This way of learning is often referred to as "modeling" or "observational learning." For example, if a child grows up watching a parent cross to the other side of the street every time a dog is approaching, the child may begin to avoid dogs in a similar fashion. Or if a child hears a news report about deadly spiders, the child may begin to display a fear of spiders. If the learning experience provokes enough fear or learning occurs repeatedly, it may eventually escalate into a phobic-level fear.[15] Of course, not everyone who has such experiences develops a phobia. This illustrates the point that it is necessary to examine how learning relates to other factors in order to more fully understand the origins of phobia.

Evolutionary Theories

The picture of the infant in the python's coil caused quite a stir. The picture was disturbing enough that some people wrote letters to the editor regarding the photograph; one person whose letter was printed in a subsequent magazine felt the photograph was in "poor taste." Apparently, looking at the picture made many people uncomfortable. It is likely that the picture was aversive because many of us have some fear of snakes; seeing a baby in such a vulnerable position makes us uncomfortable. If not snakes, perhaps we fear spiders, heights, or strangers. These are common fears among individuals without phobias, and, more interestingly, they are also common phobias.[13] When looking for similarities across these phobias, it is evident that most of the feared objects and situations are things that can actually be dangerous under certain circumstances. The observation that people frequently fear things that may actually be dangerous has led to theories about the evolutionary significance of phobias.

One such theory is that humans have become biologically prepared to more easily fear some stimuli than others because people who feared dangerous things such as snakes and heights were more likely to survive and pass on to their offspring the disposition to fear these things.[13] Although these fears are manageable for most of us, for some people the sense of fear is so strongly ingrained that it may reach the level of a phobia. Originally, this evolutionary idea was an extension of learning theories. It was believed that humans had become biologically prepared to easily learn some fears such that it might take only one scary encounter with a spider to develop a fear and avoidance of spiders. Recent research has suggested that we may actually be prepared to fear without any learning so that certain fears are actually akin to instincts.[16,17] The evolutionary theories of phobia origin appeal to many people on an intuitive level and are supported by research.[13,16]

Genetic Theories

The specific phobias are not believed to be as highly heritable as many other psychological disorders, including the other anxiety disorders. However, research indicates there may be at least a small genetic component that may predispose people to phobias.[18,19] Researchers believe that some phobias such as situational phobia and blood-injection-injury phobia can be directly inherited, while others, such as animal phobias, are more likely to be inherited via a general tendency to be fearful in a variety of situations.[20] For example, some infants have temperaments that make them more likely to withdraw from unfamiliar people or situations, and infants with this behavioral inhibition are more likely to develop a variety of phobias later in life than infants without the inhibition.[21] It is speculated that this temperament makes it less likely that the person will ever approach the thing he or she is afraid of and will thus miss out on the opportunity to disconfirm fear of that object. In a sense, he or she is always imagining the worst with no opportunity to amend that belief through positive experience.

Another way in which people may inherit a generally fearful disposition is by inheriting the tendency to feel a strong disgust reaction; some people have more intense disgusted reactions to blood or certain animals. Moreover, these reactions seem to run in families.[22] It is not yet known whether disgust is transmitted from parents to children through learning, genes, or a combination of the two. However, the disgust hypothesis is another possible way in which people may be genetically predisposed to developing phobias.

Other Biological Theories

In addition to the idea that people are genetically predisposed to developing phobias, recent research using the brain-imaging technique of functional Magnetic Resonance Imaging (fMRI) indicates that people with phobias show different responses to feared objects than people without phobias. When looking at pictures of feared things (e.g., spiders, snakes), individuals who fear these objects showed increased activity in the amygdala, a region of the brain that is widely believed to be important in human emotions.[22] Research also suggests that there is a "fast pathway" and a "slow pathway" through which fear responses travel to the amygdala.

Researchers believe it is through the fast pathways that people initially react to potentially dangerous stimuli in the environment and that the slower pathways are used to transmit conscious information in which people use reasoning abilities to deem something as threatening or nonthreatening. When working properly, the slower, more conscious pathway should have the ability to override the fast, reactive pathway. However, in phobia there may be a dysregulation of the fear pathways and the amygdala so that conscious decisions do not successfully override the initial fear reaction and thus the fear reaction is abnormally maintained.[23]

Maintenance of Phobias: Cognitive Theories

Once a lower level fear begins escalating into a more phobic form, it appears that people's imaginations run wild in a variety of ways so that the fear is maintained and even exacerbated. If people do not confront their fear, then there may be a tendency to ruminate over it. For example, people with phobias may exhibit a bias in what they pay attention to that makes them excessively aware of anything that is related to what they fear.[24-25] Doing so thereby intensifies the emotions of fear and anxiety.[26] Imagine that a person with a phobia of heights is watching a newscast in which an accident involving a mountain climber is described. The phobic person is likely to pay disproportionate attention to the mountain climbing story, think about it continually, and thereby unintentionally strengthen the fear of heights.

Another way in which phobias might be maintained or made more severe is by always assuming the worst about things that are feared.[24] In this situation, someone with a spider phobia assumes that every spider encountered is highly poisonous rather than considering that it might not be poisonous. In fact, the latter belief is the more rational belief because the majority of spiders are not poisonous, but by their nature, phobias are not rational. Preliminary research evidence supports the idea that biased attention and biased interpretations are related to prolonging phobias.[26,27,28]

Integrating the Theories

It is evident that the process through which phobias develop involves a variety of factors. In essence, understanding how and why phobias develop is really a matter of understanding why people come to have fears and, more importantly, understanding why common levels of fear escalate into phobias in some people. As is the case with many psychological disorders, it is increasingly believed that "nature" interacts with "nurture" in the development of phobias. Genetics may make some people vulnerable to developing phobias, but these genetic vulnerabilities must also interact with life experiences before phobias actually develop. For instance, although the learning theories of phobia are widely recognized as important, it is important to consider that not all people who have traumatic experiences develop phobias from those experiences. This begs the question of why some people's learned fears become phobias while other people's do not. It seems likely that the answer to this question lies in the fact that some people are more genetically predisposed to develop phobias. Therefore, it is the combination of the predisposition *and* the learning experience that leads to the phobia development rather than either of them individually.

Consider a person who does not tend to test out things she perceives as intimidating. If she witnesses a friend nearly drowning in a lake, her disposition might make her likely to avoid large bodies of water. Consequently, she will have few if any subsequent safe experiences near water and instead will continue associating water with the near-drowning incident. Her fear of water may continue to persist in her thoughts until it reaches a debilitating level and becomes a phobia. However, somebody who is more likely to confront her fears might return to the lake and thus have a "corrective" or more positive experience at the lake. Therefore, that person is more likely to circumvent the escalation of fear and avoid developing a phobia of water. This example is just one way in which the elements of thinking, learning, and genetics might interact. Researchers continue to consider and test other ways in which these individual factors interface in order to more fully understand the origin of phobias. In doing so, it may eventually be possible to prevent some fears from ever developing into phobias. Fortunately, until that time comes, effective treatments are already making it possible to greatly improve the quality of life for people with phobias. It is to those treatments that we now turn.

TREATMENT OF PHOBIAS

Many people never seek treatment for phobias. They find ways to cope with the phobia, often by avoidance. The person who fears water will simply not go to the lake, and the person who fears driving on freeways will take surface streets to his or her destinations. It is likely that treatment becomes viable only when the person is unable to find ways to avoid the feared object or situation, or when impairment or distress becomes intolerable. Even if not significantly impaired or personally distressed, some people may seek treatment when the phobia begins to negatively affect those close to the individual such as a spouse.

For the first two-thirds of the 20th century, those individuals who did seek treatment were treated primarily by psychoanalysis or other forms of psychodynamic therapy. These approaches considered intrapsychic and subconscious conflicts, mostly deriving from childhood, as the source of abnormal anxious states. The aim of these treatments was to bring the subconscious into awareness, analyze what it means, and supplant realistic appraisals for those that produce the anxiety associated with phobias. Psychoanalysis and other related forms of psychotherapy, however, did not prove to be very successful in alleviating phobic symptoms. Freud himself acknowledged the limitations of pure psychoanalysis in treating phobias and suggested that active confrontation with the fear-producing object was necessary.[29] Indeed, the most effective treatments are those that involve exposure to feared objects or situations.[9,30] The underlying assumption is that repeated avoidance of a feared object or situation causes the anxiety associated with it to be maintained and perpetuated. Controlled and repeated exposure to the feared object or situation, however, is thought to desensitize the person to it while the person learns that the feared object or situation is not so threatening after all. Certainly this was the idea behind behavioral treatments for phobia.

Behavioral Approaches

Behavioral approaches became the predominate approach to treating phobia once it was realized that psychoanalytic treatment was not terribly effective. In particular, the 1950s saw a turning away from the focus on the subconscious in the treatment of phobias to behavioral treatments that focus on overt behavior and conscious experience. Based on learning theory, these treatments typically involve prolonged in vivo (that is, real life) exposure to fear-producing stimuli in order to recondition or desensitize an individual to such stimuli.

The first and one of the most popular behavioral treatments for phobias still in use today is *systematic desensitization*, which was developed by Joseph Wolpe in 1958. Systematic desensitization involves preplanned step-by-step exposure to imagined fear-producing objects or situations. The phobic individual is first taught procedures for physical relaxation, such as progressive muscle relaxation. Next, the individual is asked to rank situations related to the phobia that cause anxiety and distress. For example, a person who fears spiders might place physical contact with a spider at the top of the list of things that make him or her anxious, and the thought of a place that a spider may inhabit, such as a barn, at the bottom of the list. Then, the phobic individual is systematically exposed to the anxiety producing object or situation in a step-by-step fashion, beginning with the least anxiety-provoking situation to the most anxiety-eliciting ones. The phobic individual is instructed to relax during each step of the process such that a relaxation response is substituted for the fear response when thinking of the feared stimulus. If the phobic individual begins to experience anxiety at any stage, he or she is instructed to go back a step in the hierarchy and practice the relaxation procedures. This process is continued until all of the steps listed in the anxiety hierarchy have been successfully dealt with.

Although systematic desensitization with imagined stimuli is practical, a number of studies have suggested that systematic desensitization interventions conducted in imagination are not as effective as when combined with real-life exposure or compared to just real-life exposure.[31,32,33,34] Additionally, it is not clear why systematic desensitization works. The original idea, known as reciprocal inhibition, suggested that because the fear response is incompatible with relaxation, the two responses cannot coexist. Moreover, it was argued that with enough practice, relaxation supplants fear as the conditioned stimulus. More recent explanations, however, have suggested that learning relaxation may simply be a coping response that people can use when, for whatever reason, they must confront the feared object or situation.

Systematic desensitization can also be paired with *modeling*.[34] In modeling, the person observes other people (the "models") responding with relaxation rather than fear in the presence of the phobic stimulus. The models may be observed in real life or watched on film. The phobic person is encouraged to imitate the model(s) and thereby learn that the feared object or situation poses little real danger. The combination of live modeling with individual imitation is sometimes called participant modeling. Modeling is an especially popular technique for working with phobic children.[35,36]

Similar to systematic desensitization, *flooding* involves the person's experiencing of fear-provoking situations but with much greater intensity and for prolonged periods of time.[37] Because avoidance of the feared object or situation exacerbates the anxiety associated with it, the goal of flooding is to force exposure and prevent the avoidance response to the fear-producing situation. To accomplish this, the therapist, rather than the phobic individual, controls the timing and content of the imagined fear-producing scenes or real-life exposures. The therapist may also describe imagined scenes as graphically as possible in order to deliberately make them as disturbing as possible for the phobic individual. The prolonged experience with the fear-producing images or real-life exposures is thought to help the individual become accustomed to these images, so that the feared stimulus eventually loses its anxiety-causing effect. Although effective, given the intense nature of this treatment, some phobic individuals do not seek out this approach, and for those who do, some may not continue.

Although behavioral techniques differ on how gradually the phobic individual is made to encounter the fearful stimulus or how long the exposure continues, phobic individuals are typically asked to experience the situation until their anxiety begins to diminish. Equipment that measures pulse rate, respiration rate, and electrodermal response can be used to determine whether the phobic person is in a relaxed state before moving to the next step in the anxiety hierarchy in systematic desensitization. With each session, the phobic individual begins to tolerate more intimate and prolonged confrontations with the threatening object or situation. Behavioral treatments can also be successfully applied individually and in groups, such as group systematic desensitization in the treatment of dental phobia.[37,38]

Virtual Reality Exposure

Virtual reality exposure (VRE) therapy is a relatively new and exciting alternative to traditional exposure-based interventions for specific phobias. Like conventional behavioral treatments for phobias, the central component of VRE is exposure to the feared stimulus. VRE, however, involves exposure to a computer-generated rather than an actual or imagined fear-producing stimulus. VRE treatments have been shown to be as effective as standard exposure therapy.[39,40]

In VRE, situations are presented as part of an interactive three-dimensional virtual environment that allows phobic individuals to become immersed enough to react to virtual scenarios as though they were real.[41,42] In order to create a realistic and interactive virtual environment, the user is typically outfitted with a head-mounted display that consists of separate display screens for each eye and stereo earphones. A head-tracking device that allows the virtual world to change with head and body motion adds to the realism of the virtual environment. In addition, VRE can be combined with tactile stimulation that furthers the realism, such as the feel of a steering wheel or a spider.

In VRE, the simulated phobic stimuli can be controlled and monitored by the therapist. Biofeedback instrumentation can also help the therapist to monitor the person's physiological responses.[42] For example, the scene might be one of walking on the roof of a skyscraper. If the phobic person's heart rate gets too high, the therapist can freeze-frame or stop the scene completely in order to help the individual to practice relaxation in an effort to counter-condition the fear and anxiety response. Furthermore, VRE is also efficient in isolating specific points of anxiety because the fear-producing scenarios can easily be repeated in the virtual environment.

Cognitive-Behavioral Approaches

Cognitive models of anxiety state that maladaptive patterns of thinking guide information processing such that a phobic person will be overly vigilant for and selectively attend to potentially threatening situations, misinterpret ambiguous situations as threatening, and preferentially recall threatening situations. These patterns of thinking are thought to maintain anxiety and avoidance by keeping threat situations salient. Thus, cognitive and cognitive-behavioral therapies (CBT) focus on these maladaptive patterns of thinking.

The goal is to help people change their reactions to their emotional arousal and also learn to deal effectively with anxiety-provoking situations. This process involves challenging maladaptive beliefs and reinterpreting the anxiety-provoking situation.[43] During the early sessions of CBT, phobic people are taught to self-monitor their thoughts, assumptions, and beliefs during anxiety-provoking situations. The therapist helps the person to understand the role of beliefs and appraisals in anxiety. During later sessions, phobic individuals are taught to reevaluate the validity of distorted thoughts and supplant them with more rational and adaptive ones.

CBT may be combined with relaxation training in order to provide phobic individuals with a strategy to reduce their symptoms in stressful situations. Also, CBT can be combined with in vivo exposure in the form of homework assignments. For example, a person with hydrophobia (fear of water) can be instructed to visit the city pool and report on the experience. Successful completion of the homework assignment can help the person to realize that he or she has control over reactions to stressful situations and that the situation is not as dangerous as originally thought.

Pharmacotherapy

There are a number of drug treatments in use today that are helpful for reducing anxiety associated with phobias. A class of antidepressant drugs called selective serotonin reuptake inhibitors (SSRIs) has been increasingly used to treat anxiety. SSRIs may work to increase the level of serotonin, a brain neurotransmitter that has been implicated in emotional disorders such as depression and anxiety. Examples of SSRIs that have been found to be especially useful in the treatment of phobia are Effexor (venlafaxine), Zoloft (sertraline), Prozac (fluoxetine), Paxil (paroxetine), and Luvox (fluvoxamine). The SSRIs are a popular choice because they typically have reduced side effects and very low addiction potential. Furthermore, the antidepressant action of these drugs is helpful in treating patients who suffer from depression in addition to phobia. Tricyclic antidepressants (TCAs) and monoamine oxidase inhibitors (MAOIs) such as Nardil (phenelzine) and Parnate (tranylcypromine) are also helpful but may also have more side effects. Antianxiety medications known as the benzodiazapines (e.g., Valium, Xanax) have also been used to treat phobias. The benzodiazapines are fast-acting drugs that reduce the symptoms of anxiety, but they have high addiction potential and are likely to cause withdrawal symptoms when stopped.

Another class of drugs called beta-blockers, used to treat high blood pressure and some heart conditions, has also been used in the treatment of anxiety disorders. Although the calming effect of beta-blockers may be beneficial for some people with specific phobias, they are not likely to be used as a first choice of treatment. Also, there is now research that suggests that the drug D-Cycloserine, used mainly to treat tuberculosis, may be an effective treatment for diminishing the fear associated with phobias.

Other Treatment Approaches

Although the focus on subconscious experience in the treatment of phobias has been largely replaced by behavioral, cognitive, and pharmacological approaches, treatments for phobias that focus on the role of the subconscious mind are still in use today. Hypnosis, for example, has been used to help people with phobias control their reactions to fear-producing situations by helping them to control both physiological and psychological responses. Through posthypnotic suggestion, phobic individuals may be taught to physically relax and find a more tranquil state of mind. Hypnotherapy may thus help a person cope with the fear-producing situation in a calm and rational manner. Although lacking in scientific support, proponents of hypnosis claim it can be used to help a person with a phobia discover the memory of an originating event, a memory that has been repressed and relegated to the subconscious. Hypnosis might thus be useful for reexamining the event that initiated the fear, therefore helping phobic people to objectively understand their anxiety and reduce their fear of losing control in future stressful situations. However, research is still needed to determine whether this is actually effective.

Eye Movement Desensitization and Reprocessing, or EMDR,[44,45] is another technique that has been used in the treatment of phobias. EMDR is based on the idea that when a person encounters a fear-producing situation, the side of the brain that produces the emotional response dominates the other side of the brain. In EMDR treatment, people are instructed to focus on a fear-producing image, negative thought, and associated body sensations while simultaneously moving their eyes back and forth, following the therapist's fingers as they move across their field of vision for 20–30 seconds or longer. Although a focus on eye movements is common in EMDR, auditory tones, tapping, or other types of tactile stimulation have also been used. This process has been suggested to facilitate the integration of both sides of the brain (left and right hemispheres). It is important to note, however, that even though EMDR is used by some practitioners as a primary treatment or as an augmentation to other treatments, little scientific evidence is available to suggest that this is effective, or that it is effective for the reasons that proponents propose.[45,46,47,48]

Treatment: Conclusions

The outlook for people with phobias in the 21st century is an optimistic one. Although there is much variability across studies regarding the ideal duration of treatment, people with specific phobias can often be relieved of their symptoms in a matter of a few weeks. For some people, a single session of in vivo exposure lasting 2–3 hours can lead to significant improvement.[49] At this point, treatments that incorporate in vivo exposure to threatening stimuli are still considered the most effective. VRE, however, is very promising because it can be conveniently administered in traditional therapeutic settings and may therefore offer a more practical alternative to in vivo exposure.

Also very promising are the advancements in drug treatments that have led to more effective reduction of the anxiety associated with phobias. Drug treatments can also be integrated with the various forms of treatment for specific phobias. For example, people with fear of flying can benefit from both medication that reduces anxiety and in vivo exposure therapy that involves visiting an airport and taking a short flight. In addition, many of the therapies for specific phobias can be conducted as group therapy, which provides the benefit of interaction and support of the group as well as overall cost effectiveness.

CONCLUDING COMMENTS

The purpose of this chapter is to provide an overview of specific phobias. To this end, we have described this problem and examined how common it is, how it develops, and how it can be treated. We believe that this chapter's title truly captures the nature of specific phobias: they are a common problem, but they are rarely treated. Perhaps people with specific phobias avoid treatment because overcoming the fear seems daunting. For people who do seek treatment, however, the prognosis is good. Indeed, when considering the range of possible disorders and the range of possible psychological treatments, behavioral treatments for specific phobias have amongst the strongest scientific support for their usefulness.[50] For those interested in further reading about the nature of specific phobias and their treatment, as well as those interested in obtaining help for phobia-related distress, we have included a brief list of resources.

SPECIFIC PHOBIA RESOURCES

www.adaa.org. This is the Web site of the Anxiety Disorders Association of America. It includes information about specific phobias and a "Find a Therapist" link.

www.aabt.org. This is the Web site of the Association for Behavioral and Cognitive Therapies. Many members of this organization have an interest in scientifically supported therapies, including those for specific phobias. The Web site includes a "Find a Therapist" link.

The Anxiety & Phobia Workbook (3rd ed.) by Edmund J. Bourne, PhD. This self-help book contains an overview of anxiety disorders and their treatments, and provides methods of coping with anxiety symptoms. The book also includes self-assessments and numerous suggestions for additional reading.

REFERENCES

1. *Webster's new universal unabridged dictionary.* (1992). New York: Barnes and Noble Books.
2. American Psychiatric Association. (1994). *Diagnostic and statistical manual of mental disorders* (4th ed.). Washington, DC: Author.
3. Roden, S.K. (2001). Blood-injection-injury phobia in a commercial aviator: A case report. *Aviation, Space, and Environmental Medicine, 72,* 1138–1140.
4. Urizar, G.G., Jr., Sears, S.F., Jr., Handberg, E., & Conti, J.B. (2004). Psychosocial intervention for a geriatric patient to address fears related to implantable cardioverter defibrillator discharges. *Psychosomatics, 45,* 140–144.
5. Kamphuis, J.H., Emmelkamp, P.M.G., & Krijn, M. (2002). Specific phobia. In M. Hersen (Ed.), *Clinical behavior therapy: Adults and children* (pp. 75–89). New York: John Wiley & Sons.
6. Meyer, C., Rumpf, H., Hapke, U., & John, U. (2004). Impact of psychiatric disorders in the general population: Satisfaction with life and the influence of comorbidity and disorder duration. *Social Psychiatry and Psychiatric Epidemiology, 39,* 435–441.
7. Greenberg, P.E., Sisitsky, T., Kessler, R.C., Finkelstein, S.N., Berndt, E.R., Davidson, J.R.T., et al. (1999). The economic burden of anxiety disorders in the 1990s. *Journal of Clinical Psychiatry, 60,* 427–435.
8. Eaton, W.W., Dryman, A., & Weissman, M.M. (1991). Panic and phobia. In L.N. Robins & D.A. Regier (Eds.), *Psychiatric disorders in America: The Epidemiologic Catchment Area study* (pp. 155–179). New York: Free Press.
9. Antony, M.M., & Barlow, D.H. (2002). Specific phobias. In D.H. Barlow, *Anxiety and its disorders: The nature and treatment of anxiety and panic* (2nd ed., pp. 380–417). New York: Guilford Press.
10. Magee, W.J., Eaton, W.W., Wittchen, H., McGonagle, K.A., & Kessler, R.C. (1996). Agoraphobia, simple phobia, and social phobia in the National Comorbidity Survey. *Archives of General Psychiatry, 53,* 159–168.
11. Watson, J.B., & Rayner, R. (1920). Conditioned emotional reactions. *Journal of Experimental Psychology, 3,* 1–14.
12. Rachman, S. (1977). The conditioning theory of fear acquisition: A critical examination. *Behaviour Research and Therapy, 15,* 375–387.

13. Seligman, M. E. P. (1971). Phobias and preparedness. *Behavior Therapy, 2*, 307–320.

14. King, N. J., Gullone, E., & Ollendick, T. H. (1998). Etiology of childhood phobias: Current status of Rachman's three pathways theory. *Behaviour Research and Therapy, 36*, 297–309.

15. Menzies, R., & Parker, L. (2001). The origins of height fear: An evaluation of neoconditioning explanations. *Behaviour Research and Therapy, 39*, 185–199.

16. Poulton, R., & Menzies, R. G. (2002). Non-associative fear acquisition: A review of the evidence from retrospective and longitudinal research. *Behaviour Research and Therapy, 40*, 127–149.

17. Hettema, J. M., Prescott, C. A., Myers, J. M., Neale, M. C., & Kendler, K. S. (2005). The structure of genetic and environmental risk factors for anxiety disorders in men and women. *Archives of General Psychiatry, 62*, 182–189.

18. Kendler, K. S., Neale, M. C., Kessler, R. C., Heath, A. C., & Eaves, L. J. (1992). The genetic epidemiology of phobias in women: The interrelationship of agoraphobia, social phobia, situational phobia, and simple phobia. *Archives of General Psychiatry, 49*, 273–281.

19. Carey, G. (1990). Genes, fears, phobias, and phobic disorders. *Journal of Counseling and Development, 68*, 628–232.

20. Biederman, J., Rosenbaum, J. F., Hirshfeld, D. R., Faraone, S. V., Bolduc, E. A., Gersten, M., et al. (1990). Psychiatric correlates of behavioral inhibition in young children of parents with and without psychiatric disorders. *Archives of General Psychiatry, 47*, 21–26.

21. De Jong, P. J., Andrea, H., & Muris, P. (1997). Disgust and fear before and after treatment. *Behaviour Research and Therapy, 35*, 559–562.

22. Dilger, S., Straube, T., Mentzel, H-J., Fitzek, C., Reichenbach, J. R., Hecht, H., et al. (2003). Brain-activation to phobia-related pictures in spider phobic humans: An event-related functional magnetic resonance imaging study. *Neuroscience Letters, 348*, 29–32.

23. Nader, K., & LeDoux, J. (1999). The neural circuits that underlie fear. In J. Schulkin, L. A. Schmidt, & A. Louis (Eds.), Fear, shyness, and social phobia: Origins, biological mechanisms and clinical outcomes (pp. 119–139). London: Oxford University Press.

24. Muris, P., & Merkelbach, H. (2001). The etiology of childhood phobia: A multifactorial model. In M. W. Vasey & M. R. Dadds (Eds.), *The Developmental Psychopathology of Anxiety* (pp. 355–385). New York: Oxford University Press.

25. Purdon, C. (1999). Thought suppression and psychopathology. *Behaviour Research and Therapy, 37*, 1029–1054.

26. Hadwin, J., Frost, S., French, C. C., & Richard, A. (1997). Cognitive processing and trait anxiety in typically developing children: Evidence for an interpretation bias. *Journal of Abnormal Psychology, 106*, 486–490.

27. Lavy, E., Van den Hout, M., & Arntz, A. (1993). Attentional bias and facilitated escape: A pictorial test. *Advances in Behaviour Research and Therapy, 15,* 279–289.

28. Watts, F. N., McKenna, F. P., Sharrock, R., & Trezise, L. (1986). Colour naming of phobia-related words. *British Journal of Psychology, 77,* 97–108.

29. Freud, S. (1955). The justification for detaching from neurasthenia a particular syndrome: The anxiety neurosis. In J. Stachey (Ed.), *The standard edition of the complete psychological works of Sigmund Freud* (Vol. 1, pp. 78–106). London: Hogarth. (Original work published 1894)

30. Menzies, R. G., & Clarke, J. C. (1993). A comparison of in vivo and vicarious exposure in the treatment of childhood water phobia. *Behaviour Research and Therapy, 31,* 9–15.

31. Barlow, D. H., Leitenberg, H., Agras, W. S., & Wincze, J. P. (1969). The transfer gap in systematic desensitization: An analogue study. *Behaviour Research and Therapy, 7,* 191–196.

32. Barlow, D. H., & Wolfe, B. E. (1981). Behavioral approaches to anxiety disorders: A report on the NIMH-SUNY, Albany, research conference. *Journal of Consulting and Clinical Psychology, 49,* 448–454.

33. Linden, W. (1981). Exposure treatments for focal phobias. *American Journal of Psychiatry, 38,* 769–775.

34. Bandura, A., Blanchard, E., & Ritter, B. (1969). Desensitization and modeling to induce behavioral, affective, and attitudinal change. *Journal of Personality and Social Psychology, 13,* 173–179.

35. Ollendick, T. H., & King, N. J. (1998). Empirically supported treatments for children with phobic and anxious disorders: Current status. *Journal of Clinical Child Psychology, 27,* 156–167.

36. Baum, M. (1970). Extinction of avoidance responding through response prevention (flooding). *Psychological Bulletin, 74,* 276–284.

37. Berggren, U., & Linde, A. (1984). Dental fear and avoidance: A comparison of two modes of treatment. *Journal of Dental Research, 63,* 1223–1227.

38. Smith, T. A., Kroeger, R. F., Lyon, H. E., & Mullins, M. R. (1990). Evaluating a behavioral method to manage dental fear: A 2-year study of dental practices. *Journal of the American Dental Association, 121,* 525–530.

39. Rothbaum, B. O., Hodges, L., Smith, S., Lee, J. H., & Price, L. (2000). A controlled study of virtual reality exposure therapy for fear of flying. *Journal of Consulting and Clinical Psychology, 68,* 1020–1026.

40. Nash, E. B., Edwards, G. W., Thompson, J. A., & Barfield, W. (2000). A review of presence and performance in virtual environments. *International Journal of Human-Computer Interaction, 12,* 1–41.

41. Regenbrecht, H. T., Schubert, T. W., & Friedmann, F. (1998). Measuring the sense of presence and its relations to fear of heights in virtual environments. *International Journal of Human-Computer Interaction, 10,* 233–249.

42. Rothbaum, B.O., Hodges, L.F., Kooper, R., Opdyke, D., Williford, J.S., & North, M. (1995). Effectiveness of computer-generated (virtual reality) graded exposure in the treatment of acrophobia. *American Journal of Psychiatry, 152,* 626–628.

43. Beck, A.T., & Emery, G.W. (with Greenberg, R.I.). (1985). *Anxiety disorders and phobias: A cognitive perspective.* New York: Basic Books.

44. Shapiro, F. (1995). Eye movement desensitization and reprocessing: Basic principles, protocols, and procedures. New York: Guilford Press.

45. Acierno, R., Hersen, M., Van Hasselt, V.B., Tremont, G., & Mueser, K.T. (1994). Review of the validation and dissemination of eye movement desensitization and reprocessing: A scientific and ethical dilemma. *Clinical Psychology Review, 14,* 287–299.

46. Muris, P., & Merckelbach, H. (1997). Treating spider phobics with eye movement desensitization and reprocessing: A controlled study. *Behavioural and Cognitive Psychotherapy, 25,* 39–50.

47. Muris, P., & Merckelbach, H. (1995). Treating spider phobia with eye movement desensitization and reprocessing: Two case reports. *Journal of Anxiety Disorders, 9,* 439–449.

48. Muris, P., Merckelbach, H., van Haaften, H., & Mayer, B. (1997). Eye movement desensitization and reprocessing versus exposure in vivo: A single-session crossover study of spider phobic children. *British Journal of Psychiatry, 171,* 82–86.

49. Öst, L.G., Brandberg, M., & Alm, T. (1997). One versus five sessions of exposure in the treatment of flying phobia. *Behaviour Research and Therapy, 35,* 987–996.

50. Chambless, D.L., & Ollendick, T.H. (2001). Empirically supported psychological interventions: Controversies and evidence. *Annual Review of Psychology, 52,* 685–716.

Chapter 13

Conclusion: How Might We Prevent Abnormal Behavior from Occurring and Developing?

Thomas G. Plante

This book series has tried to bring the contemporary world of abnormal psychology and behavior to you in an informative, updated, and understandable manner. Hopefully, you have learned much about how abnormal behavior impacts all those around us including those we care most about. The book has tried to articulate what is currently known about a wide variety of abnormal psychology topics so that you will be much better informed about these issues that are often discussed in the news and elsewhere.

After reading and reflecting on these important topics, one might wonder what can be done to minimize, eliminate, or prevent these kinds of problems from occurring. There is clearly no simple answer to this question. There are a variety of reasons why abnormal behavior emerges and develops. Some are due to biological or physiological factors such as genetics, hormonal and biochemical influences, and the exposure to both legal and illegal substances. Others are due to internal psychological conflicts associated with personality, mood, and stress mechanisms. Still others are due to the interactions of many social and interpersonal relationships with loved ones, work or school associates, neighbors, and community members. There are many different roads that lead to abnormal and problematic behavior. However, this does not mean that we can't do much more to improve the odds that abnormal behavior won't develop within ourselves and others. We clearly can make a better world for ourselves and for society if we can follow some key principles of prevention. After reading this book series and

carefully evaluating the advice of many leading experts, several important principles of prevention emerge as being especially important in preventing abnormal
behavior from either developing or getting worse. While we cannot do justice to
each prevention strategy articulated, we can at least introduce these seven principles to the reader. This list is not meant to be exhaustive or exclusive. It merely
provides some very brief reflections and observations as well as prevention and
coping principles.

AVOID ABUSE AND NEGLECT OF CHILDREN

As clearly articulated in several chapters of the series, the abuse and neglect
of children occurs at alarming and disturbing rates. Abused and neglected children are much more likely to develop certain troubles with depression, anxiety,
violence, substance abuse, interpersonal difficulties, and a host of other problem
behaviors. Once developed, these problems impact others around them and can
be passed on from generation to generation. Somehow, efforts must be increased
to minimize child abuse and neglect. Public policy experts, child protection professionals, family attorneys, politicians, mental health professionals, and others
must work closely to help children stay safe and to ensure that those entrusted
with the welfare of children (e.g., parents, teachers, coaches, child care providers)
are capable of providing the competent and effective care that children need,
which is free from any abuse or neglect. While we can't totally eliminate child
abuse and neglect, we can certainly try to minimize it by pooling our collective resources and expertise making a firm commitment to the safety and well-
being of all children. Like a lot of things, it will take a selfless commitment of
time, money, and other resources to make significant progress in this area. It will
involve working with many different community, civic, religious, educational,
law enforcement, mental health, political, and other agencies. Perhaps as former
President Nixon argued for a "War on Cancer" or former President Johnson's
"War on Poverty," we may need a "War on Child Abuse and Neglect."

MINIMIZE POVERTY

Those who are poor are less likely to have access to professional mental
and physical health care services and are much more likely to be impacted by
the stress that is associated with poverty (e.g., unemployment, poor housing,
and exposure to community violence). As poverty levels increase and the gap
between the rich and poor widens, it is likely that the psychological and behavioral problems associated with poverty will increase. Therefore, efforts to reduce
poverty will likely minimize the development of or the worsening of a variety
of abnormal psychology problems. Again, politicians, business leaders, mental

health professionals, family advocates, and others must somehow work together in order to minimize poverty both here and abroad. Perhaps former President Johnson's "War on Poverty" needs to be waged once again.

MINIMIZE EXPOSURE TO VIOLENCE

Sadly, we live in an often highly violent world. Violence is not only perpetrated during wars and in street crime but also in the seclusion and privacy of one's own home. Domestic violence, child abuse, date rape, and other kinds of violence are all too common. Furthermore, research has clearly indicated that exposure to violence through entertainment sources (e.g., movies, video games) also increases the risk of both violence and other mental health–related problems among vulnerable viewers. The entertainment industry, politicians, mental health professionals, family advocates, and others must somehow work together in order to minimize violence exposure in entertainment, in the media in general, and in both public communities and private homes.

DEVELOP AND NURTURE EFFECTIVE AND AFFORDABLE TREATMENTS (INCLUDING PHARMACEUTICALS)

The development of quality and effective intervention strategies including pharmaceutical agents has the potential ability to greatly reduce the impact of abnormal behavior, assuming these options are available to all those in need. For example, medications such as Prozac and other selective serotonin reuptake inhibitors have revolutionized the treatment of depressive disorders during the past decade and a half. These medications, while not perfect or right for everyone with depression, have greatly improved the odds of effectively dealing with a number of psychiatric troubles including obsessive-compulsive disorder, depression, bulimia, and so forth. Recent quality research using empirically supported psychological interventions has also demonstrated remarkable results for a wide variety of abnormal behavior problems. Quality behavioral and psychological interventions for panic disorder, depression, eating disorders, post-traumatic stress disorder, and many other problems are available. Research and development on affordable medications and psychosocial interventions to help those who suffer from abnormal behavior offer hope to not only those afflicted with these conditions but also to those loved ones who suffer too.

However, medications in particular can often too easily be seen as a magic pill to solve all problems. Medications can also be extremely expensive in the United States in particular. A careful and thoughtful effort to make appropriate medications available to those who can truly benefit from them will likely help to minimize the severity of abnormal behavior for not only identified patients but also for all those who are connected to them via family, work, school, or other relationships. The best available research and practice is needed to ensure that interventions that can help people with abnormal behavior are readily available and used.

ALTER CULTURAL EXPECTATIONS ABOUT BEHAVIOR

In previous decades, children rode in cars without seat belts and rode their bikes without bike helmets. Parents physically hit their children at will and in public. People were allowed to smoke wherever they wanted to do so. Women who sought to work outside of the home were considered odd or too bold. Cultural expectations about how we live our lives that have impacted social customs and expectations can be applied to abnormal behavior risk factors as well. For example, violence exposure, maintaining zero tolerance for child abuse, alcohol and other substance abuse, poverty, and so forth may help to create a society where abnormal behavior cannot flourish. Public policy can be used to help decrease the odds that abnormal behavior risks are tolerated. Cultural expectations and policy decisions can be used to ensure that those who experience particular problems seek appropriate resources. There is too often a social taboo to request help from mental health professionals about abnormal psychology related problems. This resistance and avoidance tragically often allows potential problems to become more severe and serious.

AVOID EXPOSURE TO ABNORMAL PSYCHOLOGY RISK FACTORS

While Americans demand individual freedoms, exposure to particular risks increases the chance of abnormal behavior of developing. For example, legalized gambling in some form (e.g., Indian gaming, lotteries, Internet gambling) is now allowed in just about all states and is certainly not confined to Las Vegas and Atlantic City. Bars and liquor stores are open and available around the clock in just about every city. Pornography and online gambling are available on the Internet and thus just about everyone who has a computer or can get to one can be exposed to these influences. These trends increase the odds that those who are vulnerable to developing certain abnormal problems (e.g., alcoholism, pornography, gambling) will do so. As I have heard many times, "An alcoholic probably shouldn't work as a bartender." Controlling the environment so that temptations are not available very easily would go a long way in minimizing the development of many abnormal behavior problems. Furthermore, vulnerable children and those with predilections to particular behavioral problems can all too easily access materials that can contribute to further abnormal psychology problems. Therefore, being thoughtful about the environmental influences that increase the odds of developing problems later in life should make all of us more sensitive to these influences.

MAXIMIZE ETHICS—ESPECIALLY SOCIAL RESPONSIBILITY AND CONCERN FOR OTHERS

At the end of the day, somehow we all must find a way to live together, sharing the planet and its resources. If we have any hope of living in a world that is humane and just and where abnormal behavior and problems are managed better and minimized, we'll need to maximize our social responsibility and concern for others. The ethical treatment of all persons and our efforts to make the world a better place for all will hopefully prevent or at least minimize many of the troubles associated with abnormal behavior. A global effort to support ethical interactions among all may help us better live with social responsibility and concern for others.

While abnormal behavior is likely to be with us forever, there is much that we can do as a society to minimize the possibility that abnormal behavior will develop in at-risk individuals and groups as well as to help those who experience these troubles. Mental health professionals working with others including public policy leaders, industries such as the pharmaceutical companies, and experts in many other fields can help a great deal. Can our culture and society make the commitment to do this? Let us hope so.

Index

About the Editor and the Contributors

EDITOR

Thomas G. Plante, PhD, ABPP, is professor and chair of psychology at Santa Clara University and adjunct clinical associate professor of psychiatry and behavioral sciences at Stanford University School of Medicine. He has authored, coauthored, edited, or coedited six books, including *Sin against the Innocents: Sexual Abuse by Priests and the Role of the Catholic Church* (Praeger, 2004), *Bless Me Father For I Have Sinned: Perspectives on Sexual Abuse Committed by Roman Catholic Priests* (Praeger, 1999), *Faith and Health: Psychological Perspectives* (2001), *Do the Right Thing: Living Ethically in an Unethical World* (2004), and *Contemporary Clinical Psychology* (1999, 2005) as well as over 100 professional journal articles and book chapters. He is a fellow of the American Psychological Association, the American Academy of Clinical Psychology, and the Society of Behavioral Medicine. He maintains a private practice in Menlo Park, California.

CONTRIBUTORS

Bruce A. Arnow, PhD, is associate professor of psychiatry and chief of Adult Outpatient Psychiatry Clinics at the Stanford University School of Medicine. His research interests include treatment of chronic and non-chronic major depression, the epidemiology of depression and chronic pain, and relationships between child maltreatment, adult health, and psychiatric outcomes. Dr. Arnow is author of numerous clinical and scientific papers on depression as well as eating disorders and anxiety. He is currently coinvestigator on a large multisite trial funded by the National Institute of Mental Health whose aim is to evaluate the efficacy of pharmacologic and psychosocial treatments for chronic depression.

Susan Bernadett-Shapiro, PhD, is a clinical psychologist in private practice and part-time adjunct faculty member and supervisor of group training in the Graduate Department of Counseling Psychology at Santa Clara University. She has been practicing psychotherapy as a licensed therapist for over two decades. Her specialties in clinical practice and teaching include adolescents, couples therapy, and group therapy. She has published research articles and scholarly presentations in the areas of the development of empathy and group and family therapy and has coauthored a group therapy text. Her clinical practice is in Los Altos, California.

Michael J. Constantino, PhD, is currently an assistant professor of psychology at the University of Massachusetts-Amherst. His primary research program focuses on psychotherapy process, outcome, and integration, with a particular emphasis on patient-therapist relationship dynamics. He has also developed a secondary line of research focused on the role of the self-concept in psychological functioning and psychotherapy. He has published empirical and conceptual papers in both research areas.

Candice Fischer, MS, is a doctoral candidate in the clinical psychology program at the University of Massachusetts-Amherst. She is also a licensed psychologist in Chile. Her main areas of research include the study of treatments for personality disorders, psychotherapy outcome, the integration between research and clinical practice, and the acculturation process for the Latino population. She currently holds an appointment at Harvard as a part-time trainee in the Latino Mental Health Clinic of the Cambridge Hospital.

Mary A. Fristad, PhD, ABPP, is a professor of psychiatry and psychology at the Ohio State University and is the director of Research and Psychological Services in the OSU Division of Child and Adolescent Psychiatry. Dr. Fristad's area of specialty is childhood mood disorders. She has published over 100 articles and book chapters addressing the assessment and treatment of childhood-onset depression, suicidality, and bipolar disorder (manic depression). Dr. Fristad recently edited the *Handbook of Serious Emotional Disturbance in Children and Adolescents* (2002). She has also written a book for families entitled *Raising a Moody Child: How to Cope with Depression and Bipolar Disorder* (2003). Dr. Fristad has been the principal or coprincipal investigator on over two dozen federal, state, and local grants.

Jon Grant, MD, is an associate professor of psychiatry at the University of Minnesota Medical Center and is the editor-in-chief of the *Journal of Gambling*

Studies. Dr. Grant has written over 80 peer-reviewed articles and book chapters on the phenomenology and pharmacological management of impulse control disorders, particularly kleptomania and pathological gambling. He is the author of a book on impulse control disorders titled *Stop Me Because I Can't Stop Myself* (2002) and editor of *Pathological Gambling: A Clinical Guide to Treatment* (2004). Dr. Grant serves on the editorial board of the *Annals of Clinical Psychiatry*.

Mark Griffiths, PhD, is a chartered psychologist and Europe's only professor of gambling studies (Nottingham Trent University). He has published over 130 refereed research papers, several books, and more papers and articles on gambling and computer games than any other academic in the U.K. In 1996 he was awarded a Media Fellowship by the British Association for the Advancement of Science, and in 1997 he was the Magnus Pike Fellow. In 2004 he was awarded the Joseph Lister Award by the British Association for the Advancement of Science for being one of the U.K.'s "outstanding academic communicators."

Rick E. Ingram, PhD, is currently professor of psychology at the University of Kansas. He previously taught at San Diego State University and was a core faculty member in the SDSU/USCD Joint Doctoral Program in Clinical Psychology. His research program focuses on cognitive functioning in emotional disorders and the association between cognitive functioning and vulnerability to depression. He is currently the editor of *Cognitive Therapy and Research* and an associate editor for the *Journal of Consulting and Clinical Psychology*. Along with Jeanne Miranda and Zindel Segal he is coauthor of *Cognitive Vulnerability to Depression* (1998), and with C. R. Snyder he is the coeditor of the *Handbook of Psychological Change: Psychotherapy Processes and Practices for the 21st Century* (2000).

Julie B. Jampel, PhD, a clinical psychologist at the Tufts University Counseling Center, has worked with college students for over 15 years. She also serves as lecturer on psychology in the psychiatry department at the Cambridge Hospital, a teaching hospital of Harvard Medical School. She supervises psychologists-in-training and has a private practice in Brookline and Somerville, Massachusetts. Her particular interests focus on the effects of exceptionality, developmental disabilities, intellectual giftedness, and development and adjustment from childhood through adulthood.

Martin Kantor, MD, is a psychiatrist who has been in private practice in Boston and New York City. He served as assistant clinical professor of psychiatry at Mount Sinai Medical School and clinical assistant professor of psychiatry at the University of Medicine and Dentistry of New Jersey, New Jersey

Medical School. Dr. Kantor is the author of more than 12 books, including *Distancing: Avoidant Personality Disorder, Revised and Expanded* (2003), *Passive Aggression: A Guide for the Therapist, the Patient, and the Victim* (2002), *Treating Emotional Disorder in Gay Men* (1999), and *Homophobia* (1998) all published by Praeger.

Daniel Kim, MD, is a fourth year psychiatry resident at Brown University. He has worked with Dr. Grant on various research projects concerning impulse control disorders. He is coauthor of an article currently in press at the *American Journal of Psychiatry* that examines prevalence rates of impulse control disorders in psychiatric inpatients.

Jarrod M. Leffler, PhD, is currently the post-doctoral study coordinator for the Multi Family Psychoeducational Group (MFPG) at The Ohio State University Medical Center. His research interests include childhood mood and disruptive behavior disorders, the development and application of treatment interventions for youth, treatment outcome, and consumer satisfaction.

Anna Lembke, MD, is currently a staff physician and senior research scientist at the Stanford University School of Medicine. Her research interests include comorbid substance use and mood disorders as well as the effect of altered mood states on emotion processing. She is the author of numerous clinical and scientific papers and is currently studying the safety and tolerability of smoking cessation in depressed adults.

Heather C. Lench, MA, MFTT, conducts research in the Department of Psychology and Social Behavior at the University of California, Irvine, where she is a doctoral candidate. She received training in experimental psychology and marriage and family therapy at California State University, Fresno. Her research focuses on the influence of emotions and motivation on judgments and behavior over time. She is particularly interested in the relationships between emotions and expectations for the future. She has recently coauthored a chapter in *Judgments Over Time: The Interplay of Thoughts, Feelings, and Behaviors* (2006).

David Luxton, MS, is currently a PhD graduate student in clinical psychology at the University of Kansas. His research primarily involves cognitive vulnerability toward depression with an emphasis on vulnerable self-esteem, thought suppression, and the developmental origins of cognitive risk factors. He also has research interests that focus on the physical health implications of stress and depression.

Viola Mecke, PhD, ABPP, is a clinical emerita professor in the Department of Psychiatry and Behavioral Sciences at Stanford University Medical School, emerita professor of psychology at California State University at Hayward, and a fellow of the Academy of Clinical Psychology.

She retired from private practice as a clinical psychologist and had served as consultant to several organizations for over forty years. She has authored several professional articles and books, including among them *Fatal Attachments: The Instigation to Suicide* (Praeger, 2004).

Lori Goldfarb Plante, PhD, is a clinical lecturer at Stanford University School of Medicine. She conducts a private practice in clinical psychology in Menlo Park, California, where she specializes in the assessment and treatment of adolescents and young adults. She is the author of a book addressing chronic illness and disability within the family as well as the author of numerous professional articles on eating disorders, sexuality, and sexual abuse in adolescents and young adults.

Christine D. Scher, PhD, is an assistant professor in the Department of Psychology at California State University, San Bernardino. Her research interests include cognitive risk and vulnerability in anxiety and depression and psychological measure development and psychometric evaluation. She teaches courses in abnormal psychology, behavior modification, clinical assessment, and psychotherapy theories. Dr. Scher is a licensed psychologist and maintains a small private practice in San Bernardino, California, specializing in cognitive-behavioral treatment of anxiety disorders.

Jerrold Lee Shapiro, PhD, ABMP, is professor and chairman of the Counseling Psychology Department at Santa Clara University. In addition, he is a licensed psychologist in California and Hawaii, managing partner of *Family Business Solutions,* and former president of PsyJourn, Inc., a firm that created psychological software to enhance therapy and counseling. He is author, coauthor, and coeditor of eight books including two that have won literary awards in psychology, psychiatry and nursing. Dr. Shapiro has also authored several software programs and over 200 professional papers, book chapters, presentations, and symposia. He maintains a private practice, specializing in men's therapy and couples therapy, in Los Altos, California.

Dana Steidtmann is a graduate student in clinical psychology at the University of Kansas. She received a BA in psychology from the University of Wyoming. Her research interests include causes and treatment of anxiety and mood disorders.

About the Series Advisers

Patrick H. DeLeon, PhD, ABPP, MPH, JD, is a former president of the American Psychological Association and has served on Capitol Hill for over three decades working on health and educational policy issues. A fellow of the APA, he has been active within the APA governance, having been elected president of three practice divisions. A former editor of *Professional Psychology: Research and Practice,* he has been on the editorial board of the *American Psychologist* since 1981. He has received several APA Presidential citations as well as the APA Distinguished Professional and Public Interest Contributions awards. He has also been recognized by the leadership of professional nursing, social work, and optometry. He is a Distinguished Alumnus of the Purdue University School of Liberal Arts. He has authored in excess of 175 publications.

Nadine J. Kaslow, PhD, ABPP, is professor and chief psychologist at Emory University School of Medicine in the Department of Psychiatry and Behavioral Sciences. She is president of the American Board of Clinical Psychology, -former president of the Divisions of Clinical Psychology and of Family Psychology of the American Psychological Association, past chair of the Association of Psychology Postdoctoral and Internship Centers, and associate editor of the *Journal of Family Psychology.* Her research interests and numerous publications focus on the assessment and treatment of suicidal behavior in abused and non-abused women, family violence (intimate partner violence, child abuse), child and adolescent depression, and training issues in psychology. She is currently principal investigator on grants funded by the Centers for Disease Control and Prevention on the treatment of abused suicidal African American women, the treatment of suicidal African American women. She is a licensed psychologist who maintains a psychotherapy practice in Atlanta, Georgia, for adolescents with eating disorders, adults, couples, and families.

Lori Goldfarb Plante, PhD, is a clinical lecturer at Stanford University School of Medicine. She conducts a private practice in clinical psychology in Menlo Park, California, where she specializes in the assessment and treatment of adolescents and young adults. She is the author of a book addressing chronic illness and disability within the family as well as the author of numerous professional articles on eating disorders, sexuality, and sexual abuse in adolescents and young adults.